Sites of Vision

Sites of Vision

The Discursive Construction of Sight in the History of Philosophy

edited by David Michael Levin

The MIT Press
Cambridge, Massachusetts
London, England

First MIT Press paperback edition, 1999

This book was set in New Baskerville on the Monotype 'Prism Plus' PostScript
Imagesetter by Asco Trade Typesetting Ltd., Hong Kong.

Printed and bound in the United States of America.

Library of Congress Cataloging-in-Publication Data

Sites of vision : the discursive construction of sight in the history
  of philosophy / edited by David Michael Levin.
     p.   cm.
  Includes bibliographical references and index.
  ISBN 0-262-12203-0 (hardcover : alk. paper), 0-262-62129-0 (pb)
  1. Vision—Philosophy—History. I. Levin, David Michael, 1939– .
BD214.S58   1997
121'.3—dc20   96-41860
                                                          CIP

The forming of the five senses is a labour of the entire history of the world down to the present.

—Karl Marx, *Economic and Philosophical Manuscripts of 1844*

Contents

Contents

Introduction

Our vision has, as Marx once said, a history. As a condition of nature, it has, first of all, what we might call a natural history. But it also has a human history—its history as a social and cultural construction.[1] This, of course, is the history to which Marx was calling our attention—in order to say that the tragic vision by which we have lived and suffered is not a supernatural fate or a final sentence of nature, to which we must be resigned but, rather, a gift of nature, the gift of a natural power, a natural capacity for perceptual responsiveness, that it is our responsibility to question and educate, working with the nature we have been given to construct out of its materials a different vision. To recognize that vision has a history is already to endistance ourselves from nature and begin the work of critique—and even, perhaps, to open our vision to the prospect, however distant and uncertain, of rational reconstruction and enlightenment.

In *History and Truth*, Paul Ricoeur argued for the Hegelian idea that "history becomes reflected in the history of philosophy and becomes aware of itself in the form of the history of philosophy."[2] The studies in this book take up an important and timely problematic in the history of philosophy. Considered as a whole, the book pursues the logic of two intricately interconnected lines of inquiry: (1) an examination of the history of vision as a history of the discursive construction of vision within, and consequently by, the history of philosophy; and (2) an examination of the history of philosophy, questioning the connections between this discursive construction of vision and the history of philosophy as a discourse itself constructed, to a certain extent, by the rhetoric of vision. Because of the decisive role that vision has played in the discourse of philosophy, I would claim, following Ricoeur's argument, that, in the chapters in this book, the history of vision is abundantly reflected in the history of philosophy and that it is therefore possible for both vision and thought to achieve a greater awareness of themselves in the form of the history of philosophy.

One of the principal hypotheses at stake in these studies is that if we acknowledge that the discourse of philosophy is itself a historical construction and that it has often relied on a vision-generated vocabulary and way of thinking (not only, for example, with words such as *speculation, observation, insight, reflection, evidence,* and *intuition,* and with metaphors such as *mirroring, clarity, perspective, point of view, horizon of understanding,* and *the light of reason,* but also with certain methodological concepts such as *totality, analysis, objectivity, reflective detachment,* and *representation*), even to the extent, sometimes, of drawing on an ocular vocabulary and rhetoric for the construction of a system of thought at the same time that it has constructed a model of the gaze profoundly hostile to the testimony and claims of vision, then we must also acknowledge that the use and the construction of this vocabulary needs to be examined, together with the discursive effects of such use and construction on the way of thinking that has dominated the history of philosophy.

As Richard Rorty pointed out in *Philosophy and the Mirror of Nature,* philosophical thought in the twentieth century has taken a "linguistic turn."[3] In this turn, principally inaugurated, in the analytic schools, by Frege, Bertrand Russell, and Ludwig Wittgenstein, and, in the continental schools, by Edmund Husserl and Martin Heidegger, the hegemony of vision as the philosophical paradigm of knowledge, truth, and reality was overthrown and replaced by a paradigm in which language is given the determinative role. This, however, has made it possible, as the chapters in this book show, to recognize now, and make explicit, in the vision that dominated philosophical thought for so long, the traces of its discursive construction—startling evidence that a linguistic turn had already taken place and that from the beginning language was already at work in the discursive hegemony of vision, invisibly constructing models and paradigms of vision within the framework of diverse epistemological, metaphysical, ethical, and political programs.

If vision is an unreliable source of truth, why has philosophical discourse relied so heavily on the language of vision? Why has philosophical thought adopted this language in order to construct itself? Does philosophical thought need to *see* itself? What would an affirmative answer to this question imply? When we read the texts with these questions in mind, what can we learn about how philosophy sees—or imagines—itself? And when we examine what philosophical thought has had to say about vision, noticing how such thought has constructed vision, what can we learn about how philosophy sees the world—and how it imagines it? What can we learn about the history of philosophy when we read it as a history of visions—visions of a tragic world in ruins, visions of the world in its rational reconstruction, visions of a redeemed world transformed by its enlightenment? Is there a connection between philosophical deployments of a rhetoric of vision in the reflective construction of thought and philosophical critiques of vision in epistemological projects of rational reconstruction? What interventions and alterations in our historical experience with vision may be driven by or are implicit in the logic of these critiques and reconstructions? Could it be that the philosophical gaze that engages with the history of vision is a figure of the productive imagination, an inscription of the reflective judgment in search of a principle, an ideal, toward which to elevate our sight?

In "Philosophy and the Crisis of European Man," Husserl declared that "man becomes the disinterested spectator, overseer of the world; in other words, he becomes a philosopher."[4] Reading Plato, René Descartes, Baruch Spinoza, G. W. Leibniz, George Berkeley, G. W. F. Hegel, and Husserl, the argument for the historical dominance of this thoroughly patriarchal, male-engendered conception of philosophical thought can seem compelling. Since the time of its beginning, the discourse of philosophy has for the most part either taken the visual interpretation of philosophical thought for granted or else explicitly proclaimed it. As Heidegger observed, "From the beginning onwards the tradition of philosophy has been oriented primarily towards 'seeing' as a way of access to beings and to being."[5] In order to free his philosophical thinking from the framework of this tradition, Heidegger formulated a critique of the discourse of ontology that he connected with a vision-generated epistemology and a diagnosis of the errancy typical of everyday vision. Later he moved beyond diagnosis and critique, and gave thought to the cultivation of a way of seeing that could perhaps prepare our world for the advent of a new epoch in the history of being.

In a different challenge to the tradition, Walter Benjamin declared that "the tasks which face the human apparatus of perception at the turning points of history cannot be solved ... by contemplation alone."[6] And in keeping with this criticism, he turned the philosophical gaze of the tower and the cabinet into the critical gaze of a *flâneur*, a man, like Socrates, who practices his philosophical calling on the street and in the marketplace, fully engaged in the praxis of critical dialectics, using his eyes to call our attention to things that in "normal life" we do not see, or do not want to see.[7] In 1934, as Europe was careening out of control toward the Holocaust, André Gide expressed an indictment similar to Benjamin's, writing in his *Journals*, from the depths of what he called "lamentation," this: "Wherever my gaze turns, I see around me only distress. He who remains contemplative today demonstrates an inhuman philosophy, or monstrous blindness."[8]

As early as 1927, however, John Dewey had already formulated a serious public challenge to the prevailing philosophical investment in vision. Thinking about ways to support the public use of reason and improve the functioning of the public sphere as a multiplicity of sites for democratic processes of discursive will-formation, he wrote in *The Public and Its Problems* that "the connections of the ear with vital and outgoing thought and emotion are immensely closer and more varied than those of the eye. Vision is a spectator; hearing is a participator."[9] More recently, Hannah Arendt attempted to revive this criticism of philosophical thought, arguing that "from the very outset, in formal philosophy, thinking has been thought of in terms of *seeing*.... The predominance of sight is so deeply embedded in Greek speech, and therefore in our conceptual language, that we seldom find any consideration bestowed on it, as though it belonged among things too obvious to be noticed."[10] It seemed to her that philosophers were finally beginning to question their historical reliance on a terminology drawn from the realm of vision, and that perhaps a certain shift might be taking place—a shift from the paradigm, or episteme, of sight to the paradigm, or episteme, of communication: "Since Bergson, the use of the sight metaphor in philosophy has kept dwindling, not surprisingly, as emphasis and interest have shifted entirely from contemplation to speech, from *nous* to *logos*."[11]

This is a shift that the writings of both Hans-Georg Gadamer and Jürgen Habermas have strongly encouraged. In his major work, *Truth and Method*, Gadamer appropriated the ocular experience of horizons and reinscribed it within a hermeneutics of interpretation. This enabled him to propose principles for "civilized conversation" aimed at reaching a shared understanding. In "The Entwinement of Myth and Enlightenment," Habermas argued against "the gaze of contemporary diagnosis," a "cramped optics that renders one insensible to the traces and existing forms of communicative rationality."[12] And he continues to work on the formulation of the theoretical principles that are necessary for a discursive rationality, drawing the discourse of philosophy increasingly farther from its ocularcentric rhetoric.

Is the ocularcentrism of philosophical discourse merely a continuation, then, of myth? Has it always figured in the service of enlightenment? Or does the paradigm exemplify precisely that disquieting entwinement of myth and enlightenment to which, in the wake of the Holocaust, Max Horkheimer and Theodor

Adorno called our attention? Actually, what Habermas opposes is not so much the paradigm of vision as such but rather the epistemological privileging of a reifying and totalizing vision, a gaze of domination. Defining the character of this way of seeing in "An Alternative Way Out of the Philosophy of the Subject: Communicative vs. Subject-Centered Reason," he points to "the kind of objectification inevitable from the reflexively applied perspective of the observer," whereby "everything gets frozen into an object under the gaze of the third person."[13] For Habermas, the philosopher's gaze must not limit itself to the external perspective of the observer; the philosopher's responsibility—to articulate her time in a discourse of critical reflection—also requires the adoption of a participant's gaze, a gaze capable of taking part in the exchanges of mutual recognition that accompany civilized conversation. For Habermas, then, the paradigm of the philosopher's critical gaze is not to be abandoned, but it must be inscribed within the paradigm of a discursive rationality.

In a perhaps similar spirit, Michel Foucault challenged the "sovereignty" of the philosopher's gaze—and indeed, more generally, the very idea of a "sovereign gaze." For him, as for Friedrich Nietzsche, the philosopher's assumption of such a gaze is nothing but an arrogant—and futile—historical conceit. If the philosopher must renounce his know-it-all position, must become, as Gramsci said, a "specific intellectual," then he must also give up his claim to enjoy a God's-eye vision. The imperial vision of the philosopher—contemplative, speculative, all-encompassing, proud of the ability to remain unmoved—belongs to the classical order, the world of monarchies and aristocracies. Because Foucault believed that, today, the power constitutive of the most technologically advanced states is channeled by a decentralized apparatus through a multiplicity of disciplinary regimes, he argued that the philosopher's vision can function critically only insofar as it correspondingly renounces the authority of center and totality and moves about, witnessing and registering life from a multiplicity of positions—most of all from positions of marginality, exclusion, and subordination. "What is effectively needed," he asserted, "is a ramified, penetrating perception of the present, one that makes it possible to locate lines of weakness, strong points, positions where the instances of power have secured and implanted themselves."[14]

Jacques Derrida, too, has contested the domination of vision in the discourse of metaphysics, arguing that ocularcentrism, heliocentrism, and photocentrism are responsible for, or at the least have significantly contributed to, the rhetorical forces of reification and totalization in a "metaphysics of presence." Thus, in a way that is strikingly similar to Foucault's, he has practiced a vision that subverts the vision which supports this metaphysics, deploying a gaze that deconstructs its reifications, its pretensions to certainty, decidability, constancy, totality.

There is thus an important debate taking place within philosophy regarding the role of vision and the discourse of vision in the very construction of philosophical thought. This debate is actually part of a larger cultural debate over the hegemony and character of vision in the contemporary world. In question are the nature and role of vision and the functions and effects of the discourses of vision, in the formation of individual identity, the constitution of social relations, the cultural genealogy of stereotypes, the administrative power of the state, the visibility and accountability of governmental agents and agencies, the human relationship to nature and use of the environment, and the construction of discursive sites, of places and spaces, in the public sphere. Many philosophers have contributed to the debate over these questions.

This larger debate brings out the significance of the debate taking place now within philosophy. The studies in this book explore the hypothesis that the "nature" of the visual perception (vision, sight, seeing) about which philosophers talk, and which they claim to be "describing" and critically examining, primarily in the context of an epistemology, is, and must explicitly be recognized as, a discursive construction, and indeed a historical construction in the force field of philosophical discourse. This "visual perception" is never just a simple, immediate, straightforward, unproblematic presentation of the phenomenon and experience of vision. First, it is always something the description, or account of which is arrived at in and through discourse, in and through a variety of discursive strategies and instruments. This work of construction is not the work of any one philosopher but is, rather, the product of an intricate historical discourse involving many different philosophers and their texts. Moreover, the process—the how—of interpretation, whereby philosophers are involved in the textual construction of a certain representation of vision, of sight, of visual receptivity and perception, invariably seems to involve the rational reconstruction of sight as part of a larger program, in which what is at stake is the rational reconstruction of knowledge. In other words, the accounts of vision that figure in philosophical discourse more often than not seem to be not so much faithful phenomenological descriptions or objectively accurate empirical descriptions but, rather, ideal models with a distinctively normative rhetorical function. That many of the philosophical accounts of vision are actually rational reconstructions of sight is one of the hypotheses in terms of which the studies in this book are organized.

Whether this hypothesis is right needs to be examined critically. Thus, these studies will be considering the hypothesis that some of the ways in which philosophers have represented vision in their so-called descriptions and accounts (e.g., of how visual perception takes place, what it is to see, what it is that one sees or can see, what seeing entitles us to say and claim, and how seeing and its technologies relate to, or are involved in, the achievement and production of power and knowledge) are theoretically mediated, or indeed discursively adjusted to fit into some larger epistemological, ontological, or metaphysical program of requirements—requirements for knowledge, truth, belief, certainty, objectivity, testimony, corroboration, justification.

The studies in this book reflect on the meaning and significance of this hypothesis. Let me briefly clarify the point with an example. When Maurice Merleau-Ponty articulates the epistemological conditions of objectivity, he is also involved in the construction of vision.[15] The phenomenological "descriptions" that he provides are hermeneutical and do not in fact immediately correspond to the way we typically see, the way we typically inhabit and experience our vision. As faithful renderings of what and how we usually experience vision, his "descriptions" are unquestionable failures, for our habitual experience with seeing is typically shallow, without the dimensionality of intricate awareness. The "descriptions" work, however, by setting the truth in motion, articulating an implicit, prereflective dimension of experience that is normally not recognized. In other words, the truth of his "descriptions" does not correspond to a ready-made reality, as the truths of positivism and rationalism do, but is instead always in the making—a performative achievement, a discursive construction. If the "description" is "faithful," true to the implicit dimensionality of the experience, then the words of the "description" will become true, will make themselves true, as they motivate an awareness that alters the experience, unfolding its intricate implicit structure retrospectively or after the fact. For example, it requires a certain amount of work and the discipline of hermeneutical phenomenology to experience in vision the truth of the propositions that "in so far as I have sensory functions, a visual, auditory and tactile field, I am already in communication with others," that vision is an erotic "ecstase," and that "I am all that I see."[16]

However, even explanatory accounts are presented not just to correct the "naive," unreflected-on understanding of vision that is implicit in the common cultural experience but also actually to alter the vision itself, to rehabilitate or construct a different vision, or promote a different practical relationship to vision, altering, for example, ethical viewpoints and moral attitudes, or revising the implications and inferences that people tend to draw from what and how they see.

Our vision is not just a biological endowment; it is also a capacity, a potential that can be developed and realized in a number of different ways. As soon as infants open their eyes, their vision is appropriated by culture and takes part in cultural life. Vision is socially produced and tends to confirm and reproduce the culture that brought it into being. Our vision is accordingly historical, bearing within itself a past that has figured in many different narratives, some of them significantly and irrevocably altering the culture of vision to which they spoke or within which they were inscribed. Once we acknowledge the historicity of our vision, we must also acknowledge the history within the discourse of philosophy, narratives to be told regarding the construction of our quotidian vision—the way our vision has been interpreted, elaborated, framed, constructed, and reconstructed— within the discourse of philosophy. And we must also acknowledge that there is history in the construction and reconstruction of philosophical thought itself, narratives to be told regarding the ways in which philosophical thought has reflected on itself: on its own methods of seeing things and on its numerous attempts to formulate the epistemology of vision with a vocabulary, a metaphorics, drawn, mostly without any sign of recognition or any sign of indebtedness, from the vision of its own construction.

Looking back over the history of philosophy, we are provoked to inquire whether and how it may be useful to read empiricism in the light of an interpretation that takes it to be proposing a discursive reconstruction of our everyday way of looking and seeing, a project of reconstruction that wants this reconstructed sight to be a way of looking and seeing that understands itself *as* constructed—materially and inductively constructed, atomic sensation by atomic sensation, impression by impression, datum by datum, into a perceptual inference, judgment, or idea. And by the same token, we are compelled to ask whether and how it may be useful to read rationalism as likewise the discursive construction of a vision that must understand itself *as* constructed—but in this case constructed by the application of classificatory categories to the interpretation of the sensuous material given in and by perceptual experience.

The studies in this book bring to the light some of the crucial moments in the history of discursive constructions: constructions and reconstructions of the vision at work within the texts of philosophy itself and also philosophical constructions and reconstructions of the vision constitutive of our everyday lives.

In *Walden,* Henry David Thoreau asks, "Could a greater miracle take place than for us to look through each other's eyes for an instant?"[17] In the original studies written for this book, this possibility is given a historical dimension. The contributors are reading here the different ways of seeing, and the different ways of reading and writing this seeing, that have figured in the works of some of the most important philosophers, in an attempt to understand how and why they saw and thought the world in the ways that they did. Thus, the chapters examine not only what these philosophers have said about vision but also problematize their philosophical use, almost never subject to question, of a terminology drawn from the realm of vision but often transfigured in odd and uncanny ways. This vocabulary has played such a constitutive role in the reflexivity of their philosophical discourse that it is not too far-fetched to suggest that the chapters in this book involve an attempt, literally speaking, to *see* how the philosophers in question think. There is much to learn, and much, indeed, comes to the light, if we ask: What have these philosophers said—or perhaps, rather, what have they been tempted to say—precisely because of the logic of their vision-generated terminology? If we can see through the eyes of others, we can also see through their words. And when their words, however abstract, have been derived from the way(s) that sight has been experienced and understood, then through their words we can also see into the process of thinking behind the vision. This is an original way of reading texts in the history of philosophy.

Our vision belongs as much to a future of possibilities as to an order that is past. The studies in this book also function according to Theodor Adorno's method of immanent critique. The task of philosophical thought, he maintained, is to "dissolve the rigidity of the temporally and spatially fixed object into a field of tension of the possible and the real."[18] A fruitful way of reading the studies in this book would be to take them as explorations of a field of tension that brings out new possibilities—not only for the philosophical understanding of vision and for the critical reflections of this thought in our construction of the discourse of philosophy but also for our vision itself.

When we consider the history of philosophy from Plato to Foucault, Derrida, and Gilles Deleuze, we find a significant number of philosophers deeply critical of the way in which the gift of sight has been exercised inside and outside philosophy—and correspondingly critical of the world our common vision has brought to the light. Consider, Plato. In Book VII of *The Republic,* Plato uses the myth of the cave to reflect on the question "how far our nature is enlightened or unenlightened."[19] The story that he tells is a philosophical indictment of the way of seeing common to the many. But it is also an allegory through which Plato attempts to envision a journey of the soul: the possibility of ascent from a sight lost in an illusory realm of shadows and reflections through a sight seduced by images and visible objects, and a higher sight drawn to the lights of the sky in which the divinities make themselves visible, to the moment, finally, of a glorious intellectual vision, a pure, disembodied contemplation, with the eye of the mind, of the Form of the Good, the invisible condition of all that is visible.[20] For Plato, the sensuous, sensible world of sight is "a prison-house," a world in which the many are hopelessly lost; without a contemplative vision of the Forms, their eyes wander and drift, without discipline, without knowledge, without end. "The idea of the good," he wrote, "appears last of all, and is seen only with an effort; and, when seen, is also inferred to be the universal author of all things beautiful and right, parent of light and of the lord of light in this visible world, and the immediate source of reason and truth in the intellectual; and ... this is the power upon which he who would act rationally either in public or private life must have his eye fixed."[21] The philosopher, for Plato, is one who can see what needs to be seen even in the darkness, one whose eyes are not "dazzled by excess of light," one who has learned "by degrees to endure the sight of being, and of the brightest and best of being, or, in other words, the good."[22] The philosopher is one whose sight is guided by the light of reason.

The moral significance of the allegory is clear: Plato tells the story in order to inspire as many as will listen to alter their customary vision, thereby making it possible for the soul to undertake its dialectical ascent out of the world of becoming into the realm of being: "And the soul is *like* the eye: when resting upon that on which truth and being shine, the soul perceives and understands and is radiant with intelligence; but when turned towards the twilight of becoming and perishing, then she has opinion only, and goes blinking about, and is first of one opinion and then of another, and seems to have no intelligence."[23]

Consider Spinoza. To earn a living, he turned pieces of glass into fine lenses, a technology that enabled people to see with improved vision. But in his *Ethics,* he also articulated, *ordine geometrico,* a new way of looking at the world: a vision improved by philosophical understanding. It is as if he hoped that the reader whose eyes have been taken through the logical order of his deductions will come away with a vision that is rationally disciplined. This possibility is announced within the work itself, for he says, in a passage that scholars have consistently avoided interpreting, "The more capable the body is of being affected in many ways, and affecting external bodies in many ways, the more capable of thinking is the mind."[24] This proposition does not say only that philosophical understanding can improve our vision. It also says that an altered vision—a vision with a greater readiness to being affected in many different ways by what it is given to behold—can improve understanding. Commentators on the *Ethics* invariably continue the traditional philosophical animosity toward the senses, reading Spinoza's correlation of mind and body in only one direction. Be that as it may, it is time to acknowledge that Spinoza, like Plato, and many other philosophers after him, wrote in the hope of altering the way we see and look at the world.

Consider Hegel. In one of his letters, he wrote: "In teaching philosophy in the Gymnasium, the abstract form is, in the first instance, straightaway the chief concern. The young must first die to sight and hearing, must be torn away from concrete

representations, must be withdrawn into the night of the soul
and so learn to see on this new [philosophical] level."[25] Here,
more bluntly perhaps than in his systematic writings, Hegel recognized that the work of thought is not to formulate an empirical
or merely "subjective" understanding of the sense of sight, but
rather to undertake a rational reconstruction of the spiritual
potential that is immanent within our vision. Convinced, unlike
Immanuel Kant, that in the appropriate spiritual conditions, we
are capable of an "intellectual vision" of the good and the right,
he wrote, "Intellectual intuition is alone realized by and in ethical life." And he added that what is required is that "the eyes of
the spirit and the eyes of the body [should] completely coincide."[26] This clearly articulates the arduous historical task to
which he summons our worldly eyes. Behind this summons is the
assumption that we can, and should, allow our vision to be oriented according to the compass of this world-historical mission.

Consider Nietzsche, who wrote, in *Twilight of the Idols*, that
"one has to learn to see, one has to learn to think, one has to
learn to speak and write: the end in all three is a noble culture."[27] For him, "learning to see" means "habituating the eye
to repose, to patience, to letting things come to it; learning to
defer judgment, to investigate and comprehend the individual
case in all its aspects ... the essence of it is precisely not to 'will',
the ability to defer decision."[28] He had, according to one of his
posthumously published Notes, a "profound aversion to reposing once and for all in any sort of totalized view of the world."[29]
In *The Will to Power*, this learning to see means opening up new
perspectives and new horizons.[30] It means learning not to shut
our eyes to that which we would rather not see. It means learning
to look with a steady and calm gaze that does not willfully impose its images on what it beholds, but lets what is present and
visible show itself from out of itself. Nietzsche, too, then, was
concerned with the transformation of our vision, overcoming its
"pathologies."

Consider Heidegger. In "The Turning," he observes: "But we
do not yet hear, we whose hearing and seeing are perishing
through radio and film under the rule of technology."[31] Max

Horkheimer argued something remarkably similar: "As their telescopes and microscopes, their tapes and radios become more sensitive, individuals become blinder, more hard of hearing, less responsive, and society more opaque, more hopeless, its misdeeds ... larger and more superhuman than before."[32] Both philosophers see advances in the technologies of vision, while our natural capacity for vision diminishes and atrophies in a culture that fails to encourage its aesthetic, imaginative, spiritual, and rational-critical potentials.

After articulating, in *Being and Time*, a critique of everyday vision, Heidegger draws attention to what he calls "a potentiality for seeing" in order to suggest the possibility of redemption in a "moment of vision."[33] After asking us, in *What Is Called Thinking?* "Can we see something that is told?" Heidegger writes: "We can, provided ... the seeing is more than just the seeing with the eyes of the body. Accordingly, the transposition by the leap of such a vision does not happen of itself. Leap and vision require long, slow preparation."[34] Thus he holds in *Gelassenheit* that our vision is in need of such "preparation," because it is not yet a way of seeing that is appropriate to the presencing of the horizon: "What lets the horizon be what it is [the openness of being] has not yet been encountered at all."[35] "The horizon," he writes, "is what guarantees the identity of the object throughout the exploration [by the gaze]."[36] Recognizing that "the subject-object relation ... is apparently only an historical variation of the relation of man to the thing," that the "same is true of the corresponding historical change of the human being to an ego," and that, in "the relation between ego and object there is concealed something historical, something which belongs to the history of man's nature," Heidegger attempts to question a "nature we have hardly experienced as yet, supposing it has not yet been realized in the rationality of the animal."[37]

According to the "scientist" in Heidegger's *Gelassenheit*, we have come to "see thinking in the form of transcendental-horizonal re-presenting."[38] The dialogue in this text continues with the "scholar" replying that, as we experience it, "this re-presenting ... [not only] places before us what is typical"; it also lays down a space into which we look.[39] To this, then, the "scientist" says: "You are describing, once again, the horizon which encircles the view of a thing—the field of vision."[40] Is there some way for us to experience the openness beyond the horizon—the openness that gives the horizon and clears a field of visibility for the presencing of things—without reifying it in the willfulness of a re-presentation? That, as the "teacher" points out, is the question that calls for thought.

Giving thought to the horizon of our vision, Heidegger observes that it is normally "determined only relative to objects and our representing of them" and that it is thereby reduced to being nothing but "the side of that-which-regions turned toward our re-presenting."[41] Consequently, "we do not place the appearance of objects, which the view within a field of vision offers us, into [the] openness" by grace of which alone there is a possibility of vision and horizon in the first place.[42] And yet the openness is that which surrounds us, revealing itself to us as the horizon that not only delimits our field of vision but enables us to take the measure of all that is visible. Thus, Heidegger attempts to learn how to see, in a more "thoughtful" way, a way that would "release" him into this openness—and "release" the openness from his willful perceptive grasp.[43] In releasement, he says, thinking would be "changed": instead of re-presenting what gives itself to be beheld, it would "wait" on "that-which-regions."[44] If there were to be a vision capable of such "waiting," Heidegger's dialogue suggests that it would be a vision that is thoughtful, a vision that has renounced its normal willfulness in order to hold itself open to the event of openness that first laid out for our vision the field of the visible and the invisible, the field within the horizons of which it moves. It would be difficult to understand the dialogue in *Gelassenheit* without reading it as a philosophical endeavor to think beyond our present historical vision, to see with a different vision.

Consider Merleau-Ponty. He holds that "the chiasm, reversibility, is the idea that every perception is doubled with a counter-perception, ... one no longer knows who speaks and who listens."[45] His words are, and yet also are not, an accurate phenomenological description. They can only be understood as a performative intervention, an attempt to influence our vision— to construct a different way of seeing by calling our attention to a potential implicit in our vision and enabling us to work with it and bring it out.

Consider Herbert Marcuse. For Marcuse, "human freedom is rooted in human sensibility: the senses do not only receive what is given to them, ... rather, they discover, or can discover by themselves, in their 'practice', new (more gratifying) possibilities and capabilities, forms and qualities of things, and can urge and guide their realization."[46] In other words, "the senses are not only the basis for the *epistemological* constitution of reality, but also for its *transformation*, its *subversion* in the interest of liberation."[47] Marcuse even turns to the radical potential inherent in perception and sensibility for the transformation of reason—a "shaping [of] the categories under which the world is ordered, experienced, changed."[48] Thus, carrying forward the logic of Marx's proposition regarding the historical nature of human perception and sensibility, Marcuse explicitly calls for "alternative cultural forms and practices, new ways of seeing and a new sensibility."[49]

And finally, consider Foucault. In *The Birth of the Clinic,* he asks us to question the complicity of our vision in relations of power: "But to look in order to know, to show in order to teach, is not this a tacit form of violence, all the more abusive for its silence, upon a sick body that demands to be comforted, not displayed? Can pain be a spectacle?"[50] "There are times in life," he wrote, as he neared the end of his own, "when the question of knowing if one can think differently than one thinks, and perceive differently than one sees, is absolutely necessary if one is to go on looking and reflecting at all."[51] For Foucault, this is a question of the relation between "the growth of capabilities and the growth of autonomy," or, more specifically, since vision is one of our capabilities, a question of how we can free our vision from the dominant way of looking at things. "How," he asks, "can the growth of capabilities be disconnected from the intensification of power relations?"[52] Throughout his life, Foucault attempted to answer this question. But if one of the ways in which he worked with this question involved studying how a certain kind of vision came into being and in turn contributed to the formation of our present world of power-knowledge, another way certainly involved exploring the critical potential in our vision. Thus one can see in his work the artful, strategic construction of a critical vision: a vision that cannot be captured within the hegemonic episteme, a vision through which we can at least see the world differently, if not, or not yet, in the light of redemption. "My project," he once explained, is "to contribute to changing certain things in people's ways of perceiving and doing things, to participate in this difficult displacement of forms of sensibility and thresholds of tolerance."[53]

To the extent that Benjamin is right, that "there is a history of perception that is ultimately the history of myth," it would not be inappropriate to regard these philosophical studies as critical illuminations of that mythology—an ideological formation.[54] But when we consider the metaphoricity that haunts philosophical discourse, forming its thought in the very images of vision, making its only cognitive sense depend on our sense of sight, we must also resist the temptation to regard the discourse of philosophy, to which these studies belong, as one of pure illuminations, pure theoretical reason produced in the dispassionate light of contemplation, a discourse capable of casting such a light as could dispel all the spirits and shadows of mythology. What the light of history shows, we have learned, it shows only with adumbrations. There is no light without shadows, without darkness and concealment. And in this acknowledgment, there is perhaps a lesson for history already inscribed in the field of our vision.

In a short study on Heraclitus, Heidegger maintains that, as beings gifted with a capacity for vision, we have been "entrusted" to the lighting that keeps and shelters us within its revealing-concealing gathering. But he also holds that the meaning of this lighting has been entrusted to our vision in such a way that our very "essence" [*Wesen*] unfolds and is fulfilled only in its recollection of this lighting and what it has given us. Thus he comes to an interpretation regarding the fragment attributed to Heraclitus: "Gods and men belong in the lighting not only as lighted and viewed, but also as invisible, bringing the lighting with them in their own way, preserving it and handing it down in its endurance."[55] The gods may have vanished, but we mortals are still inhabiting the earth, measuring out the length of our lives in the light and warmth of the sun. And some among us have not only been kept and sheltered by this lighting. Some, acknowledging the entrustment, have also given thought to this lighting—and seen in its gift a claim on our vision that has moved them to question the habits, routines, assumptions, and conventions through which we see and reflect on the visible world.

One way to think about the chapters in this book might be to read them as "bringing the lighting with them in their own way, preserving it and handing it down in its endurance." Questioning the vision by which we have lived, questioning its history, its technologies, and its potential; questioning the discursive construction of vision in the history of philosophy—and, with a reflexive turn, questioning the very materials of vision that have been appropriated by philosophical thought in the history of its discursive construction of itself.

If we as philosophers fail to give the gift of critical thought to the vision of our culture, to its history and its future possibilities; if we fail to examine the vision that the discourse of philosophy promotes with its descriptions, explanations, and epistemologies; if we fail to reflect on the world our vision has made, or made visible, how shall we answer to those who, like Benjamin, may someday accuse philosophical thought of tolerating, or even producing, "seers whose visions appear to them over corpses"?[56]

Of course, not many of us—those of us who have been gifted with the capacity to see—think of ourselves as seers. This thought brings out the striking ambiguity, or say the tension, in our word *vision*. The word can refer not only to sight, to visual perception, but also to a certain moral capacity; a vivid, articulate, imaginative understanding of the world, of life, of reality; a deep sense of what really matters; a clear realization of ultimate concerns, and of how our world must be related to these concerns; the capacity to think about things with a sense of how they all hang together, how everything comes together to form a whole; and the capacity to imagine a different and better world, life, reality. A seer is one who can speak of, with, and out of "a vision": one whose sight is informed by a vision. Such a vision is not only different from sight; it is also different from a view, a viewpoint. The difference is a question of largeness, of reach and range—and also the presence or absence of a sense of the matter in its wholeness. But it is also a question of openness, and consequently of a certain vulnerability, generosity, and sense of justice—taking this last term in its ancient meaning, according to which it refers to a sense of order, measure, and limit.

The history of vision to which the discourse of philosophy has contributed may not be a history constructed out of visions in this most elevated sense. But I argue that the philosophers examined in this book do not just see what they see and record their reflections on what they can or cannot see. Rather, they are thinkers who have looked at their world and seen it as no others have seen it: thinkers who have seen with, or in the light of, a certain understanding of what it is to see, what sight really is, what its conditions, limits, and possibilities are, and what it can, or should become, that is much deeper, and or anyway different from, the understanding that informs the ways of seeing that have prevailed in the world. These philosophers have at least this in common: all are estranged from ordinary vision, or from prevailing habits; they are moved by some discomfort, or by a sense of the uncanny, something invisible to others, to engage in critical reflections on ordinary vision, ordinary sight, and are engaged in a project of (re)construction: the articulation of a different vision, a different way of seeing things. For some, it is a question of the correct and the incorrect, of appearance and reality, deception and truth; for others, it is a question of the visible and the invisible; and for still others, it is a question primarily of reification, and the end of domination and violence. For some, it is a question of bringing sight in line with science; for some, it is a question of drawing out what is playful and poetic in our capacity for vision; for others, it is a question of an ethics of lucidity or a politics of subversion.

For many of the contributors to this collection, the political dimension of the visualism that has ruled over the discourse of philosophy is of paramount significance—and even perhaps of some urgency, insofar as philosophy is not only a reflection on the ideals and conditions of society but also, inevitably, a reflection of these ideals and conditions—a reflection that, if it is not subject to critical questioning, can end up merely serving to reinforce existing social and cultural forces. Thus, we need to give thought to the ways in which the rhetoric of vision, which philosophical discourse has for too long uncritically adopted, can disempower, alienate, and marginalize members of gender, racial, and ethnic groups that are not strongly oriented by the ocularcentrism of the dominant culture. As Bernard Hibbitts points out in "Making Sense of Metaphors: Visuality, Aurality, and the Reconfiguration of American Legal Discourse," there are "profoundly divisive social implications" in the metaphors on which a discourse chooses to depend.[57] When we take the cultural resonances of language usage into account, to describe thought as "reflection" and knowledge as "seeing with clarity" is not a normatively neutral discursive practice.

The chapters in this book examine some of the philosophers who have made, or attempted to make, some kind of important difference in the history of vision, exposing our habits, dispositions, practices, and institutions to an array of discursive contestations.

In chapter 1, "From Acoustics to Optics: The Rise of the Metaphysical and the Demise of the Melodic in Aristotle's *Poetics*," Christopher Smith proposes a reading of the *Poetics* that not only challenges the extreme cognitivism, and therefore the commitment to ocularcentrism, that has prevailed from the very beginning in the interpretation of this work, but also reveals, by an immanent critique that reads the text hermeneutically as a palimpsest of meanings, the presence in Aristotle's thought of some deep tensions, conflicts, and contradictions—problems Smith attributes to the philosopher's incomplete shift from a thinking that acknowledges the importance of the auditory to a thinking firmly committed to the priority of vision. Reading the *Poetics* after Nietzsche, Smith extends to this text Nietzsche's deconstruction of the opticality in Greek tragedy—and in the interpretations of Greek tragedy prevailing in his time—as well as Nietzsche's iconoclastic argument that the origin of this theater was Dionysian ritual, song, and music. Smith argues that although Aristotle's thought is predominantly visual, there still are traces of an earlier acoustical vocabulary and a way of thinking much closer to listening; and he attempts to bring out an "understanding of tragedy as the self-contradictory turn away from tragedy's acoustic and melodic underpinnings . . . , a turn that for all its self-contradictoriness has defined the subsequent course of Western thought." "Hence," he says, "in going back to this text, we reach a decisive moment in the development of Western metaphysical thought, when the optical has come to prevail, but not without leaving traces of the 'earlier' acoustical experience that it would displace."

Smith finds in Aristotle's text a complex, ambiguous, incompletely settled synthesis of earlier, pre-Platonic understandings of tragedy and later, post-Platonic understandings. The conception of tragedy that understands it to be a theatrical representation for spectators looking on at a certain spatial and psychological distance conceals traces of an earlier, more archaic conception that understands it as a ritual enactment for an audience immersed in an experience of music and voices. According to Smith, this betrays a momentous historical shift in which the *logos* and its rationality—a detached, dispassionate, theoretical mode of insight—silently displaced the participatory pathos of a musical mode of experience. This privileging of seeing over hearing, the logical over the tonal, involved, Smith says, profound shifts in the way *mimesis* and *katharsis*, the theatrical demand for emotional participation, were to be understood and experienced. It also meant the triumph of written culture over the older culture of speaking and listening, and the privileging of learning by detached mental representation or envisioning over learning by mimetic physical participation, a deacoustification of language, whereby onomatopoetic namings were replaced by visible signs for things beheld theoretically. Ultimately, therefore, the domination of vision meant the hegemony of a different conception of rationality—one that thinks itself disembodied, timeless, and unchanging and that takes pride in its emotional detachment, its ability to remain untouched and unmoved by what it sees. In the early years of Western philosophy, Plato turned the philosophical vocation into a theoretical discipline, a strenuous effort to achieve an intellectual vision of the eternal Forms. In his bold and surprising interpretation of Aristotle's *Poetics*, Smith convincingly retrieves from the ruins of the text a moment of great significance when Aristotle conformed his thought to the discursive hegemony of his teacher's ocularcentrism—a moment when the history of vision itself was in the process of being discursively made.

In chapter 2, "Aristotle on Specular Regimes: The Theater of Philosophical Discourse," James Porter examines the discursive logic of the vision-generated tropes and figures at work in Aristotle's thinking, especially in his *Metaphysics*, *Ethics*, and *Politics*, deploying strategies of reading—critical, hermeneutical, and deconstructive—that are similar to those used by Smith.

Porter's work significantly clarifies how, as Charles Taylor puts it, "*visions* of the good may be connected to certain forms of domination." According to Taylor, this "was obvious in certain cases, e.g., the warrior ethic of fame and glory plainly exalted men and gave a subordinate and largely ancillary role to women. But various forms of more lofty, seemingly universal spiritual *outlooks* may also foster inequality and the suppression of supposedly lesser beings. Allegiance to certain kinds of hypergoods leads to a suppression of 'nature', and this introduces relations of domination within us. These relations then become fatally *reflected* in those between people."[58] But whereas Taylor connects domination only with the assumption of a sovereign good, Porter's analysis of Aristotle's *Politics* demonstrates a connection between domination and visuality in the relationship of citizens to the ethical source of their political life—and indeed a connection between domination and the character of the vision in terms of which the sovereign good is brought to the light and granted authority over comportment and the conditions of life. (Notice the words I have italicized in quoting Taylor.)

Calling attention to a familiar system of figures and tropes that in many ways has been constitutive of philosophy since its very beginning—the system of terms that come from the realm of visual perception—Porter analyzes what he calls the "stylisms of thought" operative in Aristotle's texts and brings to the light their theoretical and practical effects, their metaphysical and political significance. According to Porter, many features of Aristotle's thinking fall into place when his philosophy is viewed as a discipline and method for organizing the "perceptual field," reconstituting the objects within any domain, so that they can be controlled from the commanding perspective of the discipline that oversees it. Like Plato's *Republic*, the *Politics* formulates a typology of political systems and a theory of their evolution. But it is in addition an attempt, again like Plato's, to formulate the true theory—or, quite literally, the appropriate philosophical gaze—that should govern the exercise, the *techne*, of power. On Porter's reading, Aristotle's text comes into focus not only as a critical examination of theories of power generated by vision but also as a reflection on the operations of power, a reflection that anticipates Foucault's analysis of the theatrical and panoptical modes of power. Reading the *Politics* in this light, we see, through Aristotle's eyes, that repression works by keeping subjects under constant public surveillance, subjecting them to normative conditions of visibility. We see that, in tyrannies, the political space is externally organized as a perceptual field dominated by an inescapable administrative presence. According to Aristotle, there are two techniques by means of which the tyrannies he considers are able to control their populations. One of these techniques turns the people of the state into objects of the administrative gaze and disperses the source of the gaze to prevent its detection and verification. With the other technique, the people are collectively constituted as the subject of the gaze, but the focus of their gaze is dispersed by directing it to a dissimulated object. Thus, whereas the first technique involves controlling the population by the constant visibility of the threat of violence, the second technique involves controlling the population by a theatricality that perpetually deceives. The first technique controls by the highly visible appearance of manipulation; the second controls by deception, the invisible manipulation of appearances.

Porter shows Aristotle's thought as strongly influenced by vision. It also shows his thought to be aimed at guiding the civic body to a theoretical vision. Finally, it brings to the light, at the level of both theory and technologies, the complicity of vision in the politics of domination and shows this complicity already determining political thought in the "theoretical" works of Aristotle.

Chapter 3, by Catherine Wilson, is titled "Discourses of Vision in Seventeenth-Century Metaphysics." Thinking about Descartes, Nicolas de Malebranche, Spinoza, and Leibniz, all of whom took a lively and sustained interest in optics, physics, physiology, and the latest technologies of vision, Wilson points out that, contrary to what many people would be led to believe, "it is in the so-called rationalist philosophers that we find the fullest exploitation of empirical theories of vision, an awareness of the curious effects of perspective and the ubiquity of illusion, and the most strenuous use of illuminationist metaphors for the acquisition of knowledge." By contrast, early modern empiricists like John Locke "had as little use for the puzzles and problems of the appearance-reality distinction which optics generates as they do for the notion of an 'inner light,'" and in spite of their professed empiricism, their determination to recognize and legitimate "experience" as the source of all knowledge, in actuality they were not very consistently committed to "empirical evidence" as we think of it today, nor were they much interested in scientific experimentation and the latest technologies of vision.

In Wilson's account, focused on Descartes (1596–1650), Malebranche (1638–1715), and Leibniz (1646–1716), there is a surprising explanation for this paradox, this irony: "The contrasting richness of rationalist discourses of vision is a function of the essentially *redemptive* aspirations of metaphysics, which is dedicated to showing the miraculous under the ordinary, the whole in place of the fragments." Thus, contrary to the historically prevailing view, systematic metaphysics encouraged and supported the new sciences and technologies at least as much as, if not indeed even more so than, the doctrine of empiricism.

Nevertheless, Wilson is cautious about applying the thesis of ocularcentrism and positing anything like a "scopic regime" in regard to the seventeenth century, for, as she says, "within the rationalist texts themselves, there are doubts and anxieties, retreats and rebellions, exceptions and redescriptions, which threaten what Martin Jay has termed 'Cartesian perspectivalism.'" Wilson formulates and examines three received doctrines about visual experience and its meaning in seventeenth-century metaphysics.

The first of these doctrines concerns the logic of vision: the mind as camera obscura, a private, inner theater for the screening of representations. The second doctrine concerns the morality of vision: the "Platonic-Augustinian effort to transcend and repudiate embodiment" by privileging sight over the other senses and subordinating corporeal vision to the sovereignty of "intellectual vision," or "intuition." The third doctrine concerns the politics of vision. The "attempt by metaphysics to describe God's surveillance of the world, or the world itself," from the viewpoint of eternity was accompanied by an attempt to model the absolute state based on a new, more "rational" theory of power—power exercised not through "arbitrary feudal terror" but through the administration of visibility and the visibility of administration, "well-organized, bureaucratic modes of terror." Wilson's analysis accordingly shows that the seventeenth century's "engagement with visuality" not only "produced scientifically important discoveries in optics and the theory of light, the anatomy and psychology of vision," as well as "new knowledge of the microworld and the distant cosmos"; it also was responsible for giving "philosophical and scientific authority to erroneous and coercive epistemologies" and for implicitly recognizing grounds and technologies for the legitimation of the panoptical, totalitarian state.

In her concluding summation, Wilson accounts for the contradictory legacy of seventeenth-century rationalism, its queer mixture of rich and provocative insights, together with egregious conceits and fantasies, by noting that the "rationalist philosophers move between a conception of vision which they construct as a phenomenon of embodiment ... and a conception of vision which they construct as an intellective act."

In her subtle readings of some major seventeenth-century texts, Wilson takes us inside some of their visions, visions of beauty and terror, visions of the sublime and the ridiculous; but she also articulates the invisible undercurrents of thought, the second thoughts and counterproposals, the hesitations, doubts, and inner contradictions that traverse the texts. In readings that bring these texts back to life and make them lively, Wilson demonstrates their enduring significance for contemporary concerns of thought.

In Chapter 4, "How to Write the History of Vision: Understanding the Relationship between Descartes and Berkeley," Margaret Atherton examines the theories of vision proposed by Descartes (1596–1650) and Berkeley (1685–1753) and argues for new readings of their philosophical content and their historical relationship. Pointing out major problems in Descartes's account of vision, Atherton goes on to show how Berkeley's theory emerged from his recognition of these problems and his attempt to resolve them. According to Atherton, the demonstration that there is an immanent, problem-solving logic that connects their two theories suggests a historical narrative regarding the history of vision that differs from the currently prevailing narratives.

In the course of developing her critical analysis of the two philosophers' theories, Atherton establishes the grounds for her doubts concerning the usefulness and accuracy of the narrative, identified now with Richard Rorty and Martin Jay, that portrays Descartes as "a quintessentially visual philosopher" whose ocularcentrism inaugurated "the dominant scopic regime of the modern era" and that makes Descartes "emblematic" of an entire period, "an age that assimilates knowing to seeing, so that knowing is described as gazing with the mind's eye on mental representations that mirror the external world." In addition to challenging this narrative as an accurate account of Descartes's theory and a useful account of his historical significance, Atherton criticizes the narrative for neglecting the existence of an alternative account of vision in the work of George Berkeley—an account that, at the beginning of the eighteenth century, contested major elements in Descartes's theory, and, in the history of vision, "virtually replaced Descartes's as the prevailing account of the nature of vision." Finally, in opposition to the narrative method that emphasizes total epistemic and ontological ruptures, radical discontinuities in history, Atherton also establishes the grounds for a narrative that recognizes instead an "ongoing conversation."

According to Atherton, Descartes deployed no fewer than three different and conflicting models to explain vision and its knowledge—a mechanistic model, a picture theory, and a model that grounds vision in intellectual judgment—as he struggled unsuccessfully to understand how seeing can be both a physiological event and an intellectual act. A "major goal" of Descartes's writing on optics was to argue against the picture model and its camera obscura: "against those who believed that we see by means of little images ... that resemble the objects in the world to be seen." But Descartes's knowledge of the physiology of vision convinced him to carry this iconoclasm further. Holding "that what we see, so far from being a picture copying an exterior world, in fact bears no resemblance to that world at all," he is eventually drawn to the conclusion that "it is the mind which sees, not the eye." If he once thought that, for all he could tell, what his eyes see may be deceptive, he eventually comes to believe that what the eye itself actually perceives is necessarily a false representation of the world. The logic of his account finally compels him to hold that the body inevitably records a distorted image of an exterior scene. Vision cannot be trusted. Thus, as Atherton shows, he could not entirely twist free of the picture model of vision, even though he realized that the camera obscura could never tell the whole story. For Descartes, the truth about our visible world is a construction achieved by geometrical reasoning.

Atherton's Berkeley began his reflections on vision with a keen understanding of the deep tensions in Descartes's account. And being both a philosopher and a theologian, Berkeley, the bishop of Cloyne, wanted not only to achieve a new understanding, something more rationally satisfying and more scientifically adequate; he also wanted to "restore" the dignity of vision. In the philosophically familiar domain of theory, of course—but also, one must surmise, in everyday life as well. Atherton's reading focuses on the strictly philosophical significance of Berkeley's project, but it enables us also to get a sense of its larger significance—say, its redemptive, utopian, theological dimensions. On Atherton's reading, we see Berkeley undertaking a discursive (re)construction of vision, restoring vision to its truth—perhaps as an organ capable of seeing the world in its true light, as the glorious divinity of God's creation.

In any case, Berkeley abandoned Descartes's pictorial model, with its assumption that, in vision, what we see is a picture that misrepresents a nonpictorial world and ventured a different model entirely. The theory that he proposed represents vision as (or as like) a language. In relation to the particular problems with which Descartes was struggling, what recommends this model is the fact that, in a language, the signs do not (or do not have to) resemble their causes and objects—the things they signify. But there were other grounds for Berkeley to find the language analogy appealing. Atherton observes that "Berkeley's theory is predicated on ... the notion of the innocent eye." Indeed: "The device of the blind man made to see is used by Berkeley throughout his account of vision in order to help the reader to become restored to a state of visual innocence. It is a central element in his work." In other words, Berkeley's theory of vision is not only a discursive (re)construction of the vision that figures in the discourse of philosophical theories; it is also a discursive effort to (re)construct the vision through which we dwell in the world. And not only that: it is also, finally, a discursively effected (re)construction that brings to the light the discursive nature of vision.

Atherton points out some surprising—and very attractive—features of Berkeley's theory. Berkeley found that he could make use of the language analogy to formulate a theory of learning that would avoid the problems generated by Descartes's intellectualism and go a long way to explaining how, by sight, we actually perceive distance, size and situation. Just as we have to learn (empirically) the meaning of words—the relation between words and what they signify—so we have to learn (empirically) the meaning of the connection between smallness and faintness and distance. Moreover, this learning process essentially involves tactility and motility; in other words, it essentially involves the body. Thus, whereas Descartes's model of vision turns the one who sees into a detached spectator, a subject who views or observes the world from a disembodied, disengaged, and essentially dehistoricized position, Berkeley's model brings out the intimate relationship between seeing and touching, and it recognizes, at least implicitly, that the one who sees is a practical subject, an agent bodily and practically involved in the world.

Atherton observes that *The New Theory of Vision* is "almost completely free" of theological references and considers that the support the theory rendered to the theological picture of a benevolent God and a providential nature was not in fact the lesson that subsequent readers took from the language analogy. "Berkeley's theory of vision, as it survives in the nineteenth century, is entirely secular in form." This is a tribute to Berkeley's cast of mind: whatever theological significance contemporaries could draw from his theory, Berkeley himself kept his eye on the available scientific evidence and proposed his theory as the best philosophical account of this evidence. Thus, there are, as Atherton shows, reasons internal to the logic of the epistemological problematic that would make Berkeley's insight—that vision is best understood as (or as like) a language—useful and compelling. And yet among some of his contemporaries, the theory would also have suggested certain theological sources and grounds, themes adding for a while to the attractiveness of this theory. In some circles, Berkeley's theory would certainly have been understood in the light of the idea that Nature is a Book written by God in a visible language that we are capable of reading. Atherton notes that although the idea that Nature is God's Book and that we are made capable of reading it was already a very old one in Berkeley's day, Berkeley introduced some new angles. In arguing that nature is a language that can be read, he was denying that natural signs represent by means of resemblance, but he was also calling attention to the fact that it is only through experience—processes of learning, acquired skills—that we connect seemingly arbitrary signs with what they signify. In many ways, then, the vision that Berkeley constructed—a discursive vision—can still speak to us in a way that Descartes's vision surely cannot.

In chapter 5, "Embodying the Eye of Humanism: Giambattista Vico and the Eye of *Ingenium*," Sandra Rudnick Luft retrieves the thought of Giambattista Vico (1668–1744) for a utopian vision that would speak to our time. The story her Vico wants to tell is about the increasing "rationalization" of the human, a process that was already underway in the philosophical thought of ancient Greece and was dramatically advanced by Descartes, for whom the being of the human being was essentially reduced to the identity of a theoretical, epistemological subject. This prioritizing of knowledge, especially the disengaged knowledge of theoretical contemplation, involved subordinating the formation of philosophical discourse to the hegemony of vision—and it meant that doing (*praxis*) and making (*poiesis*) were correspondingly devalued.

Introducing her study of Vico and bringing out the significance of Vico's humanism for our understanding of the present historical situation by taking as her initial point of reference Heidegger's interpretation of the history of Western philosophy and his diagnosis of Western culture, Luft writes, "Heidegger's critique of modernism's enframing of the world as picture at the twilight of the age is matched by one which foresaw the dangers inherent in the objectifying eye of intellect at its dawning.

Giambattista Vico was among the first to sound the alarm against the totalizing tendencies of the system inherent in Cartesian philosophy, against that 'unlimited power for the calculating, planning and molding of all things' which Descartes's optical conception of philosophical method ensured."

According to Luft's reading, which departs from prevailing interpretations, in *Nuova Scienza*, his last work, Vico not only challenged the Cartesian theory of knowledge and formulated a compelling humanist response to its rationalism—a response that led to the development of the human sciences in the nineteenth century. He also repudiated Cartesian subjectivism for the sake of a humanism in which the being of the human being in its true dimensionality would be recognized and encouraged to find expression. "The understanding of being-human that he finally achieved," she writes, "was his way of saying to his age that [in Heidegger's words] 'Being a subject as humanity has not always been the sole possibility belonging to the essence of historical man.'" In order to make his new humanism convincing, Vico constructed a narrative, a story of poetic origins, showing that *humanitas* was not given, but made—a historical achievement of *poiesis*.

According to Vico, this *poiesis*, this making, "was not the activity of subjects, nor of subjectivity, but of language," because language has "the [greatest] power to make what did not exist in nature and thought, the power of setting up a world." Vico's *poiesis* was also a way of seeing, "but its vision was not that of the eye of the soul or rational intellect. It was the imaginative, inventive vision of corporeal beings." (In Latin, the word for this inventiveness is *ingenium, ingegno* in Italian.) Thus: "The eye of *ingenium* did not represent or enframe what it saw." Nor was it driven to objectify and totalize. It was, rather, an imaginative, poetizing eye, an eye that makes what it sees, a truly utopian eye—an eye, therefore, very different from the eye of intellect that figures in the processes of rational judgment.

Luft holds that, "because of his critique of rationalism and its method, and his relation to the rhetorical tradition, Vico seemingly escaped the ocularcentrism of the tradition" to arrive at a uniquely poetic and rhetorical, or discursive, conception of vision. Luft points out that Vico promised the turn from one kind of vision to another in his explanation of the frontispiece that appeared in the original edition of his *Nuova Scienza*. But as Luft shows, one of the things that gives Vico's humanism its contemporary relevance is his understanding in that work of history: "The *factum* of making was recovered from the *certum* of history: the certainty his age desired would not be found in rational concepts, but only in [the making of] history."

Moreover, according to Luft, Vico argued that "causes in the human world are not only historical, but poetic." This, she claims, was the "master key" of this thought—and it meant, as he himself stated, that "the nature of institutions is nothing but their coming into being at certain times and in certain guises." For Vico, "Knowledge was as subject to this genetic principle as were all other institutions. As a *factum* of making, knowledge was itself conditioned by the process of its making.... 'Knowing,' for Vico, was an activity of making social customs and institutions in the concrete historical world." Moreover, "Vico went beyond concern for a formative process within human history to raise even more radical questions about the very setting up of that historical world." Seeing had to be both originary and ontological. "It had to be originary in seeing what did not already exist in nature or in reason and making fictive images. But it also had to be ontological, in that those fictive images would constitute the real world for the seers—the only world they could inhabit."

Luft contends that this new conception and new way of seeing was essentially a "metaphoric vision," a discursive vision utterly different from the vision of Descartes's *Optics* and his methodological works in philosophy: "The metaphoric seeing and making which Vico attributed to the poets was an event in the world, an act of violence," which forced into connection what did not yet exist that way in either nature or thought. Luft also shows that this inventive vision, a vision that is, for Vico, a language, eloquent and communicative, was to participate in the making of a new social and cultural order: "The first way of being was that of Cartesian subjects, cut off from their own imaginative natures and from the *sensus communis* of social beings: it was the existence and optics of beings incapable of civic life."

Vico "did not hold out much hope for preventing a fall into that barbarism of detached and disembodied reflection." But he certainly thought that if we followed a different pedagogy, one that taught the inventive vision, and visionary language, of the imagination, rather than the vision of the Cartesian "eye of judgment," we might be able to achieve the dream of the Rinascimento—a true humanism. Vico called his *Nuova Scienza* a *Rational Civil Theology of Divine Providence* because he thought of it as a radically new vision of the human possibility. And if it was ultimately, for him, a tragic vision, Luft suggests that that was because his recognition of the constructed origin of the human world made him to that degree more keenly aware of the fragility of human institutions, the limitations of cultural horizons, and the fallibility of the human mind.

In *The Phenomenology of Spirit*, Hegel (1770–1831) declared that "the Unhappy Consciousness itself *is* the gazing of one-self-consciousness into another, and itself *is* both, and the unity of both is also its essential nature."[59] He also observed that "the activity of dissolution [*Scheidens*] is the power and work of the understanding, the most astonishing and mightiest of powers, or rather the absolute power ... the monstrous power of the negative [*ungeheuer Macht des Negativen*].... The life of the Spirit is not the life that shrinks from death and keeps itself intact from devastation, but rather the life that endures it and maintains itself in it. It wins its truth only when, in utter dismemberment [*Zerissenheit*], it finds itself. It is this power, not as something positive, which looks away from [*wegsieht*] the negative; ... on the contrary, Spirit is this power only by looking the negative in the face and lingering with it. This lingering [*Verweilen*] with the negative is the magical power that converts it into being."[60] In the next chapter, " 'For Now We See Through a Glass Darkly': The Systematics of Hegel's Visual Imagery," John Russon draws the history of vision into the ruins of the history of *Geist*, carefully looking for dialectical signs, or at least a few traces, hinting at the future of a dawning new Enlightenment. "Hegel's philosophy," he says in his conclusion, "is a philosophy of vision, but of a vision which has its own path of dialectical development." In this chapter, Russon takes the reader step by step through what he calls Hegel's "dialectic of reflection."

Russon contends that our culture is in dire need of a radical critique of the primacy of the "reflective ego" and its vision—its vision of culture and its culture of vision. He argues that such a critique, challenging this ego's delusions—its groundless assumptions, for example, about epistemic superiority of daytime vision, the virtue in clear-sightedness, and the need to disengage vision from all its entanglements with sensory experience, emotion, temporality, and history—and finally giving appropriate recognition to the truth in darkness, in the subterranean, the nonreflective and the embodied, is "at the very heart of Hegel's philosophy," and that, because of the essential connection between the domination of the "reflective ego" and the domination of a certain vision, Hegel's conceptual analysis is "mirrored in a systematic use of visual imagery." Russon shows, moreover, that his numerous but commonly overlooked rhetorical use of vision-generated images and metaphors—his reliance on references to the sun, the dawn, daylight, twilight, the night of the soul, light and darkness, clarity, insight and blindness, reflection, speculation, and enlightenment—corresponds in suggestive and thought-provoking ways to "distinct positions and logical roles along the path of knowledge," beginning with the immediate vision of sense-certainty and its "external reflection" and ending with the absolute vision of speculative thought. According to Russon, the history of Reason, in Hegel, is a story of alienation and reconciliation told in the rhetoric of vision: there is, in fact, a deep complicity between the logic of sight and the logic of the reflective ego, in that "each portrays its object as an alien and self-subsistent reality."

"For Hegel," says Russon, even "the very immediacy of our vision is [in fact a product of mediation] *constructed* through the tradition: social practices which indoctrinate us into a particular vision, a particular set of images, a particular set of visual expectations." And in the story Hegel wants to tell, it is to the

achievement of this vision, the disengaged vision of the autonomous "reflective ego," that the overzealous rationalism of the
Enlightenment, well intentioned yet also in a certain way excessive and distorted, urged us—at least in one of the moments in
its own dialectic. But this, he points out, is the vision of an
observer who experiences himself as totally external to the visible
world; strives to live as if he were a totally self-contained, self-
sufficient, monadic substance, independent and impermeable;
and considers his virtue to consist in the stoic ability to remain
unaffected by anything he sees. Thus, in "external reflection,"
self and other exist in a state of "mutual externality."

Consequently, Russon argues, in regard to the Enlightenment
portrait of the autonomous rational ego, that "Hegel's phenomenological description of . . . the self-reliance of the rational being
as it functions as a hegemonic cultural ideal shows that the social
institutions built exclusively around this ideal destroy themselves
precisely because, by recognizing as valuable *only* what universally and necessarily belongs to all human beings *qua* rational,
this cultural ideal negates the value of all human particularity,
and thus ends up negating the very basis of our self-identity."

According to Russon, Hegel saw the rituals of religion and
everyday life as serving a necessary function. Russon follows
Hegel's narrative of the Spirit's dialectical journey to knowledge,
giving particular attention to Hegel's view that the ego's "reality"
is "the product of the labor of a communal subjectivity struggling to find for itself an identity," and therefore to the function
of religion and the moment of its *Aufhebung*, its sublation or
sublimation, in "absolute knowing." On Russon's reading, Hegel
considered religion to be an extremely important stage on this
journey, because it is "a system of ritualized practices which
establishes for a community an immediate sensible certainty—a
faith in the immediacy of one's vision." In other words, in ritualized life, "we establish for ourselves as members of a community a shared sense of who we are." But he points out that Hegel
also formulated a strong critique of religion, understanding how
it "offers both a context in which individuals can develop, but
also a situation that fails to see its own significance and is

oppressive in its conservatism." The community founded in ritualized life is without critical self-reflection, essentially "idolatrous," worshipping "a set of *Vorstellungen* that are the images
within which the 'rationality' of our existence is enacted."

The tension within ritualized life consequently brings to consciousness the spiritual need for the "absolute knowing" of
"speculative" metaphysics. Speculative thought is a "vision of a
universal humanity." Obviously, therefore, it is radically different
from the vision constitutive of ritualized life. But it is also radically different from the vision of the Enlightenment, because its
universality is not formal and abstract, is not disengaged from
particularity. The transition from religion to "absolute knowledge" is articulated, in Hegel's narrative, by a corresponding
transition from the religious imagery of light and revelation to
the philosophical imagery of speculation, indicating "the perfected vision which apprehends the universal light of concrete
reason as both the ground and the goal of even our darkest
activities." Thus, according to Russon, Hegel's philosophy puts
an end to the egocentric gaze that has been given pride of place
in "reflective philosophy" and can be read as discursively constructing a vision that is "inherently multicultural"—a truly
"enlightened" vision that is precisely what we need as we enter
the twenty-first century.

Russon concludes that "the truth, for us, will always be expressed in images, in metaphors, but equally, our existence as
reflective beings means that our task will always be to see how the
images a community uses to articulate the truth do offer a route
to establishing a universal communication based on the shared
human project of rational self-understanding." The "absolute
knowing" of speculative thought is therefore a political vision
inspired by a "utopian" or "redemptive" Spirit. And its dream,
according to Russon, is "a cross-cultural communication that
seeks not only to enlighten but to be educated by the other into
a new language of self-consciousness within the context of a
mutual pursuit of free rationality."

But how are we to understand Hegel's use of a rhetoric drawn
from vision when it figures in a discourse—for example, in his

lectures on the history of philosophy and his lectures on the philosophy of history—that claims to represent the philosophical truth? What is the "epistemological" status of such rhetoric? Does his use of such metaphoric language compromise the claims of speculative thought? In chapter 7, John H. Smith speaks about "Sighting the Spirit: The Rhetorical Visions of *Geist* in Hegel's *Encyclopedia*." Smith wants to contend that "although Hegel's philosophy develops a clear priority of the conceptual over the visual, (as in his emphasis on *Begreifen* over the contemporary notions of *intellektuales Anschauen*), the problem of how to visualize the Spirit persists in crucial and ironic ways even in his later, more abstract philosophical systems." This, Smith observes, is a major problem because, since the Spirit exists in the world, Hegel must be able to give us images of it and we must be capable of seeing it. Smith points out, however, that the demonstration of Spirit is an extraordinarily tricky matter, and in any case it cannot be done directly: "we and he must be very careful not to *reduce* Spirit to the visible" or in any other way give it priority over the conceptual. It should not be surprising, then, that the clarity of Hegel's thought must be rendered obscure by "a series of basic tensions between images of seeing and concepts of invisible thought"—tensions that Smith shows he could only resolve dialectically "by using the rhetorical strategy of simultaneously depicting and then negating the visual in order to render the 'Spiritual' indirectly visible *through* the negation."

Focusing on Hegel's reflections in the *Encyclopedia*, where he discusses "visions" of a distinctly "pathological" nature— "intuition," clairvoyance," visions" aroused by animal magnetism—Smith's contribution displays Hegel's dialectical treatment of vision and shows how Hegel "argues for, and rhetorically performs, a different kind of visualization"—the one he called "speculation." In this way, we can see how Hegel's text was constructed to enable its readers to participate concretely in a vision of the Spirit: a speculative vision discursively, dialectically, constructed with the cunning of Reason: *die List der Vernunft.*

Smith's analysis concentrates on "Hegel's argument that phenomena (appearances, *Erscheinungen*) of a particular sort can make a visualization of the ideal possible (*zur Anschauung bringen*), a visualization that in turn creates a confusion of the viewer's [taken-for-granted] categories of understanding, so that a different kind of viewing—a *spekulative Betrachtung*—becomes necessary." The possibility of this "shift of vision" depends entirely, however, on Hegel's rhetorical strategies, techniques, and devices, which, ironically and paradoxically, captivate our attention with "amazing and dazzling visions," wondrous events in the realm of the visible that our normative understanding "cannot grasp or even believe," only to use them dialectically—ultimately, after they have served their purpose, he negates them, for they are, after all, "pathological" phenomena—to deconstruct our framework of epistemological and ontological assumptions and release us from the bondage of everyday vision and the immediacy of its sense certainty, making us realize that there is a deep and undeniable spiritual need for the vision of speculative thought, the "sighting" of the Spirit.

Smith explains that the whole point of reflecting on these paranormal "visions" is that, even though—and indeed, precisely because—they "represent the Spirit in a state perilously undifferentiated from nature," they serve to weaken the grip, the normative authority, of the categories of the understanding by which we normally live. "Ironically," says Smith, it turns out that "the only way to come to see speculatively is to learn to see what is not there." But, of course, as Smith shows, to persuade readers to relinquish some of their deepest perceptual norms and see what is not there requires of Hegel all of his considerable rhetorical skills. " 'See the reality of these visions,' Hegel seems to be saying, 'so that in seeing it you will accept the negation of [the heretofore unquestioned] reality they entail, and thereby change your notion of reality.' " The dialectical journey on which Smith's Hegel takes his readers accordingly transports us into the realm of the "feeling-psyche," the realm of darkness, sleep, and dream— a realm of undifferentiated unity that already gives us precious intimations of the speculative unity of the objective and the subjective. Smith's contribution follows the discursive cunning of Hegel's thinking as it strives to open our eyes to the splendor and nobility of speculative vision.

Chapter 8, "Perspectives and Horizons: Husserl on Seeing the Truth," by Mary Rawlinson, examines the visuality of Husserl's phenomenological language, bringing out the deep tensions and contradictions in his commitment to a certain ocularcentrism. Believing, as he says in *Ideas* I, that we need to "learn to see what stands before our eyes," Husserl turned this conviction into a boldly new phenomenological method and an extremely ambitious phenomenological program rigorously committed to the disciplined exercise of the "mental eye."[61]

Perhaps even more than Descartes, the philosopher who influenced him the most, Husserl was an ocularcentric thinker. But there are unresolved tensions, and indeed even contradictions, in this philosophy, because his commitment to a certain rationalism and transcendental idealism simultaneously compels him to depend on and privilege the experience of vision, the seeming immediacy and presence of the gaze, and yet also to reconstruct the nature of vision so that it will be capable of supporting the rationalism of a transcendental metaphysics.

Husserl's rationalism not only blinds him to the assumptions he makes about the nature of vision—assumptions, moreover, that cannot be sustained by a phenomenology not already committed to such a project; it also involves him in a double, and doubly dubious, philosophical movement, whereby with one hand he borrows resources from visual perception—the very same perception that he will subsequently "reject," suspending its sense of contact with reality in an *epokhe* of theoretical doubt—while with the other hand, he undertakes a reconstruction of this borrowed vision that will culminate in the assertion of a purified mental gaze capable of securing absolute and apodictic transcendental knowledge. Rawlinson consequently begins her chapter with a quotation from Merleau-Ponty: "Even the mind's eye has its blind spot."

Rawlinson penetrates the thinking behind Husserl's fatal attraction to vision, exposing the process through which Husserl attempts his discursively generated "translation" of "real" vision into the metaphorical space of an idealized and idealizing vision; along the way, she brings out what is most problematic in a vision claiming to be free of shadows, free of perspectivity, free of horizontal delimitations, free of the mirror play of reflections, and free of all possible illusions—a vision whose claims to immediacy, presence, and an absolute freedom of movement Husserl affirms as the normative paradigm for knowledge, truth, and reality—the paradigm by which even the "real" perception of everyday experience in the "natural attitude" is to be judged.

Carefully following the trajectory of Husserl's thinking, from his vision of philosophy as a presuppositionless science grounding the ontologies of logic, mathematics, geometry, and the objective sciences in the meaning-giving, meaning-constituting acts of transcendental subjectivity to his radical phenomenological suspension of the "thesis" of the life-world, Rawlinson casts a strong critical shadow over Husserl's great enterprise, questioning and problematizing the system of visual terms on which he depends, making it visible as an intricate web of metaphors in which, beyond the possibility of escape from their ultimate ruination of his dreams, Husserl gets himself hopelessly entangled.

Attracted to mundane vision because of some characteristics he assumes—quite mistakenly—that it possesses and enjoys, yet also, as a philosopher thinking in the tradition of rationalism and idealism must be, deeply dissatisfied with the manifest limitations and vulnerabilities of such vision, Husserl struggles, as the narrative in this chapter shows, to transfer to philosophical theory the power, immediacy, presence, and self-certainty of mundane vision, while at the same time protecting it from the incompleteness and inadequation that essentially characterize it. Husserl's strategy thus requires, as she points out, "its own blindness." In spite of this blindness, in spite of his ultimate disownment, Husserl nevertheless provides an excellent picture of perception in action, accurately articulating the enactment of perception in terms of the experiences lived through by the embodied subject and its intentionally structured field. Thus, for example, his account of mundane visual perception boldly contests and radically rewrites—or say discursively reconstructs—the conventional philosophical understanding of our perceptual relationship to the unseen parts of visible objects, insisting against the weight of tradition that it is not a question of inference or induction but involves, rather, a prepredictive, prelogical, prereflective intentional sense. Husserl's careful, patient, detailed phenomenological descriptions of mundane visual perception, some examples of which Rawlinson provides, were, and still are, unequaled models of phenomenological method, exhibiting the power and the truth of this method.

As Rawlinson brings out, the phenomenological description of mundane vision is, for Husserl, merely a preliminary step, making it possible for him to define an altogether different vision: the essentially omnipotent vision of the transcendental Ego, freed of all mundane interests, all worldly limitations—an abstract gaze released, he thought, even from time and from the finality of death time inevitably brings. Thus, it was in the "eidetic vision," the *Wesensschau* of the transcendental Ego, that Husserl's obsession with vision found its moment of consummation. But as Rawlinson points out, this victory—if that is what it may be called—is won at a very high price, for this vision is haunted by the ghosts of the Other, the ghosts of all those whom its seemingly undeniable solipsism has unilaterally banished from its world. Thus, she says, "The other can be presented as another ego only insofar as he is 'the same.'" Tracing the discursively generated reconstruction of vision in Husserl's phenomenology, what Rawlinson shows us is that although, in the end, the transcendental ego can see only itself, for Husserl "it would [thereby] see everything."

In his *Philosophical Investigations,* Wittgenstein says: "We find certain things about seeing puzzling, because we do not find the whole business of seeing puzzling enough."[62] In chapter 9, "Ducks and Rabbits: Visuality in Wittgenstein," William James

Earle argues that Wittgenstein's work should be read as an endeavor, among other things, to free philosophical thought from the hegemony of vision—a "worldview" that in one way or another has determined it since Plato—and put an end to treacherous metaphors from the zone of vision, as well as misleading assumptions about the nature of vision and dubious arguments in which the mischief of vision somehow always figures.

And yet in the *Investigations*, Wittgenstein admonishes philosophers with the counsel, "Don't think, but look!" What is involved in looking? What would be the difference, here, between thinking and looking? In Umberto Eco's *Il nome della rosa*, there is a search for a missing book of great importance. In the course of this search, the man who represents enlightenment in an age dominated by the feudal mentality has occasion to clarify a common distinction: the one between looking and seeing. Here is the dialogue:

—Allora dovrebbe essere ancora là. Ma non c'è.
 —Un momento. Noi diciamo che non c'era perché non lo abbiamo trovato. Ma forse non lo abbiamo trovato perché non lo abbiamo visto dov'era.
 —Ma abbiamo guardato dappertutto!
 —Guardato, ma non visto. Oppure visto ma non riconosciuto.[63]

 —*Then it should still be there. But it isn't.*
 —*Wait! We say that it's not there because we haven't found it. But perhaps we haven't found it because we haven't seen it where it was.*
 —*But we've looked everywhere!*
 —*Looked but not seen. Or rather seen, but not recognized. (my translation)*

What is the difference between looking and seeing? Is this a "natural" difference or something we have discursively constructed? And what is involved in "recognition"? Is it a constituent of the act of seeing? Or is it an inference, a purely cognitive act, performed on the basis of the "visual evidence"? As Earle shows, these questions generate problems that, for later Wittgenstein, can be resolved only by close philosophical attention to the intricate grammar of our discourse.

With regard to the question of ocularcentrism—the hegemony of vision in our cultural paradigm of knowledge, truth, and reality—Earle argues that Wittgenstein disliked, and explicitly rejected, the use of grand narratives in philosophizing—an attitude implying that, although he never explicitly recognized ocularcentrism and never discussed it, he would have been opposed to it as an interpretation or explanation of the history of philosophy and the history of vision, and indeed would have opposed it with equal force as the premise of a philosophical argument. For related reasons, Wittgenstein also rejected philosophical oversimplification and reductionism, thinking that assimilates all things (entities, phenomena, situations, experiences) to one kind of thing (entity, phenomenon, situation, experience), twentieth-century versions of the doctrine of immutable species. And this he did explicitly. Thus, says Earle, for Wittgenstein, there is "no *Zeitgeist*, no World-Spirit, no *Weltanschauung*, no episteme, no Spirit of the age, no Western philosophical tradition, no 'key cause,'" making perfect sense out of our culture. Wittgenstein would consequently have had no use for Heidegger's interpretation of Western history, according to which modernity is "the age of the world picture," an epoch in the history of being toward the pictorial, enframing character of which Western civilization was already disposed from the very beginning.

In spite of this attitude, expressed unequivocally in his later writings, it might still be thought nevertheless that Wittgenstein's *Tractatus Logico-Philosophicus*, written at the beginning of his philosophical work, is in fact a text unquestionably influenced by, and belonging to, the tradition of ocularcentrism; it could be argued that it makes sense only if read as a work conceived by and addressed to a certain mental or intellectual vision—a work that assumes our mental capacity for picturing something to ourselves.

Earle argues, however, that "there is, in fact, next to nothing about vision, the visual, or visibility in the *Tractatus*. 'Picture' or *Bild*, which sounds visual, always refers to representations or models viewed purely abstractly in terms of their isomorphism (or, in the case of *false* propositions, isomorphism-failure) with the reality they purport to picture." But is the matter of Wittgenstein's relationship to ocularcentrism so easily settled? Earle quotes P. M. S. Hacker as commenting that "the *Tractatus* provided a complex and non-trivial logico-metaphysical *explanation* of the pictoriality of thought by way of the doctrines of isomorphism and atomism. Agreement between thought and reality was held to be agreement in form, and an elaborate atomistic logic and metaphysics was delineated to explain isomorphism." In other words, Hacker concludes, "Pictoriality doesn't mean more than 'representationality.'" But what exactly does this mean? In what sense does "representationality" entirely escape visualism—escape not only its substance but its rhetoric? And how can we understand "isomorphism," and even "logical space," without in any way assuming a pictorial, vision-like, or image-producing mental activity? Earle cites a later comment by Wittgenstein: "Here instead of harmony or agreement of thought and reality, one might say: the pictorial character of thought. But is the pictorial character an agreement? In the *Tractatus* I had said something like: it is an agreement of form." After considering the reflections of several eminent scholars on Wittgenstein's so-called picture-theory of propositions and propositional meanings, Earle concludes that "Wittgensteinian pictures have no more to do with visual pictures than logical space has to do with the ordinary three-dimensional space we move around in." Whether this reading settles the question will no doubt remain a matter for continued debate. Earle's conclusion still permits one to argue that "logical space" is a projection the possibility of which is dependent, or say "parasitic," on a prior practical understanding of the space we bodily inhabit, and that Wittgenstein's *Tractatus* propositional pictorialism is similarly dependent on our prior experience with making and seeing pictures.

As for the discussions of matters that, prima facie, are "about" vision—the diagram of the eye in a visual field, for example—Earle contends, "In any case, it seems obvious that nothing here has a special connection with *seeing* or *visual* experience." Thus, for example, the discussion of the eye and the visual field is "really" to be read—or is "better" read—as an argument about the grammar of reflexive pronouns and the logic of our conception of the self, while the discussion of the Neckar cube is "really" to be read—or is "better" read—as an argument against Russell's analysis of simple and complex facts. In any case, whether or not we read the *Tractatus* as a work generated by a certain vision, Earle shows that it cannot be denied that Wittgenstein eventually abandoned the *Tractatus* way of thinking in his later work. In his later writings, what changed most fundamentally was his conception of philosophy itself. Philosophy became "whatever we can use in the 'battle against the bewitchment of our intelligence by means of language.' Philosophy clears away misunderstandings, assembles reminders for particular clarificatory purposes, generates perspicuity or *Übersichtlichkeit*, and its methods are like therapies, its treatments of questions like the treatments of illnesses." So, if Wittgenstein's thinking is sometimes articulated in the rhetoric of vision and seems at times to be preoccupied with questions of vision, that is only because he is fighting fire with fire.

Focusing on Wittgenstein's discussion of "seeing as," "noticing an aspect," and "the dawning of an aspect," Earle argues that, even here, Wittgenstein's interest was not in vision as such, or even only in the contrast between the *grammar* of our ordinary way of talking about seeing and its objects and the *logic* of the accounts of vision that philosophers have proposed, but rather more in showing how proper respect for the grammar of the language we ordinarily use in talking about our experience with sight can dissolve our philosophical perplexities about larger, more central epistemological problems, of which the philosophical accounts of vision are merely instances or exemplifications. This, Earle asserts, "is not a matter of becoming aware of a difference in our visual experience. Scrutinizing our experience will always, in Wittgenstein's book, get us nowhere."

According to Earle, then, Wittgenstein's interest in the duck-rabbit picture and the sudden gestalt-switch it induces, as well as in the other cases of visual perception he examines, is "really" to be understood in terms of his attempt to demonstrate that philosophical perplexities and aporias can best be handled by contextualizing them in the practical situations, the "forms of life" he calls "language games." The relevance of this linguistic turn to the concerns of this book is that the "grammatical" approach enables Wittgenstein to deconstruct a framework with some very tenacious ideas and assumptions, dominant for a long time in the epistemological systems of both rationalism and empiricism, regarding the nature of seeing—ideas and assumptions that philosophical thought, departing from "common sense" and "ordinary language" usage, discursively constructed and that have played a significant, rather mischievous role in the philosophical elaboration of theories claiming to account for knowledge, understanding, belief, deception, illusion, learning, and so forth. Although many of these ideas and assumptions that Wittgenstein attacks are clearly dependent on an ocularcentric way of thinking—a function of a vision-generated and vision-based logic—it seems that Wittgenstein never thematized or challenged this logic as such. And yet it must be acknowledged that, in his later writings, he singled out for especially sharp and sustained attack four of the major, vision-generated tenets that disfigure the epistemologies to which he was heir. In other words, without challenging ocularcentrism as such, he nevertheless challenged many of the philosophical constructions of vision—the predominant ways philosophers have interpreted, described, and explained vision—and unequivocally rejected the common philosophical uses of vision in the construction of theories of knowledge—above all, and in particular: (1) philosophies that rely on the psychology of introspection and intuition and model the activity of the mind on vision; (2) the picture-theory of the mind, for which the mind is an inner theater or screen, mental activity is a form of seeing, and ideas and meanings come in the form of images; (3) the assumption that self-knowledge is a form of self-observation and that the justification of such knowledge follows the logic of third-person reports; and finally, (4) phenomenalism, the theory holding that the perception of "external objects" is the outcome of a process of interpretation, an inference based on the direct and immediate perception of private intensional objects called "sense data." Thus, however one interprets the *Tractatus*, there can be no question that by the time of the *Philosophical Investigations*, Wittgenstein was a major advocate for what subsequently has been described as the 'linguistic turn,' and that this turn is, above all, a turn away from vision as the paradigm of knowledge, truth, and reality.

Chapter 10, by Yaron Ezrahi, is on "Dewey's Critique of Democratic Visual Culture and Its Political Implications." In "The Idea of an Overlapping Consensus," John Rawls declared: "The maxim that justice must not only be done, but be seen to be done, holds good not only in law but in free public reason."[64] It cannot be reasonably denied that the justice of modern democratic institutions must be in the public's eye. If power is to be legitimate, it must be rendered public—open to the rationality of scrutiny, debate, and participation. This is a fundamental axiom of liberalism, and it is at the very heart of social contract theories. But the question is: Just how much of a role, and what kind of role, should the condition of visibility be granted in our contemporary technologized world, in particular, with regard to the further democratization of the state, the flourishing of a lively, democratic public sphere and the formation of a critical public, and the rational institutionalization of administrative accountability? This is a question about the contribution of vision and visibility to public morality, democratic politics, and an adequate civic epistemology.

Ezrahi examines Dewey's critique of the Enlightenment's "spectator theory of knowledge" in order to show how this critique enabled Dewey to challenge the "scopic paradigm" of democratic politics, with its "presupposition that public actions and their consequences are, or can be, transparent to critical democratic citizens," and to formulate a theory of democratic politics in which he proposes a radically different understanding of "the very nature of authority, action and accountability in the modern democracy." According to Ezrahi, the "dimensions of Dewey's break with the established spectatorial model of democratic politics can be supported by reference to Tocqueville's influential articulation of the place of sight in the American democracy nearly a hundred years earlier."

Ezrahi contends that Dewey's challenge to the hegemony of vision in democratic political theory and democratic politics is easy to overlook: first, "because his vocabulary is still rooted in classical Enlightenment metaphors"; second, "because in some respects the shift is less than complete"; and third, because "Dewey's writings show at times a tendency to romanticize the Enlightenment ideal of government fully visible to the public." Ezrahi argues, however, that in spite of these problems, these tensions, "Dewey's shift away from spectatorial democratic politics is ... decisive and significant." According to Ezrahi, Dewey's thinking addresses itself to a "spreading, late-twentieth-century distrust of the earlier Enlightenment faith in the possibility of visually manifest rationality in public affairs." And Dewey's worries about the "eclipse of the public" are especially relevant at this time, when a media-run politics of images is becoming increasingly theatrical, while the mechanisms that really determine public policies, actions, and their consequences become more and more opaque, more and more invisible. Ezrahi's analysis thus shows that Dewey's work is a timely and thought-provoking answer to our increasingly urgent, increasingly recognized need to find a democratic successor to ocularcentric politics: a theory and praxis of political power, responsibility, and participation that would promote and protect rational processes of democratization in the public sphere—just as, in very different historical conditions, the ocularcentric theory and praxis of the Enlightenment once did.

Calling attention to Dewey's 1929 work, *The Quest for Certainty*, Ezrahi shows that Dewey's attempt to move beyond the spectator theory of politics was "not unrelated" to his dissatisfaction with a spectatorial conception of scientific knowledge and his effort to formulate a more rationally adequate account of experimentation and observation in the sciences. In that work, Dewey laid out his objections to the model of knowledge based on disengaged vision and proposed a model based on interaction, recasting the "outside spectator" as an "inside participator."

In Dewey's discussion of his hopes for a flourishing public sphere, and in particular, a more participatory form of democracy, Ezrahi discerns three major arguments for the new model of politics he wanted to propose: (1) that "relations between the causes and consequences of public actions in the modern industrial society have become increasingly more complex and more invisible to the wider public"; (2) that "seeing and observing is not a merely passive recording of external objects, but rather an active, productive process of engaging, selecting and organizing visual experience"; and (3) that communication—speaking and listening—is actually "more instrumental than seeing in the formation of public opinion and in substantiating and legitimating sociopolitical participation."

Ezrahi agrees with Dewey's critique of ocularcentric politics—quite moderate in comparison with the antiocularcentrism in contemporary French thought—and appreciates Dewey's attempt, deeply embedded in the American tradition of liberalism, to formulate a model of politics based on free and rational interaction, on the freedom and rationality of speaking and listening. But he shows that Dewey, like Rousseau, cannot satisfactorily resolve the problem of "how meaningful conversation can take place in the larger society beyond the boundaries of local communities, in which individuals can engage in ongoing face-to-face relationships." This, perhaps, is the point where Habermas's theory of communicative action carries forward Dewey's theoretical efforts to strengthen, expand, and democratize the public sphere, promoting the activities constitutive of good citizenship, opening up the public sphere to the justice of more rational, more democratic, more egalitarian processes of decision making and opinion formation, protecting the freedoms of the public sphere from the excessive power of the state and the pernicious effects of corporate capitalism.

After a comparison of Dewey's critique of ocularcentric politics with the recent critique advanced by French philosophers—a comparison followed by an explanation for the extreme hostility of the French—Ezrahi concludes his study with the reflection that "Dewey's importance as a twentieth-century democratic thinker resides ... in the degree to which he has gone beyond this classical vocabulary of the democratic discourse on culture and politics", beyond the vocabulary of both the Enlightenment and the French critics of the Enlightenment. While discursively deconstructing the hegemony of vision in our modern paradigm of knowledge, truth, and reality, Dewey was also attempting a discursive reconstruction of the way we see, the way our vision functions. "In the final analysis," says Ezrahi, "Dewey's critique of the scopic paradigm of democracy, which Tocqueville enunciated so clearly, is one more step in the emancipation of democratic politics from the grip of hierarchical and oppressive cultural forms inherited from the predemocratic era."

One more step—which means that other steps must follow, for this historical process must be a continuing one. The very concept of enlightenment demands that the promise in the goal, in the end, never be identified with an already achieved state. This demand, however, draws us into the problematic of the next chapter. In one of Vitaliano Brancati's short stories, there is a character whose experiences in life draw him into the penumbra of a disquieting observation: "La sproporzione fra la portata della nostra vista e quella della nostra mano fa nascere le chimere e provoca le grandi disillusioni" ("The distance between the reach of our sight and that of our hand gives rise to phantasms and provokes great disillusionments").[65] This observation has material and indeed political implications. Does progress toward social enlightenment require the guidance of a political vision? Could such a political vision avoid the turn that leads into the abyss of terror or despair?

In chapter 11, "Materialist Mutations of the *Bilderverbot*," Rebecca Comay reflects on the dialectical complexities involved in the radically new, secularized, and materialist interpretation that Benjamin and Adorno give to the ancient suspicion of images and to the law of their prohibition—a prohibition at the very heart of Jewish theology. That the Jewish ban on images was connected with the emergence of monotheism, and thus with an attempt to put an end to "idolatry," seems clear enough. But how can the iconoclasm in this theological history be appropriated for a critique of the function of representation in the modern world? How can it be used in a critical social theory to interpret the nature and development of late capitalism? How can it give support to dialectical materialism?

Comay begins her reflections by pointing to the connection that Benjamin and Adorno see between the theological ban on images, intended to avoid the danger of idolatry, and their own reluctance to picture in any positive way the world that would follow in the wake of capitalism. For them, the danger that must be avoided is a secular form of idolatry, a false materialism, a regressive positivism: identifying utopia with the existing political order. Drawing out the implications of her reading of Benjamin's first thesis on history, a thesis formulated in terms of some very provocative images—the "theological" dwarf and the puppet of "historical materialism"—Comay's commentary brings out not only the complexity of Benjamin's thinking but also its dialectical ambiguity: "To celebrate the unfettered progress of the 'apparatus'—Social Democracy, from one side, Stalinism, from the other—is in itself to fall prey to the transcendental illusion which would hypostatize the absolute as already there."

Pointing out the elective affinities between Benjamin's and Adorno's analysis of the danger and earlier formulations of the problem in Kant, Hegel and Marx, Comay observes, "This is fetishism: to depict redemption as a logical extension or continuation of the present is effectively to confuse noumenal with phenomenal and thus only to confirm one's own immersion in the imaginary. Every 'ideal of liberated grandchildren' cannot but fail, in this sense, to function ideologically: the very faith in a better future secretly prolongs and sanctifies the given, offering placating pictures that would only distract the viewer from the most urgent imperatives of the day. Thus idolatry: the substitution of the existent for the possible." For Benjamin and Adorno, the philosophers of the Enlightenment fell victim, in spite of their sagacity, to a tempting illusion: confident that the light of Reason could give them a certain vision, they honored the false god of progress—a god that subsequent history has shown to be nothing but a terrible illusion. As Benjamin and Adorno see things, if there is still an unredeemed utopian potential for happiness, its promise can be safeguarded only so long as we deny that it can be adequately represented in the present.

The danger in producing images of utopia that reconcile us to the fate of prevailing conditions must be weighed against the danger in refusing to imagine alternatives to oppression, an end to misery and violence—or against what is perhaps the most extreme danger: denying the very possibility that the conditions of damaged life could someday be otherwise. If there is risk in trusting an imagination that could fail, in spite of good intentions, to free itself from the *adequatio ad rem*, there would seem to be equal danger in the absence of images that would represent, and bear witness to, the need for a different world, the *Sehnsucht nach dem ganz Anderen*, images that would simultaneously demonstrate what is wrong with our social order and affirm the hope that things could be different.[66] A certain positivism, surrendering to the given social reality, haunts both the production of utopian images and the renunciation of such images. But can the imagination be productive? Can it ever really free itself from the prevailing social conditions of production? Can it avoid being the deceptive re-production of prevailing social forces? Is there a way out of this double bind? Can a critical social theory dispense with the imagination? Can a theory of society function in a critical way without a vision of something better—without a vision of ends? Does the avoidance of imagination impair the critical, theoretical functioning of Reason, reducing it to an instrument that reflects only on means, not ends? (The connection between vision and the word *theory*, derived from the language of ancient Greece, should not be forgotten here.)

Although apparently not familiar with the thought of Benjamin and Adorno, Foucault followed a trajectory of thinking that led him to a similarly iconoclastic position. Concerned about utopian imagination turning into a "gaze of power" and about the importance of not settling "for the affirmation or the empty dream of freedom," he consistently argued against "global, totalitarian theories" and urged the adoption of a certain "positivism," a certain "historical-critical" and "experimental" methodology.[67] In a 1971 interview, given the title, "Revolutionary Action: 'Until Now,'" Foucault declared: "I think that to imagine another system is to extend our participation in the present system." And in replying to an interlocutor who suggested that what is needed may be "a utopian model and a theoretical elaboration that goes beyond the sphere of partial and repressed experiences," Foucault said: "Why not the opposite? Reject theory and all forms of general discourse! This need for theory is still part of the system we reject." What he proposes is to base resistance to oppression on "actual experiences rather than the possibility of a utopia. It is possible," he says, "that the rough outline of a future society is supplied by the recent experience with [psychotropic] drugs, sex, communes, other forms of consciousness, and other forms of individuality. If scientific socialism emerged from the *Utopias* of the nineteenth century, it is possible that a real socialization will emerge, in the twentieth century, from *experiences*."[68] In Foucault's words on the question of utopian images one can discern the struggles of many other thinkers coming before him, notably those of the Frankfurt school philosophers—except that the matter is more complex for Benjamin and Adorno, and the interpretation of their position is correspondingly more shaded by equivocation.

Thus, as Comay says, we find in Benjamin's "Theses on History" the "familiar catalog of renunciations—the historian as the prophet facing backward (Schlegel), the modern Orpheus who now stands to lose his Eurydice by looking ahead (Jean Paul). The angel of history catches not even a glimpse of the future to which his back is turned.... No image, similarly, inspires the revolutionary: neither 'the ideal of liberated grandchildren' nor the 'utopia 'painted in the heads' of the Social Democrats." As Comay suggests, Benjamin stated the position very tersely when he wrote: "Whoever wants to know how a 'redeemed humanity' would be constituted, under what conditions it would be constituted, and when one can count on it, poses questions to which there is no answer. He might as well ask about the color of ultraviolet rays."

"But," Comay writes, "how can a materialist prohibition against images be enunciated?" Because of the way prohibition incites desire, Comay asks: "Is there not something profoundly contradictory about the very representation of the law forbidding representations of the future? Would not the law inevitably transgress itself in its very pronouncement?" These questions strike at the very heart of radical politics. As she observes, "the very renunciation of images threatens precisely once more to determine the future as a tabula rasa or blank slate receptive to the arbitrary projections of the present day." This would mean the self-defeating reaffirmation of the "homogeneous empty time" of classical physics and the factory assembly line of capitalism.

Reflecting on Scholem's suggestions concerning the interpretation of redemption in Judaism, Comay observes that the hermeneutic approach to the texts of Judaic theology and the correlative privileging of language (the symbolic) over vision (the imaginary) effectively forecloses the temptation to identification inherent in all visualization, and hence the likelihood of an idolatrous confusion of the Same and the radically, absolutely Different. These considerations lead Comay into a discussion of the debate over *schöne Schein*, the consoling image of a redeemed world, and the relation between truth and beauty. Benjamin and Adorno resumed this debate, formulating the question of the fate of art in the context of the dialectic of Enlightenment. Comay's contribution takes the reader into the dialectical subtleties of this problematic.

Like Dewey, Hannah Arendt called into question the hegemony of vision in the discourse of philosophy; and also like Dewey, she came to "wonder why hearing did not develop into the guiding metaphor for thinking," especially in regard to the realm of the political.[69] In chapter 12, "Hannah Arendt: The Activity of the Spectator," Peg Birmingham examines Arendt's critique of the construction of vision in the history of philosophy and brings out an implicit dimension of the argument that other readings of Arendt have overlooked: one in which the paradigm of vision is not so much rejected as it is reconstructed and reformed, making it capable of assuming a vital, critical function in the realm of the political. Readers of Arendt will be familiar with her questioning of the vision-paradigm and her entertainment of the idea that listening and speaking would be a much better paradigm. But readers seem not to have noticed that Arendt's critique of this paradigm and her brief speculations about making language the new paradigm are only part of her project: the other part, drawing on her retrieval of the historical role of the spectator-judge in the public events of ancient Greece, is a rehabilitation of the critical potential in vision. Seeing is not necessarily believing, nor is it necessarily a form of resignation. According to Birmingham, what Arendt's return to the lifeworld of the ancient Greeks brings to the light is a practice of vision that is much more than a simple, uncritical perception of the given—a vision, in fact, that is the exercise of a capacity for critical reflection and judgment. Reading Arendt, Birmingham reminds us that looking and seeing can take place in a spirit of suspicion as well as in a spirit of trust, that they can meet what is to be seen with questioning as well as acceptance, and that they can be endistancing as well as receptive.

Birmingham's chapter begins with Arendt's observation, in *Life of the Mind*, that a paradigm shift of major proportions has taken place within philosophy: a shift, as she puts it, "from contemplation to speech, from *nous* to *logos*." But Birmingham proceeds to show that on a more comprehensive reading, Arendt's reflections suggest that her position is more intricate than the one this observation, taken by itself, seems to represent. This is the case, according to Birmingham, for two reasons: first, because, in an interpretation of the history of philosophy that begins to bring out what previously remained implicit, Arendt shows that *nous* is never found without an accompanying *logos*, which means that philosophical vision—what the ancient Greeks referred to using the words *theoria* and *theorein*—was always implicitly conceived, from its very inception, as discursive; thus, second, her reading of the history of philosophy suggests that, from the very beginning, *nous* itself was not understood in terms of a purely contemplative vision, passive, docile, and solitary, but was implicitly understood quite differently as the public, theoretically grounded judgmental activity of an engaged spectator. Birmingham's reading carries forward Arendt's work, elaborating and making even more explicit Arendt's adumbrations of this implicit construction of vision in the history of philosophy.

Birmingham maintains that there is a certain tension between the argument Arendt makes in *The Human Condition* and the argument she makes in *Life of the Mind* in regard to the construction of vision in the philosophical interpretation of *nous*. In *The Human Condition*, it seems that Arendt argued that the philosophers' contemplative vision of eternal, timeless being was a silent, speechless vision, a vision that emerged from, and was meant to displace, an earlier, very different vision: a vision of divine immortality achieved by a community of spectators actively participating in public ceremonies, theatrical events in which the great deeds of gods and mortals were made visible—through speech, through the telling of stories—in all their immortal splendor and glory. In *Life of the Mind*, however, it seems that she recognized in Aristotle's *aletheuein* a *nous* whose vision needed to be articulated in words. And this led her, according to Birmingham, to the realization that, all along in the history of philosophy, there has been another paradigm of vision, of *theoria* and *theorein*: a construction of *nous* and its vision as discursive, public, active, and participatory, the theoretically guided activity of publicly rendered judgment. Bringing out Arendt's incompletely articulated recognition of this other construction of vision, little recognized in contemporary readings of the history of philosophy, Birmingham is able to elaborate the significance of a practical *theoria*, a spectatorial vision in the context of Arendt's political philosophy. Briefly stated, she shows how, in Arendt's later work, vision is constructed—once again, and yet, in a sense, only now, for the first time—as a faculty ideally embodying the exercise of critical judgment.

Reflecting on Arendt's discussion of Kafka's parable, "He," Birmingham points out how she uses this story to rethink and reconstruct the vision of the spectator, severing thinking not only from a vision that is detached, contemplative and mimetic but also from a vision that is private, solitary, and introspective, connecting it instead to a vision that is responsibly engaged, timely, and responsive to the needs of the times. The philosophical vision that, with Birmingham's assistance, Arendt's thought reconstructs does not gaze up to eternal and necessary forms, universal truths; situated in its time, actively participating in the "now" of historical happening and in the space of public discourse, it looks after the singular and the contingent. And thus, as an embodiment of critical judgment, a being-in-the-world through which thought and action are not split apart but brought together, it is also a vision alert to conditions that call on us to change our customary ways of seeing.

Chapter 13, my own, is entitled "Keeping Foucault and Derrida in Sight: Panopticism and the Politics of Subversion." In the interview, "Body/Power," Foucault declared: "What's effectively needed is a ramified, penetrative perception of the present, one that makes it possible to locate lines of weakness, strong points, positions where the instances of power have secured and implanted themselves."[70] If this is an accurate description of the gaze that Foucault learned to practice, it could be said with equal accuracy to describe the character of the gaze that is discursively constructed in the philosophical writings of Derrida. Both philosophers engage in a discursive critique of vision, the rhetoric of vision, and the domination of vision in our cultural paradigm of knowledge, truth, and reality. In the work of both philosophers, this critique is not confined to the discourse of philosophy but refuses such delimitations, such arbitrary divisions between what is inside the philosophical discourse and what is outside it. For both, the critique moves "outside" this discourse to take the form of a subversive practice—a politics of strategic visual positions, alternative visions, countervisions.

Foucault saw that the power of the state and its culture no longer imposes domination by means of a "sovereign gaze": its power of panoptical surveillance is dispersed, disseminated, and maintained instead by a vast network of disciplinary regimes that subjects impose, more or less freely, more or less consciously, on themselves. He reasoned that since there is no longer a sovereign gaze located at the center of power, the politics of resistance and freedom requires a strategic gaze: one that is correspondingly decentered and multiplied and consequently faces the power whose oppressiveness it refuses to accept at all the local points of pressure. Foucault's answer to the dissemination of power, the most contemporary modus operandi of oppressive power, is, then, a philosophical gaze that discursively produces a multiplicity of critical and subversive gazes, gazes strategically stationed throughout the field of power and forming networks of perspectives and viewpoints for the projection of strategies of resistance. Derrida's gaze, the gaze of the philosopher, is similarly strategic in its functioning, resisting and subverting oppressive forms of power by multiplying its positions, perspectives, and viewpoints. Derrida saw a historical connection between our metaphysics of presence and the character of the gaze that has inscribed itself into philosophical discourse, and from the ocularcentrism of metaphysical discourse he reasoned that if this gaze is in any way responsible for a metaphysics of presence, then his gaze can only break the spell of ocularcentrism and the domination of this metaphysics if it refuses to be centered, refuses permanence, refuses stability, refuses predictability. Derrida's answer to the hegemony of vision and its metaphysics of presence is an aleatory gaze, one that moves about freely and unpredictably, leaps about, suddenly showing up where it was least expected, multiplies itself incessantly, proliferating viewpoints, compels recognition of the absent, the excluded other, and makes differences—and an undecidable difference.

Both Derrida and Foucault deploy vision, a gaze they discursively construct, as a critical weapon—not only against the dominant cultural vision, the gaze whose character is dominant today, but also against the domination of vision in a cultural and political *episteme* to the construction of which the discourse of philosophy has significantly contributed. "In effect, they not only practice a politics of subversion, using vision itself to resist the willful character of vision, its dreams and images of domination, its ethics of sameness, its politics of violence, its metaphysics of presence; they also use their vision to examine the limits and antinomies of vision—and the rationality of vision with this type of character."

As early as, and perhaps in part because of, his work on Husserl, Derrida could see deeply rooted connections between ocularcentrism, the metaphysics of presence, and a politics of repressive identity. He could also see the double bind these connections impose. His animadversions accordingly take the form, the style, of an ironic double gesture, a "textualization" of the philosophical gaze in an "optical" writing that plays with the metaphorics of light and vision in order to effect a discursive deconstruction of vision: "He uses (his) writing to appeal (in both senses of the term) to our vision, only to seduce it into acknowledging dissemination, invisibility, absence, alterity— vision's inevitable failure to achieve metaphysical totalization and plenitude."

Foucault, and Derrida too, saw a politics hidden in the domination of vision. For Foucault, the politics that is allied with the hegemony of vision and the metaphysics of presence is a technopolitics of "invisible surveillance, disciplinary regimes of supervision, the totalitarian administration and authoritarian control of vision and visibility. Panopticism." For Derrida, as for Adorno, it is more a question of the violence inherent in the logic of identity. If ocularcentrism is involved in the domination of the metaphysics of presence, it is also complicitous in a certain politics. Thus, Derrida tries to show us, tries to make us see, that our ocularcentric metaphysics of presence reflects and reinforces an ocularcentric politics of presence: pressures to conform, intolerance of difference, oppressive forms of inclusion, injustices of exclusion.

The argument developed in this chapter accordingly suggests, in drawing its conclusion, that the subversive deployments of the gaze that illuminate the discourse of these two philosophers constitute significant adumbrations of our present need for a postmetaphysical vision.

The final chapter, by Dorothea Olkowski, is on "Difference and the Ruin of Representation in Gilles Deleuze." According to Olkowski, the history of the West for Deleuze seems to be dominated by a vision of power willfully bent on submitting everything it sees to a representational order—an oppressive order that is hierarchical, totally determinate, unalterable, and intolerant of real difference. Deleuze believes, moreover, "that visual representation has always been linked to the development of the Western metaphysical framework, [a way of thinking] that imposes and guarantees a particular kind of order and truth." Above all, and in particular, he maintains that "visual representation is used to justify certain types of rooted social and political as well as philosophical regimes."

Olkowski finds this narrative persuasive, but her reflections turn around a certain perplexity, for she is struck by an apparent "disjunction between the claim that space has a history and the fact that theories (and in most instances practices) of representation have tended to remain constant, faithful to the Euclidean, geometrical-optical metaphors of the modern period—which themselves fall back on Aristotelian representational schemes." In other words: "If the so-called history of space has not coincided with the dominant mode of vision derived from Greek cosmology and Renaissance science, and consequently has not affected the hegemony of representation, this incongruity needs to be accounted for."

Olkowski's discussion of this problematic is set in motion by a crucial question: whether vision is necessarily, essentially, and by its very nature reifying and representational, or whether reifying objectification and representation are instead only the identifying characteristics of a particular, historically constructed vision and a particular, historically constructed experience-conception of space—a vision and a space that consequently could be otherwise constructed. Convinced that the representational character of vision is neither a random historical fact, and in this sense inexplicable, nor a teleological necessity, preordained and therefore inalterable, Olkowski reflects on the philosophical thought of Deleuze in order to articulate "the conceptual schema that constitutes such a vision" within a critical perspective that can contribute to the eventual "ruin" of representation. Beyond this, her efforts to understand the historical construction of representational vision are exercises of imagination that point toward "alternative modes of vision."

As Olkowski shows, there are significant historical connections between the hegemony of a normative notion of difference framed originally in terms of Aristotle's metaphysics, the normative hegemony of a representational vision, and an oppressive political culture and economy. "The discovery that Deleuze makes," she writes, "is that visual representation has been constituted, in Western philosophy and visual practice, in terms of the Aristotelian framework." "According to Deleuze, it is Aristotle who, to a far greater degree than Plato, refused to recognize difference and is thus responsible for the establishment of the hegemonic reign of representation." For Aristotle, the articulation of differences must begin with, must be conceived by reference to, something common to all the particulars, "something *identical* whereby they differ." The differentiation of differences is possible only "in terms of identity with regard to a generic concept. What gets constituted in Aristotle is thus the very ruin of difference. There is and can be no concept tolerant of difference, for difference is always inscribed within the genus, the concept in general, and difference is no more than difference within identity." And with the domination of vision and the regimentation of representationalism, difference as such is excluded—and therefore also alteration, movement. Olkowski surmises that this may be why, "following *Différence et répétition*, Deleuze engages in numerous efforts to analyze visual representation as a particularly restricted form of imaging" and that "this first analysis remains the heart of all his other thinking on the question."

Olkowski accordingly gives considerable attention to the way that Aristotle's metaphysics determines his logic of categorial identity and differentiation. This focus serves to bring out the significance of Deleuze's larger philosophical project. According to Olkowski, Deleuze introduces a "nomadic" style of vision, a "catastrophic" vision, discursively constructed to "destabilize" and "ruin" representation, decentering its order, contesting the very principle of its authority, subverting its hierarchy, warping its linearity, interrupting its continuity, cracking its rigidity, setting its rigid structures in motion, multiplying its points of view, opening its system to the other, the different—all that it would exclude and deny.

Making explicit the political implications of Deleuze's "nomadic" style, Olkowski says: "Functioning according to a vision that imposes the order of representations, the state is an *organism* that: appropriates a military war machine to serve its political needs; regulates bands or clans, as conquerors imposing law on the conquered; reduces the scientific model of problems and accidents that condition and resolve them to a model based on the distinction of genus and species or essence and properties; defines thought as either the *imperium*, i.e., the 'whole' as final ground of being, or as the 'republic', i.e., a system in which the 'sovereign' subject figures as legislative and juridical ground." In contrast to the resident obedient to the order of the state, Deleuze's metaphorical nomad "is," as Olkowski puts it, "always deterritorialized, always a heretic or a criminal. The nomad, who only ever moves, whose very home is mobile, is thus distributed in a space without borders or enclosure." Engaging the tropes, the discursive, metaphorical configurations of Deleuze's thought, Olkowski demonstrates that "it is Deleuze's project to point to other ways to see, to open up the field of our vision to the nomadic *nomos* that creates wandering distributions of assemblages, distributions whose univocity and consequent tolerance of differences hold out more hope for truly democratic institutions."

Notes

1. Max Horkheimer elaborated on Marx's point thus: "The objects we perceive in our surroundings—cities, villages, fields, and woods—bear the mark of having been worked on by man. It is not only in clothing and appearance, in outward form and emotional make-up that men are the products of history. Even the way they see and hear is inseparable from the social life-process as it has evolved over the millennia. The facts which our senses present to us are socially preformed in two ways: through the historical character of the object perceived and through the historical character of the perceiving organ." Thus: "At the higher stages of civilization, conscious human praxis unconsciously determines not only the subjective side of perception but, to an increasing degree, the object as well." See "Traditional and Critical Theory," in *Critical Theory* (New York: Seabury Press, 1972), pp. 200–201. But if our vision, our capacity for seeing, is historical, it is precisely not a "fate," a mere event of nature, but a

Introduction

disposition that is at least partially subject to our volition, our second-order desires, our reflexive, self-critical rationality—and is thus a matter that calls on our responsability. One would expect that, precisely at the higher stages of civilization, it would be regarded as both rational and desirable that we attempt, as much as possible, to bring to consciousness—to a critical consciousness—the unconscious determination of the "subjective side of perception" by "conscious human praxis," and that we attempt, moreover, to transform the "subjective side of perception" in accordance with enlightened norms and ideals. The chapters in this book may be read as contributions to this project.

2. Paul Ricoeur, *History and Truth* (Evanston: Northwestern University Press), p. 63.

3. Richard Rorty, *Philosophy and the Mirror of Nature* (Princeton: Princeton University Press, 1979).

4. Edmund Husserl, "Philosophy and the Crisis of European Man," in Quentin Lauer, ed., *Phenomenology and the Crisis of Philosophy* (New York: Harper & Row, 1965), p. 172.

5. Martin Heidegger, *Being and Time* (New York: Harper & Row, 1962), p. 187.

6. Walter Benjamin, in *Illuminations* (New York: Schocken Books, 1969), p. 242.

7. See Susan Buck-Morss, *The Dialectics of Seeing: Walter Benjamin and the Arcades Project* (Cambridge: MIT Press, 1989).

8. André Gide, cited by Maurice Blanchot in *The Space of Literature* (Lincoln: University of Nebraska Press, 1982), p. 215.

9. John Dewey, *The Public and Its Problems* (Athens, Ohio: Ohio University Press, 1954), pp. 218–219.

10. Hannah Arendt, *The Life of the Mind* (New York: Harcourt Brace Jovanovich, 1978), pp. 110–111.

11. Ibid., p. 122.

12. Jürgen Habermas, *The Philosophical Discourse of Modernity* (Cambridge: MIT Press, 1987), pp. 128–129.

13. Ibid., p. 297.

14. Michel Foucault, "Body/Power," in *Power/Knowledge: Selected Interviews and Other Writings, 1972–1977* (New York: Pantheon, 1980), p. 62.

15. Maurice Merleau-Ponty, *Phenomenology of Perception* (London: Routledge & Kegan Paul), p. 68.

16. Ibid., pp. 353, p. 377; Merleau-Ponty, *The Visible and the Invisible* (Evanston: Northwestern University Press, 1968), p. 452.

Introduction

17. See Carl Bode, ed., *The Portable Thoreau* (New York: Viking Press, 1964), p. 266.

18. Theodor Adorno, "Sociology and Empirical Research," in *The Positivist Dispute in German Sociology* (London: Heineman, 1981), p. 69.

19. Plato, *The Dialogues of Plato* (New York: Random House, 1937), 1:773.

20. Ibid., p. 775.

21. Ibid., p. 776.

22. Ibid., pp. 777, 779. See also bk. VI, especially pp. 761–772.

23. Ibid., bk. VI, p. 770.

24. Baruch de Spinoza, *Ethics* (New York: Hafner Publishing Co., 1949), p. 249.

25. G. W. F. Hegel, *The Letters* (Bloomington: Indiana University Press, 1984), p. 280. The letter in question is dated October 23, 1812.

26. Hegel, *System of Ethical Life and First Philosophy* (Albany: State University of New York Press, 1979), p. 143.

27. Friedrich Nietzsche, *Twilight of the Idols* (Baltimore: Penguin Books, 1968), p. 6. Also see *Daybreak: Thoughts on the Prejudices of Morality* (New York: Cambridge University Press, 1982), p. 203.

28. Nietzsche, *Twilight of the Idols*, p. 6.

29. Nietzsche, *The Will to Power* (New York: Random House, 1968), p. 262.

30. Ibid., p. 330.

31. Heidegger, *The Question Concerning Technology and Other Essays* (New York: Harper & Row, 1977), p. 48.

32. Max Horkheimer, *Dawn and Decline: Notes 1926–1931 and 1950–1969* (New York: Seabury Press, 1974), p. 162.

33. Heidegger, *Being and Time* (New York: Harper & Row, 1962), p. 397.

34. Heidegger, *What Is Called Thinking?* (New York: Harper & Row, 1968), pp. 232–233.

35. Heidegger, *Discourse on Thinking* (New York: Harper & Row, 1966), p. 64.

36. Ibid., p. 67.

37. Ibid., p. 78, p. 79.

38. Ibid., p. 63.

39. Ibid.

40. Ibid.

41. Ibid., pp. 64, 72–73.

42. Ibid., p. 73.

43. Ibid., p. 72.

44. Ibid., p. 74.

45. Merleau-Ponty, "The Intertwining—The Chiasm," in *The Visible and the Invisible* (Evanston: Northwestern University Press, 1968), p. 264.

46. Herbert Marcuse, *Counter-Revolution and Revolt* (Boston: Beacon Press, 1972), p. 71.

47. Ibid.

48. Ibid., p. 63.

49. Marcuse, *One-Dimensional Man: Studies in the Ideology of Advanced Industrial Society* (Boston: Beacon Press, 1964), p. 165.

50. Foucault, *The Birth of the Clinic: An Archaeology of Medical Perception* (New York: Random House, 1975), p. 84.

51. Foucault, *The History of Sexuality*, vol. 3: *The Use of Pleasure* (New York: Pantheon, 1985), p. 8.

52. Foucault, "What Is Enlightenment?" in Paul Rabinow, ed., *The Foucault Reader* (New York: Pantheon, 1984), p. 48.

53. Foucault, "Questions of Method," in K. Baynes, J. Bohman, and T. McCarthy, eds., *After Philosophy: End or Transformation?* (Cambridge: MIT Press, 1987), p. 112.

54. Benjamin, *Gesammelte Schriften*, volume 6: *Fragmente vermischten Inhalts, Autobiographische Schriften* (Frankfurt: Suhrkamp, 1985), p. 67.

55. Heidegger, "Aletheia (Heraclitus, Fragment B 16)," in *Early Greek Thinking* (New York: Harper & Row, 1975), p. 121.

56. Benjamin, *Gesammelte Schriften*, vol. 3: *Kritik und Rezensionen* (Frankfurt: Suhrkamp Verlag, 1972), p. 259.

57. Bernard J. Hibbitts, "Making Sense of Metaphors: Visuality, Aurality, and the Reconfiguration of American Legal Discourse," *Cardozo Law Review* 16, no. 2 (December 1994):237.

58. Charles Taylor, *Sources of the Self: The Making of the Modern Identity* (Cambridge: Harvard University Press, 1989), p. 100.

59. G. W. F. Hegel, *The Phenomenology of Spirit* (Oxford: Oxford University Press, 1977), § 207, p. 126.

60. Ibid., p. 493.

61. See, e.g., Edmund Husserl, *Ideas: General Introduction to Pure Phenomenology* (London: Collier-Macmillan, 1962), pp. 94, 107, 109, 173; § 57, p. 156; § 84, p. 223; § 92, pp. 246–249; § 137, pp. 353–354.

62. Ludwig Wittgenstein, *Philosophical Investigations* ((New York: Macmillan, 1953), p. 212e.

63. Umberto Eco, *Il nome della rosa* (Milano: Bompiani, 1980), p. 370.

64. John Rawls, "The Idea of an Overlapping Consensus," *Oxford Journal of Legal Studies* 7, no. 1 (1987):21.

65. Vitaliano Brancati, "Trampolini si imbatte in una donna alle soglie del Giardino Bellini," in *Sogno di un valzer e altri racconti* (Milano: Bompiani, 1982), p. 157. Translation mine.

66. These words, "longing for the radically other," are Max Horkheimer's and figured in a conversation he had with Helmut Gumnior in 1970. See Horkheimer, *Gesammelte Schriften* (Frankfurt: Suhrkamp, 1985), 7:385–404. His appeal to this "longing" echoes in certain ways Kant's appeal to an "enthusiasm" for revolution in *The Conflict of Faculties*.

67. Foucault, "What Is Enlightenment?" in Rabinow, *The Foucault Reader*, p. 46; Foucault, *Power/Knowledge: Selected Interviews 1972–1977* (New York: Pantheon, 1982), p. 80.

68. Foucault, "Revolutionary Action: 'Until Now,'" in *Language, Counter-Memory, Practice: Selected Essays and Interviews* (Ithaca, N.Y.: Cornell University Press, 1977), pp. 230–231.

69. Arendt, *The Life of the Mind*, pp. 110–111.

70. Michel Foucault, "Body/Power," in *Power/Knowledge*, p. 62.

1

From Acoustics to Optics: The Rise of the Metaphysical and Demise of the Melodic in Aristotle's *Poetics*

P. Christopher Smith

Um dies zu begreifen, müssen wir jenes kunstvolle Gebäude der apollinischen Kultur gleichsam Stein um Stein abtragen, bis wir die Fundamente erblicken, auf die es begründet ist.
—Friedrich Nietzsche *Die Geburt der Tragödie aus dem Geiste der Musik*[1]

We owe an enormous debt to Friedrich Nietzsche's extravagant but brilliant *The Birth of Tragedy Out of the Spirit of Music* for calling to our attention the origins of Greek tragedy in Dionysian rituals. Nietzsche alone, in his brazen radicality, succeeds in taking down the visual and intellectualist surface of Greek tragedy and in exposing for us the acoustical foundations beneath it, and this two millennia after Plato's very nearly successful efforts to obliterate these acoustical foundations once and for all and, with them tragedy, as such. My thesis here is that Nietzsche's deconstructive strategies can be extended even to the theory of tragedy put forth in Aristotle's *Poetics*, and with startling results. Rather than seeing the *Poetics* as a consistent theory of tragedy, after Nietzsche we can see it as the seminally inconsistent and tense intertwining of earlier, pre-Platonic ritual understandings of tragedy and later, post-Platonic intellectualist understandings. Put another way, we can take down the *Poetics'* own Apollonian superstructure and lay bare the Dionysian ritualistic foundations hidden beneath it. We can penetrate behind Aristotle's ultimate conception of tragedy as re-presentation for spectators (*theôretes*) looking on from a distance, to an earlier understanding, still present in the *Poetics*, of tragedy as ritual re-enactment for an audience (*akouontes*), themselves caught up in the rhythms and cadences of the voices that they hear. This, of course, is to reverse the direction that the *Poetics* actually takes, away from the acoustical and toward the optical.

This palimpsest in the *Poetics* of post-Platonic understandings superimposed on pre-Platonic ones is discernible even in the basic vocabulary with which Aristotle works. Consequently, though Aristotle himself does not distinguish, for instance, between *mimêsis* as ritual re-enactment, which is its earlier sense, and *mimêsis* as educational portrayal or re-presentation of a thing's typical features, which is a later overlay, we must make such a distinction if we are to get beneath the surface of the *Poetics*. And in like fashion we must distinguish, though Aristotle never does, between *katharsis* as ritual expiation for our misdeeds and *katharsis* as cognitive lustration or clarification of potentially destabilizing passions. In other words, where Aristotle would seem in his exposition of tragedy to have suppressed lingering traces of ritual experience undergone acoustically, and where he would displace such acoustical experience with theoretical insight, it is our task, with Nietzsche, to suspend the principle of noncontradiction and to restore what has been suppressed and displaced, to its place alongside what it contradicts.[2]

I will seek first therefore, to disclose the original acoustical exerperience still discoverable in *Poetics* behind the decisive and fateful turn taken there to the visual, theoretical and metaphysical. I will argue, specifically in regard to the *Poetics*, that Aristotle's thought is predominantly visual, to be sure, but, remarkably, in part still acoustical. Hence, in going back to this text we reach a decisive moment in the development of Western metaphysical thought when the optical has come to prevail but not without leaving traces of the "earlier" acoustical experience that it would displace. For if in the *Poetics* the withdrawal to a "divine" *apathes theôria*, an unaffected beholding, has always already been made, our original existence "in the world" is nonetheless not entirely suppressed, our existence, that is, with and among other people, in oral-aural interaction with whom we undergo and communicate the things that happen to us and are felt by us—the *pathêmata* and *pathê*. In the *Poetics*, we are not quite yet the "unmoved movers" that we aspire to be in the pursuit of pure *theôria*, not quite yet the pure, dispassionate agents who undergo nothing more as patients (compare EN X, 1177a12 f., *Metaph.* XII, 1072b15 ff.). We are not quite yet onlookers who see from a distance and no longer hear the voicings (*phônai*) of the play that would draw us into their melodic cadences and rhythms. Once these acoustical and melodic foundations are more clearly laid out before us, I will be able, second, to reconstruct Aristotle's optical and metaphysical understanding of tragedy as precisely what it is: a self-contradictory turn away from tragedy's acoustical and melodic underpinnings, a turn that for all its self-contradictoriness has defined the subsequent course of Western thought.

I

"Tragedy," says Aristotle, compactly summarizing his argument,

is the imitation of an action (*mimêsis praxeôs*) worthy and complete. It is of limited size with each of the forms of pleasing speech used separately in its various parts. It is imitation not by reporting but imitation of people doing things, which, by compassion and fear, achieves the *katharsis* of such passions undergone as these (*tôn toioutôn pathêmatôn*). I call speech pleasant that has rhythm, pitch and melody, whereas I mean by "in forms used separately" that some [tragic effects] are achieved with only meter but others, in turn, with melody. (*Poetics* 1449b24–32)

In regard to the continuing earlier pre-Platonic and premetaphysical dimension of the *Poetics* it is most striking here that Aristotle bases his exposition of tragic poetry on a rehabilitation of *mimêsis* as dramatic reenactment in voice and dance (see also 1447a13 f.), and this despite Plato's previous withering critique of just such *mimêsis* in the *Republic*. A review of just a few key passages in the *Republic* suffices to make clear just how sharply Aristotle breaks with Plato on this point and how conservative and retrospective his own reappropriation of traditional *mimêsis* really

P. Christopher Smith

is. For thematic in the *Republic* was the thesis restated at the beginning of Book X that the *mimêsis* of tragic performance, far from having any psychological benefits, brings about the "ruination ... of the thinking of those hearing it if they do not have the remedy against this ruination, namely insight into how such things [imitated] really happen to be" (595b). And whereas at least here in Aristotle's *Poetics* melody, meter, rhythm, and pitch are said to be crucial for the cathartic effect, in the *Republic*, these acoustical, musical elements of poetic imitation, once stripped away, turn out to have been only the cover for the imitator's own lack of insight (601a). Indeed, the acoustical musical elements of tragic *mimêsis* are, to take Plato's provocatively absurd analogy, comparable to the colors when someone paints a picture of a bit and reins and then tries to pass the painting off as a real bit and reins and, worse, as proof of his or her insight into what a bit and reins are really like. In fact, the colors are mere pleasing ornamentation with nothing real behind them, and so too are the "meters, rhythms and intonations" in voice with which the acoustical artist works.

But even this powerful analogical argument is not enough for Plato, for by itself it would divert us from the real danger at hand, to which he would direct us. The actual point he wants to make is that the acoustical imitations in meter, rhythm, and pitch that we hear are much more disastrously misleading than any colors that we see could ever be. The auditory and not the visual is, after all, the primary means of communicating and sharing the *pathos* or the feeling that someone is undergoing, and hence the auditory can influence our "thinking something through," our *dianoia*, in a way that nothing visual ever could. For whenever we set about thinking something through, whenever we deliberate or take counsel about something (see 604c), a fierce struggle, an *agôn*, is joined between what is best and worst in us, between what is rational and irrational, between the reasoning (*logos*) that we do actively and the feelings (*pathê*) that we undergo passively. The reasonable side of us, Plato's Socrates says here, displays a constant disposition of character "always at one with itself." But the unreasonable side, the complex of our feelings, is of multiple and various character. Hence this *agôn* between the active and passive is ultimately between what would hold us together as one integrated personality and what, in driving us to distraction, would cause us to dissolve and go to pieces (604e). In a stable person "law and reason" prevail over feeling and prevent this disintegration (604b). But precisely this predominance of *logos* over *pathos* is undermined by the acoustical nature of vocal poetic imitation in meter, rhythm, and pitch (see 603b). Unlike the visual, the melodic-acoustical goes directly to the feelings and only reinforces their domination of us. "It is plain," says Socrates here, "that by nature the imitative poet does not aim at such a [rational] part of the soul ... rather, he concerns himself with the part given to agitation, the unstable part, for this is the part easily imitated" (605a). And it is by just this imitation or *mimêsis* that he introduces "ruination" to the soul.

Seen against the background of Plato's radical proposals, Aristotle's talk of a *katharsis* of the things that we experience passively, of the *pathêmata*, a *katharsis* achieved by allowing ourselves to undergo such *pathê* or feelings as compassion and fear, is strikingly traditional. And in fact, to Plato's unrelenting critique of performative *mimêsis*, Aristotle responds not only by taking *mimêsis* as the single basis for his positive analysis of epic, tragic, and comic poetry but even by praising it as an essential and distinctively human component of the learning process (1448b6–19). How, we must ask, is this possible?

One key to Aristotle's rehabilitation of performative *mimêsis* is his perpetuation of the earlier, tragic understanding of *manthanein* or learning expressed in Aeschylus's *pathei mathos*, or "learned by having undergone."[3] The point is that in learning by *mimêsis*, we have learned, precisely not as in the Platonic paradigm of mathematics, that is, by looking on as something is demonstrated, but rather by feeling something directly with our own body, as it were. We have learned by undergoing something that happens to us and with us experientially. Learning here is not theoretical; it is not the learning of someone unmoved who beholds what is displayed before him or her; rather, it is an intensely involved learning by doing, learning by *mimêsis praxeôs* or imitation of an action. "Imitating is innate in human beings," says Aristotle; "and exists from childhood on, and they differ from other animals in that they are the most imitative and do their first learning by imitation (*tas mathêseis poieitai dia mimêseôs tas prôtas*) (1448b5–9). In poetry and tragedy this imitative learning is accomplished by reenactment.

It is not to be overlooked, of course, that Aristotle has already begun shifting the sense of imitation and learning here from something acoustical and involved to something visual and detached; the very next lines (1448b10 ff.) turn to learning the general characteristics of something by seeing—*horan, theôroun*—a painted representation of it, thus confronting us with a marked ambivalence on Aristotle's part, to which we must return later. But that he has not abandoned the earlier understanding of learning by *mimêsis* as physical reenactment, and that he has never completely lost Aeschylus's tragic sense of learning, the sense of becoming "learned by having undergone," is made clear by the perpetuation in his definition of tragedy of an ancient idea of *katharsis* by ritual reenactment (see the citation of 1449b24 f., above). In the back of Aristotle's mind there is, in other words, still an idea of learning not just as a matter of cognition but as recognition (*anagnôrisis*), and such learning as this means undergoing a change in how one feels. Learning remains for Aristotle the *katharsis* of, and expiatiation for, our wrongdoing. It is just this release to which the *manthanein* of Aeschylus's *pathei mathos* alludes, the learning of his "learned by having undergone." Here the *katharsis* has to do with *sôtêria*, with deliverance and salvation, as in the *sôtêria dia tês katharseôs* or "salvation through *katharsis*" of which Aristotle speaks, in regard to Euripides' *Iphigenia at Aulis* 1163 (see Aristotle 1455b15).

I am indebted to Aryeh Kosman's extraordinarily illuminating piece, "Acting: *Drama* as the *Mimêsis* of *Praxis*," for calling attention to this crucial phrase in Aristotle.[4] In contrast to very convincing "cognitivist" interpretations of *katharsis* in Martha Nussbaum, Jonathan Lear, and others (as we will see they are right too), Kosman argues equally convincingly that the *Poetics* is to be taken as an extension of the *Ethics* into the realm of our unforeseeable and unpreventable wrongdoing. Whereas in the *Ethics*, he points out, we learn of cognizant, reasoned restraint of our passions and cognizant, reasoned guidance of our deliberations to a choice of what is right, decent, and good, in the *Poetics* we learn of the limits to our cognition and reasoning. And we also learn of the unknowing and inevitable transgression of what is right, decent, and good that results from these limits. With Oedipus at Colonus or Orestes, we, the audience of the tragedy, learn, by what happens with our own body, what it is like to undergo the penalty for our transgression, but also what it is like to experience release from that penalty, to experience *katharsis*. In what he or she undergoes, the *pathêmata*, the tragic hero atones for our own misdeeds, and we, in reenacting these *pathêmata* and this atonement ourselves, are set free. Citing Cyril of Jerusalem's "*têi mimêsêi tôn pathêmatôn autou koinônêsantes alêtheiai tên sôtêrian kerdêsômen*," in support of his argument—that "sharing in his sufferings in imitation we might gain salvation in truth"—Kosman suggests that some different traces of this same Dionysian ritual *katharsis* by reenactment are still to be found in early Christian understandings of the celebration of baptism and the Eucharist.[5]

It is crucial for our recovery of the acoustical foundations in Aristotle that any such *mimêsis* as reenactment leading to *katharsis* and *sôtêria* is precisely not to be effected in the medium of paintings that we see but in voice (*phônê*) that we hear, and voice, to be sure, that is not in the single meter and monotone of Plato's preferred sober narration (see *Rep.* 397bc) but that, on the contrary, is richly rhythmical and tonally inflected. This the *Politics*, if not the *Poetics*, makes unequivocally clear in the *locus classicus* for Aristotle's understanding of the *katharsis* of the *pathê*:

For we see some held under the sway of such emotions [as pity and fear] and who, as a result of sacred melodies, when they make use of them and plunge their soul into an orgiastic state, are set right as if they happened to have undergone healing and *katharsis*. And those must indeed undergo this same thing who feel pity and who fear, and who generally feel the other passions in the measure that falls to each of these, and there must come to pass for all some kind of *katharsis* and pleasant alleviation. (1342a7–15)

Indeed, the whole argument here turns on the fact that music is not just pleasant adornment; rather we also learn character from it, that is, we experience the passions and acquire thereby an appropriate disposition toward them:

Furthermore those hearing imitations all come to share in the same felt experience (*eti de akroômenoi tôn mimêseôn gignontai pantes sumpatheis*) apart [from the speech and through] the rhythms and melodies themselves.... For contained in rhythms and melodies are likenesses of anger and gentleness, further, of courage and temperance, and all the opposites of these, as well as all the other dispositions of character, likenesses that most closely correspond to the true nature of these. And this is made plain by what [these rhythms and melodies] do, for we change in our soul when hearing them. (1340a13–23)

and

From these things it is plain that music is able to produce a kind of character in the soul. (1340b11–12)

Importantly, Aristotle points out here, at least, that visual depictions are at best only signs (*sêmeia*) of character and hence are not imitations of it (1340a33), whereas melodies themselves are imitations of character (1340a39–40). Furthermore, he adds that one cannot acquire the character merely by looking on as others reenact it; rather, one must participate in being "a communicant in the deeds" (*koinônêi tôn ergôn*) (1340b24). This makes clear why the instructional *mimêsis* is primarily acoustical. Like sound, indeed, *as sound*, it must be undergone, experienced, and responded to with one's whole psychosomatic being, even in gestures and dance. Put another way, learning character is a function of listening to, hearing, and rehearsing physically what we hear someone telling us.

These obvious challenges to Plato are certainly the most dramatic evidence of Aristotle's perpetuation of an earlier priority of hearing over seeing, but there are subtler traces of this priority that we should not neglect. For instance, we find that in the *Poetics* Aristotle establishes a quite un-Platonic continuum between the "voices" of the flute and the lyre and the human voice of poetry insofar as all of these imitate precisely in meter, rhythm, and pitch, which are the components of melody (1447a19 f.). To be sure, the human voice does differ from the "voice" of an instrument in that it develops significant speech (*logos*) out of these components of melody, but even so, this significant speech still remains embedded in its acoustical medium and is not yet severed from the latter in the way that it would be, for instance, when we signify the Platonic forms, and when the voiced sound that we make no longer bears any intrinsic relation to the idea that we would communicate.

Moreover, even if Aristotle does, on occasion, speak of plain speech or prose in distinction from verse (1447a29), as if to say that voicing in rhythm and meter might be divorced from speech after all, this, in fact, does not in the least imply that voiced pitch—acute (high), grave (low), and middle (see 1456b32)— would be extrinsic. For even in prose, the pitch determines whether an utterance (*logos*) is, for instance, indicative, as in *didomen* ("we give") or imperative, as in *didômen* ("let us give"). We note in this regard the passage at 1456b9 f. on the forms or "gestures of diction" (*schêmata tês lexeôs*), namely "the command, the plea, the narration, the threat, the question, the answer," which are specifically said to be the special subject matter of the art of dramatic, verbal reenactment (*hupokrisis*), and the passage at 1461a25ff. on *prosodia* or intonation. Obviously what something sounds like in the voicing of it is intrinsic even to plain speech, too, and not just poetry.

And even with regard to voicing in rhythm and meter, quite apart from pitch, Aristotle often speaks as if these too, far from belonging only to poetry, had a natural and intrinsic correlation with the logical content of what we say, or what is more, as if in tragedy, at least, that logical content, even had musical origins. For instance, Aristotle, in full agreement with Nietzsche, sees an intimate connection of tragedy with dithyramb as well as flute playing (1447a14–15) and with Dionysian phallic songs and processions (1449a10–11), and he acknowledges that tragedy has its beginnings in the satyr plays (1449a23).[6] To be sure, he adds that in starting from these origins, Aeschylus then began the shift from tragedy based in the chorus, which Aeschylus reduced in size, to tragedy based on *logos* or the protagonists' argument and speech. Accordingly, Aeschylus raised the number of protagonists from one (a single epiphany of Dionysius) to two. And as a further step in this development of the dialogical out of the musical, Sophocles, Aristotle continues, added yet a third protagonist (1449a16–18). We should note, however, that this development per se does not yet imply any separation of the logical from its natural embeddedness in the musical, the tonal, metric, and rhythmic. On the contrary, the shift in emphasis in Aeschylus and Sophocles to the logical is said to require an appropriate change from one meter to another. As tragedy and its diction became less satyric and comic and more solemn, says Aristotle, "the meter changed from [trochaic] tetrameter to iambic. For at first one used tetrameter on account of the poetry's being satyric and more dancelike. But once the diction [of the protagonists] came to prevail, nature itself found the appropriate meter" (1449a19–20). And later we find, similarly, "the heroic is the most stable and profuse of meters ... while iambic and tetrameter are the most moved, tetrameter for dance and iambic for action.... Nature itself teaches how to choose what is fitting in this matter (1459b37–60a 5).

Thus even a primarily logical diction still remains in the musical, acoustical setting natural for it, namely, iambic verse. And iambic, as Aristotle himself notes, is far from being purely logical and acoustically, affectively neutral. On the contrary, it has a definite acoustical "feel" or *pathos* to it. Originally it was, in fact, the natural meter in which people "derided each other (*iambizon allêlous*)" (1448b33).

In regard to this continuing embeddedness of the logical in the tonal, we should note, finally, that Aristotle speaks not just of the diction of the protagonists but also of the diction of the chorus. "The parode," he says, "is the entire first diction of the chorus (*lexis ... chorou*)" (1452b23). Plainly in regard to the diction of the chorus, the logical content cannot be separated from its acoustical setting and ground, and insofar as the diction of the protagonists arises out of the midst of the surrounding chorus, a continuum is established—in Aristotle as well as Nietzsche—

reaching from the diction of the protagonists, itself inflected, back to the lexical intonations of the chorus. Indeed, precisely in seeking to maintain this continuity Aristotle objects to Agathon's and others' misuses of the chorus as an arbitrary *embolima*— something just "tossed in" here and there. In this, he says, Aeschylus and Sophocles were better than Euripides, for the chorus "is to be taken as one of the players and must be a part of the whole and must take part in the action" (1456a25–33). In keeping with this observation (1452b19–23), Aristotle lists all the parts of a tragedy in reference to the melodies of the chorus: the prologue is what comes before the entrance of the chorus, the episodes are what occur between the melodies of the chorus, and the exodos is what comes after the last melody of the chorus has been sung. Thus an earlier understanding of human experience is perpetuated in Aristotle's *Poetics* in the continuing embeddedness there of what is said, of *logos* and *lexis*, speech and diction, in the voiced song of the chorus.

The acoustical foundations of the *Poetics* exposed here have important implications for those listening to tragedy. For only as listeners, *akouontes*, do they remain taken up and involved in an experience that they feel and undergo. Only as listeners do they remain under way in the midst of what occurs without yet having construed it in some sort of optical mapping of it from above. Indeed, it follows from the very stucture of the *pathêmata*, of the experiences felt and undergone by the tragic hero and participated in by the audience, that voice is the only medium in which to communicate them. For unlike a sight, voice—music, *to melos*— is always undergone and never susceptible to distanced observation. Unlike a sight, which leaves the viewers safely at a distance, a voiced sound draws the listeners out of self-possession and into physical communication in gesture and dance. Last in the chain of physical communicants taking part in the poetic event as it is told—sung—by the poet and retold and reenacted by the chorus and actors, is, of course, the audience, who "learn by having undergone," which is to say, by hearing, and not by seeing at a distance. Thus to the extent the *Poetics* remains acoustically based, the very thing that Plato sought to banish, the submission of the audience to the passions that come over it in acoustical experience, is recovered. It is recovered, however, only ultimately to be buried and lost again.

II

In the end Aristotle is far too much a Platonist to stay with this earlier understanding of learning by undergoing and the priority it gives to acoustical experience, and this is clear even when he treats musical *katharsis* positively, as he does in the *Politics*. *Katharsis* is effected best, he points out there, by a kind of music, which, insofar as it is just voice, the voice of the flute, and not at all speech, is purely acoustical and precludes communication of "envisionable" thought and logic altogether; after all, as opposed even to the lyre, with the flute it is impossible to play and speak simultaneously (1341a24–25). Indeed, the flute, we read now, "is *not* for character building, for, on the contrary, it is orgiastic," and, hence, to be used "on those occasions when looking on (*theôria*) is able to effect *katharsis rather than learning* (*mathêsis*)" (1341a21–23) (emphases added). In other words, the flute, though supremely cathartic, is not instructional; we do not learn character or anything else from it. And what is more, though the flute can provide beneficial *katharsis*, we now read that it cannot even do this for the one playing it or for someone caught up in the sound of it, rather only for someone who is just "looking on."

The distinction of *katharsis* from learning that emerges here is even more sharply drawn in regard to the appropriate use of harmonies and meters; some of these are considered "ethical" and of use in character building, and these we are to engage in ourselves. These, we might say, are "manthanic" or instructional. But others are held to be only cathartic and are to be "heard" by spectators, so to speak, but not performed personally, for their effect on the soul would then be too strong (1342a1 f.). And in fact it now turns out that the *katharsis* by "sacred melodies," of which we heard previously (see *Pol.* 1342a7 f.), belongs to precisely this category of the dangerously excessive.

With this divorce of melodic *katharsis* from *mathêsis*, and with the concomitant ban on direct participation in melody making, it is clear that Aristotle has already begun to move away from *manthanein* as participatory *mimêsis*, or at least to restrict it severely. In regard to the *melos* of the flute and Phrygian modes and meters—the choral dithyramb, in particular—we are no longer to learn by partaking in an acoustically transmitted event that we feel and undergo in imitative reenactment of it ourselves. That would only make us vulgar and cost us our status as free men (see 1340b7 f., 1341a9 f.). No wonder, then, says Aristotle, that Athene, as the tale goes, found a flute and threw it away, "For education by the flute contributes nothing to thinking something through (*dianoia*), whereas we attribute to Athene science and art" (1341b6–8). Surely with this privileging of *dianoia* over an acoustical experience undergone, Aristotle is not confronting Plato but siding with him.

And in fact, along with the tendency to rehabilitate the earlier dramatic *mimêsis* that Plato had condemned, there is in the *Poetics*, too, this contradictory and very Platonic tendency away from learning by mimetic physical participation and toward learning by detached mental envisioning. As we have seen, it is said early on there that we learn by the engaged imitation exemplified in tragedy, for "Imitating is innate in human beings and exists from childhood on. And they differ from other animals in that they are the most imitative and do their first learning by imitation" (1148b5–9). But, as already noted, there is a striking ambivalence in this passage, for if Aristotle initially had in mind learning by the *mimêsis* of reenacting someone's actions, *mimêsis praxeôs*, plainly he has also already turned here to learning by a very different *mimêsis* of representation, that is, by portrayal of a thing's essential features. And this learning comes not at all by our own temporal, heard, voiced, embodied reenactment of an action but by viewing at a distance visual imitations in space such as painted images. For in explaining his point he now continues, "We take pleasure as viewers (*theôrountes*) of the most exact likenesses of even those things that we find most painful to look at themselves, such as grotesque wild animals and corpses.... For people delight in seeing likenesses because it happens that in viewing them they learn (*manthanein*), and reason syllogistically, what each is, what sort of thing it is" (1448b10–17). If Plato, with his deliberately absurd analogy of the painting of a bit and reins, did not take the visual imitation seriously, Aristotle certainly does. Indeed *mimêsis* now means re-presentation for him and has forfeited its original sense of dramatic re-enactment.

Crucial here is the shift to a new kind of *manthanein* and *mathêsis* from which the pathetical dimension of Aeschylus's *pathei mathos*, "learned by having undergone," is eliminated. Learning is no longer learning from within experience as things happen to us "there" *in* the passage of time. Rather learning now is learning from *above* time and place, learning that has as its "object" rational comprehension of the *eidos* of things or "what" (*ti*) they "look" like. Learning is "getting the picture" of things. And in this new learning, the seat of cognizance and apprehension, the *psuchê*, is no longer down "there" in the body, no longer caught up in undergoing its sensations of the physical world, and no longer itself enacting the imitation from within the event.[7] Rather, from a distance, it looks on and sees what is arrayed before it. In effect it is no longer an audience that hears at all but a spectator that sees. In other words, the acoustical has been displaced by the optical.

We should note, too, that a de-acoustification of language itself follows necessarily from this removal of the *psuchê* from experience undergone bodily and relocation of it at the vantage point of a detached onlooker. Originally, words, as names or *onomata*, were taken to be voiced onomatopoetic imitations of acoustical experience, and to be sure, there are still obvious traces of this phonetically based language in Aristotle's discussion of speech and diction in the *Poetics*. But these traces are, we now see, largely covered over.

With the removal of the *psuchê* from acoustical experience, words must become significations of the new reality and being that this *psuchê* now "sees" before it; words, this is to say, become signs for the "look" or *eidos* of things beheld theoretically. Audible *onomata*, onomatopoetic namings, that to begin with were thought to imitate the sound of a thing, must now be seen as *sêmeia* like "2" or "<," that is, voiceless visible signs of what, in essence, the thing "looks like," visible signs signifying its visible "*eidos*" or form, its "look." Today, after Derrida, we would say that, consequently, *graphein*, marking in visual space, must no longer be based in *legein* or speaking in acoustical time but given its own priority. And in his *Poetics*, even Aristotle himself seems to be torn between thinking of language primarily as spoken and primarily as written.[8]

This tension is most obvious in Aristotle's account of the verbal component of tragedy, *lexis* or diction (1456b9 f.). From the beginning, his exposition here is oriented away from voiced speech even if, as the derivation of *lexis* from *legein*, to talk, suggests, he still makes voiced speech his point of departure. To begin with, at 1456b3–8 he has already relegated considerations of diction's role in engendering the *pathê* to the *Rhetoric* since in the tragedy, which is the concern of the *Poetics*, the *pathê* will also be engendered by something else besides speech, namely, the *sustasis* or composition of the play. This in itself makes clear that in the *Poetics* the voiced sound of what is said will now be of only marginal interest. For it is by voiced sound that diction communicates the *pathê*, but for the *Poetics*, at least, this function of diction is now incidental. And indeed, here in the *Poetics* dramatic elocution is divorced from diction and relegated to a separate discipline of acting or *hupokrisis*, which Aristotle apparently did not even deem worthy of a study of his own (see 1456b9–10).

Hence it is all the more striking that Aristotle still proceeds to base his account of diction on words as they are voiced. The basic elements or *stoicheia* of diction—it is wrong to call them "letters," which, of course, are written—are, he says, *voiced* sounds, namely the vowel, half-vowel, and mute, the *phôneen, hêmiphônon* and *aphônon*: "A vowel has an acoustical voice (*akoustikê phônê*) without resistance [of lips, throat, teeth, or tongue]; a half-vowel, such as S and R, has an acoustical voice along with such resistance; and a mute, such as G or D, as just this resistance by itself, has no voice at all but acquires an acoustical voice [if made] along with the elements that do have one" (1456b22–31).

P. Christopher Smith

With words, *onomata*, compounded of these vocal elements, however, the shift from mimetic sound to eidetic signification becomes obvious. The indivisible syllables are said to be a voicing precisely without significance, a *phônê asêmos* (1456b35), but the words and the utterance (*logos*) made up of these are said to be a "compound significant voice" (*phônê sunthetê sêmantikê*) (1457a12, 24). And with that the acoustical tone yields in importance to the meaning signified—and, I would contend, what we hear and undergo, to what we see and comprehend.

In fact it turns out that from the start Aristotle has always subordinated diction to *dianoia*—subordinated how something sounds to what the speaker, having "reasoned something through," has in view. By itself this would not necessarily imply that acoustical communication in voice had been displaced by a pure conceptualization and eidetic logic best communicated voicelessly in writing. For *dianoia*, says Aristotle, is concerned with "whatever it pertains to speech (*logos*) to provide, part of which is demonstration and refutation, *and part of which is providing for the feelings undergone such as pity or fear or rage and the like*" (1456a36–b 1) (emphasis added). Still, he goes on to say that "the excellence of diction lies in its clarity and not being lowly" (1458a18), which means, of course, that the sound of the poet's words should have a certain distinction about it in order to raise the words above the merely pedestrian, but significantly, that this elevation is now our only concern with how they sound. What *pathos* might be communicated by the way they are voiced is not a concern, for the first task is to communicate clearly (*saphôs*) the thought behind the words, the *dianoia*. The first task, that is, is to communicate clearly *ti hôs estin ê ouk estin*, "how a thing is, or is not, what it is [in essence]" (1450b12) and to show clearly what it is "in general" (*katholou*) (1450b28–29). Indeed, "diction," says Aristotle, "is expatiation (*hermeneia*) by means of putting things into words" (1450b13–14).

With this reduction of tragic diction to clear expatiation, Aristotle has effectively contradicted his initial definition of tragedy as the "imitation of actions" rather than the "reporting" of them (1449b24–27). From the start, he has, in fact, already returned to Plato's privileging of narration over *mimêsis* (see *Rep.* 392d f.) all the while he would have rehabilitated *mimêsis* against Plato's attack.

That he has is as obvious at the end of his *Poetics* as it is at the beginning. When evaluating the relative merits of tragedy and epic, Aristotle, in his typical dialectical fashion, starts with a concession to his opponents, who favor epic over tragedy. Often, he allows, "vulgar" reenactment does count against tragedy, and the epic precludes this vulgarity precisely because it is reporting and not imitation by actors on stage (1449b12). But, he responds, "the tragedy must be able do what is proper to it without [bodily] motion, just as the epic can, for in the reading of tragedy it is made plain what sort it is" (1462a17–18). Hence, he concludes, if some restrained motions and forms of dance are permissible accoutrements for tragedy (1462a9), the gyrations of indiscrete flute players—and even those of the poet Pindar—prove to be not merely unnecessary but objectionable (see 1461b30 f.). Indeed, an unmoved, uninvolved *reading* of tragedy would be fully sufficient: "The power of tragedy [to achieve its cathartic effect] also exists without a protagonist and performers," says Aristotle (1450b18–19), and "what is fearful and pitiful can, to be sure, be generated from the visual staging (*opsis*), but also solely from the [playwright's] composition (*sustasis*) of the actions" (1453b1–3).

Not surprisingly, when Aristotle makes this point that a reading without reenactment can achieve the tragic effect, he completely neglects the fact that such a reading, even if no longer a performance, would still be out loud and heard by the reader and audience, and that this hearing is something felt and undergone bodily and hence not a matter at all of just "getting the picture" intellectually. His entire emphasis now is on the logical composition or *sustasis*. To be sure, he adds, "it is necessary that the story be so composed that, without seeing the actions that came to pass the one hearing of them trembles and pities at what happened, as someone hearing the story of Oedipus would undergo this (*an pathoi*)" (1453b4–7). But remarkably, Aristotle overlooks the acoustical dimension of what he has just said. His point is only that one can dispense with *hupokrisis* and *opsis*, enactment and visual staging, and still see the logic of the composition.

By this account even the tragic *katharsis* of fear and pity, which in the *Politics* was said to result from something like becoming entranced by sacred melodies, and which surely was physical acoustical experience felt and undergone in the imitative motions of one's body, now becomes a matter of intellectual insight. Far from being the result of one's own ritual reenactment of the redemptive sufferings of another, *katharsis* of fear and pity now comes from detached observation of what these are in essence when someone else undergoes them. *Katharsis* becomes a seeing and knowing these *pathê* for what they are—a seeing and knowing precisely by onlookers who, if affected vicariously on one level, ultimately sense that on another level they are really removed and unaffected. Whereas in the soteriological experience of *katharsis* one reenacts the passions of another in order to be redeemed from the debt of one's inevitable transgressions, *katharsis* now results from sensing one's own transcendence in cognition.[9] Not mimetic participation but detachment is the principle here.

The characteristic substitution of spatial size (*megathos*) for temporal duration (*mêkos*) in Aristotle's conception of tragedy follows naturally from this shift away from the passion of acoustical experience and to the sovereign autonomy of envisioning. For time, with its measures by beats in meter, rhythm, and tempo, is the dimensional form of the acoustical, the content of the later being tone, timbre, and pitch. But space, with its measures of height, width, and depth, is the proper dimensionality of the visual, the content of the later being color and shape. Of course, Aristotle does not deny that the tragedy does have a temporal duration and he compares it with epic in precisely this regard, since the epic can go on for an unlimited time (1451a15 f.), whereas the tragedy's duration cannot exceed the retention of the audience.

Still, Aristotle conceives of the tragedy predominantly in spatial, visual terms. As is well known, he likens tragedy to a living thing, the beauty and unity of which consist not only in the right spatial relationship of its parts to each other—here is where the composition or *sustasis* comes in—but also in its having not just any size but the size that is right for it:

> For the beautiful consists in the size and the arrangement (*en megathei kai taxei*), on account of which neither the smallest living thing of all would be beautiful nor the largest. For in the first case our envisioning (*theôria*) of it would be confused, the time for its occurence being nearly imperceptible. And in the second case our envisioning does not happen all at once, rather the unity and wholeness of the envisioning eludes the one who envisions. (1450b36–1451a5)

Despite the reference to time here, it would be wrong to say that Aristotle means what he says about envisioning the spatial size of the tragedy only metaphorically and that his primary focus really remains on its acoustical temporal duration. In the first place, the recurring references to *theôria* or envisioning in this passage are not abandoned at all when he continues his analysis of the tragic; rather, they become definitive. Second, his emphasis here, and henceforth continues to be, on the *taxis* and *sustasis* of the parts, their placement and coplacement. Even if taken metaphorically, place, location in space, is the paradigm, not the temporal sequence. The concern now is with how a thing that we "see," albeit intellectually, is put together. Internally its parts must be fitted together *logically*, and externally it should have a limit or *horos*, and this, as the origin of the word in *horan* or "seeing" suggests, is "in view," which is to say comprehensible as a whole (1451a6).

Though there is some ambiguity at first (see 1450b26–30), in Aristotle the beginning, middle, and end of a well-composed story are ultimately not to be experienced and undergone acoustically in time. Rather they are to be understood as parts of a unified "living being" of which we have an overview (1459a19–20). Thus it is precisely *not* as if the tragedy were like a melody that began out of silence at some time past, came over us, and at its climax enthralled us in the symphonic interweaving (*symplokê*, *desis*) of its voices, only then for these, having transformed us, to fade away into dissolution (*lusis*) and inaudibility. Rather, says Aristotle, like the "living thing," the tragedy is to be envisioned

P. Christopher Smith

all at once (*hama*), present, in view, in its entirety. In short, we are not to hear tragedy anymore but to get a logical "picture" of it, much as Plato would have taught us not to *hear* melodies and undergo them in time but to *look* over and beyond them to the idea of them—*apoblepein pros tên idean*, as he would say—and to envision the ever-present, static logic of the harmonic laws governing them (see *Rep.* 531ab).

This is why in Aristotle the primary task of the poet is not at all to compose in "pleasant and appropriate meters," though he should do this too, but to tell "what is possible either according to likelihood or necessity" (1451a39). In other words, the poet's story must have a logical line to it or plot, for the past and particular treated by the historian is credible even if we cannot see the logic of it, but the possible and universal treated by the poet is credible only if we can (1451a39–b8).

Crucial here are the logical terms "according to likelihood" and "according to necessity." The first is said of dialectical arguments about what is "susceptible of being otherwise," and the second is said of scientific arguments that demonstrate what has to be so and cannot be otherwise. We see, in other words, that the organic unity of the tragedy is now modeled on reasoning and the logical relationship of antecedent and consequence. The end, says Aristotle, must follow from the beginning and middle "out of necessity," or as what happens "for the most part" (1450b30), where "for the most part" substitutes here for "according to likelihood." Even Homer is praised because he omits events not in a logical sequence, events, that is, which are neither likely (*eikos*) nor necessary (*anakaios*), one as a logical consequence of the other (1451a24–29). Thus ultimately the tragedy and even the epic are to be intellectually viewed as written arguments and not heard, felt, and undergone as musical occurrences. Meter and, we may presume, pitch and melody too, are in fact wholly ancillary.

As we have heard, even fear and pity, the *katharsis* of which the tragedy should provide, will arise from the logical composition (*sustasis*) of the story and precisely not from any experience the audience undergoes (1453b1–3). For this reason the "compli-

cated" storyline involving reversal and recognition are preferable in Aristotle's view to the "simple" storyline, where the
"binding" and "unraveling" lack the logical coherence that a
properly constructed reversal and recognition display.

This is striking, for the reversal and recognition, he tells us,
are, for the one undergoing them, the conversion of an intended
result into precisely the opposite of what was expected and fore-
seen. For instance, Oedipus had expected to be made happy by
the news of who he is, and he had expected the fear for his wife
to be relieved, but just the reverse happens (1452a23–27). For
Oedipus, then, what happens violates and disrupts the logic of
his thinking. What he undergoes is *for him* entirely illogical and
intrudes from beyond the horizons of his finite comprehension.
But exactly this should not be the case for us, who are no longer
communicants in the reenactment of the *pathê* and *pathêmata* he
experiences, but who look on from above and see the logical
"likelihood" or even "necessity" of what for him is a bolt out of
the blue. Whereas before, in commiseration with his fear, we
might have experienced compassion for him and felt saved from
our own fear by this very compassion, now we are removed from
feeling any passion at all. Again, the soteriological *katharsis* of
expiation by reenactment has become Plato's *katharsis* of purification by metaphysical abstraction.

No wonder, then, that in the end music and melody have
become for Aristotle mere incidental adornments that produce
only a secondary "pleasure," and that the "power of tragedy" to
effect *katharsis* is said to exist even "without protagonists and
performers" (1450b18). In contradiction to Kosman's contention that the *Poetics* carries the *Ethics* over on to the new ground
of human finitude and error, the *Poetics* could also be said only to
repeat what happens in the *Ethics*: in the end our engaged action
and the inevitable involvement in wrongdoing that comes with it
give way to the highest good of metaphysical *theôria*, of dispassionate, unmoved looking on (see EN 1177a11 f.). In the end
Aristotle, like Plato, flees the possibility of having something
happen to him. Like Plato he too shies away from the stream of
time that, like a melody, comes over us, in order that he might

find safety in a distanced beholding that alone would ensure *autarkeia*: full self-possession and independence.

Notes

1. "To grasp this [Dionysian origin] we must take down that artful edifice of Apollonian culture stone by stone, as it were, until we catch sight of the foundations on which it is based" (*Die Geburt der Tragödie aus dem Geiste der Musik* (Kröner, Stuttgart, 1976), §3, p. 57. Henceforth "GT"). (Translations of German and Greek throughout this chapter are my own.) With this strategy of interpretation Nietzsche paves the way for Martin Heidegger's "Destruktion" and, in turn, Jacques Derrida's "deconstruction," both of which will figure in my reading here of Aristotle's *Poetics.*

In keeping with Heidegger's "fundamental ontology," I will try to penetrate beneath later Platonic, metaphysical overlays in this work to "fundamental" layers of an earlier, "more inceptive" thinking "closer to the origin"—*ein anfänglicheres, ursprünglicheres Denken.* It is the young Heidegger, I would also note, who alerts us to Aristotle's striking ambivalence at the beginning of the *Metaphysics* in regard to which is the primary form of *aisthesis* or perception, seeing or hearing: having opened with the assertion that it is seeing (*horan*) that most of all makes us knowledgeable and displays to us the differences among things, Aristotle proceeds to say next, remarkably, that it is hearing, *akouein,* that distinguishes those animals that can learn, *manthanein,* from those that cannot (*Metaph.* 980a22 f.; see Heidegger, *Platon: Sophistes,* Gesamtausgabe 19 [Frankfurt: Klostermanna, 1992], p. 70).

However, Heidegger, whose primary concern at this time (1925) was with phenomenological clarification of what the world *looks* like, immediately loses track of the traces of an earlier acoustical experience that are left here in Aristotle. Hence, in my reading of Aristotle's *Poetics* I will depend more on Nietzsche's singular insight that the earlier way of thinking has musical origins and was primarily acoustical. See in particular GT §6, p. 67 f., on Schiller and the origins of the poetic word *in einer musikalischen Stimmung,* in a musical voicing or mood. (Could Heidegger have gotten his word *Stimmung* from this text?)

With Derrida, I will seek to display the contradictions into which Aristotle's only apparently coherent analysis of tragedy collapses when elements of tragedy he would relegate to the interstices and margins of his exposition are highlighted.

2. If A. O. Rorty's fine collection, *Essays on Aristotle Poetics* (Princeton: Princeton University Press, 1992), is any indication, what is missing in contemporary Aristotle analysis is insight into Aristotle's intrinsic self-contradictoriness. Despite what Heidegger's "Destruktion" and Derrida's "deconstruction" might have taught us, and despite, too, the patent irreconcilability of the different interpretations in Rorty's book, the governing principle of its Aristotle interpretations still seems to be that every text must be a unified whole logically consistent with itself. I have tried to show here what advances might be made if this principle of noncontradiction is jettisoned.

3. H.-G. Gadamer alerts us to the profound significance of this saying from Aeschylus (*Agamemnon,* 177) in his appropriation of it for a theory of experience as *Erfahrung.* See Gadamer, *Wahrheit und Methode* (Tübingen: J. C. B. Mohr, 1965), p. 339, and my own *Hermeneutics and Human Finitude* (Bronx, N.Y.: Fordham University Press, 1991), pp. 175n9, 190, 274.

4. See Rorty, *Essays*, pp. 51–72, in particular, p. 67. Kosman brings to the light a soteriological dimension of *mimêsis* and *katharsis* in Aristotle that completely eludes and contradicts the equally well-argued cognitivist explanations of these given in Rorty by Martha Nussbaum in her "Tragedy and Self-sufficiency: Plato and Aristotle on Fear and Pity" (pp. 261–290), for instance, and by Jonathan Lear in his "Katharsis" (pp. 315–340). And if the principle of noncontradiction is followed, either Kosman's analysis or theirs must be discarded. I suggest instead that we keep both sides of this contradiction in play and discard instead the principle of noncontradiction.

5. See Cyril of Jerusalem, *Mystagogical Catacheses* II.5 in *St. Cyril of Jerusalem's Lectures on the Christian Sacraments*, ed. F. L. Cross (Crestwood, N.Y., St. Vladamir, 1986) and cited by Kosman in Rorty, *Essays*, p. 68.

6. See GT § 7, pp. 79–87, on the satyr chorus as the soil and ground (*Boden*) from which tragedy arose, in particular, where Nietzsche asserts, "The tragedy grew upwards upon this foundation" (80) and "The satyr chorus of the dithyramb is the saving deed of Greek art" (82).

7. Though E. Havelock is, in my view, guilty of some quite incredible over-simplifications—for one, the thesis that Homer is to be read as an oral encyclopedia of information—his *Preface to Plato* (Cambridge: Harvard University Press, 1963) does contain some remarkable insights that would corroberate, and be corroborated by, the "Destruktion" of metaphysical thought in Heidegger and, before Heidegger, in Nietzsche. Particularly useful is chapter 11, "*Psyche* or the Separation of the Knower from the Known" (pp. 197–214), in which Havelock argues, here convincingly, that with the transition from an oral, acoustical culture to a literate, visual one, the word *psuchê* shifts its meaning from the "life" in the body to the personality, soul, or self as the seat of moral decision detached from the body and removed from bodily experience. In regard to the *psuchê*, too, Aristotle involves himself in remarkable contradictions insofar as he preserves the earlier, pre-Platonic understandings of it while at the same time elaborating Plato's psychology of disengaged contemplation.

8. Derrida does not see that Plato's turn from the acoustical to the visual would ultimately involve assigning priority to visible writing, which is statically present in space, over audible speaking, which is evanescent in time. After all, if the *eidos* or "look" of "2" is something that we see with the mind's eye, the primary physical sign for it should be visible to the bodily eye, as in fact it is; the voiced sound we make when we say "two" or "*deux*" is entirely incidental. One might ask, then, if Plato's "metaphysics of presence" can be deconstructed without getting behind the tradition of language as visible signs and back to the original language of audible musical voice, human and instrumental. Nietzsche is better than his followers on this count too. In a later criticism of his own *Birth of Tragedy*, he writes, "It should have sung, this 'new soul,' and not talked" (see "An Attempt at Self-criticism," GT § 3, p. 33).

9. The cognitive reading of *katharsis* is thus fully justified. But so was Kosman's soteriological reading. See note 4 above.

2

Aristotle and Specular Regimes: The Theater of Philosophical Discourse

James I. Porter

The application of methods of literary analysis to philosophical discourse, a recent trend most brilliantly instanced by a critic like Paul de Man, tends to isolate recognizably literary and rhetorical structures (figurative language, motifs, narratives, and so on) as a way of displacing the basis of philosophical argument. In principle, the point that nonliterary discourses rely heavily on literary or rhetorical devices is well taken. It is, however, a point whose significance can easily be overstated. The single-minded focus on literary devices, to the exclusion of the discursive logic of a philosophical text, actually serves to decontextualize and eventually distort the successive moments of the text. Often reduced to a phrase or a word, these quickly acquire, in their naked isolation, a disproportionate synecdochal and foundational significance in relation to the text, which ultimately must give way, as Paul de Man puts it, to "the disruptive power of rhetoric," that is, to language itself, which proves to be the ultimate ground, and ruin, of all philosophical discourse.[1] On an approach like this, not only does the philosophical text as a whole (its texture) suffer a certain neglect, but the differences between philosophy and literature are blurred, courtesy of an overquick, purely formalistic reduction of the one to the other. The specificity of philosophical discourse at this level is indistinguishable from that of literary discourse. Both are the beneficiaries of linguistic form, but then what discourse is not?

One solution to this impasse might be to consider the *discursive* role of tropes and figures in philosophy. These ought to be viewed, first, as elements or relays in a chain that is motivated, if not exactly determined, by conventions and procedures that are in the first instance philosophical. In Roman Jakobson's terms, metaphors in a philosophical text acquire a metonymic, syntagmatic function in the course of their being projected from the vertical axis of substitution onto the horizontal axis of contiguity, from metaphor to statement and meta-statement. By *syntagmatic*, however, I mean something more than grammatical syntax. I mean discursive logistics, the grammar and rhetoric of metaphorical thought. Tracing the history of such projections in a philosophical text can in cases reveal not just the metaphysical *impensé* of a system, but its unexpressed or even muted logic and the pragmatic ways in which this logic is realized. There is more to the performativity of a philosophical text than its express or tacit disavowal (or avowal, for that matter) of literary contamination.

Bringing to light the forces at work in philosophy reveals something beyond its surface forms alone (here, its rhetorical figures and tropes). Not even Friedrich Nietzsche, the immediate inspiration behind the contemporary rhetorical model of reading texts, was content to bring his critique to a halt once he had exposed, to his satisfaction, the "aesthetically justified" nature of philosophy. Nietzsche's critical methods are not literary, at least not reductively so, nor are they an attempt to demystify texts by exposing the literary bases of purportedly nonliterary discourses. The aesthetic features of, say, philosophical writing for Nietzsche papers over a far more potent violence of thought, in the same way that the Apollinian realm of light and appearances conceals, through its very limpidity, its own harsh politics of cruelty and suppression (*The Birth of Tragedy* § 4).[2]

In a similar spirit, I propose to reconsider a familiar system of cognate figures and tropes, one that in many ways has been constitutive of philosophy as a discipline from its first beginnings. These stem roughly from the realm of perception (theory, theater, vision, supervision), and they converge in a troubled but suggestive pattern at the intersection of a few texts from the

Aristotelian corpus. I shall be less concerned to undertake a stylistic analysis per se than to analyze a certain style of thought, which can only be read off the discursive map of a text, from within the theater of philosophical discourse.[3]

I

This *tractatus politicus* ... deals with the grand *politics* of virtue, the ways and means by which virtue leads to *power*. ... It is intended for the use of those whose interest lies in learning, not how one becomes virtuous, but how one *makes* virtuous—how virtue is made to dominate. I even intend to prove that to desire the one—the domination of virtue—one must in principle *not* desire the other; one automatically renounces becoming virtuous oneself.

—Nietzsche, *Kritische Studien Ausgabe. Werke* vol. 13, p. 25 (*The Will to Power* § 304, trans. Kaufmann and Hollingsdale; modified)

Philosophical discourse in Aristotle is best viewed as a theorization of the visual, a fact readily derived from the opening paragraphs of his *Metaphysics*, but one that gathers in force when we turn to other, less obvious contexts, especially his writings on ethics and politics. The methodological overlap evident, for instance, in the *Metaphysics'* and *Politics'* opening pages is so striking that one is compelled to take seriously, almost literally, every occurrence of the perceptual metaphor (light, vision, clarity) in Aristotle's discourse—for instance, the invitations to "consider" (*skopein*), "look" (*blepein*), "see" (*horan*), "contemplate" theoretically (*theorein*), and so forth—surely the most frequent characterization of philosophical activity in Aristotle (as it was in Plato).

Starting from the perceptual metaphor, one can observe a bifurcation in the related conceptual bases of two kinds of philosophical activity in Aristotle. The first is philosophy considered *as a discipline* and method for organizing the perceptual field. Philosophy so understood is the immediate product of a theorization of the visual, namely, the quasi-metaphor of perception itself (the kinds of philosophical seeing named just above). Philosophical activity in the second sense is philosophy considered *as a theory of discipline*. A subdiscipline of First Philosophy, it inevitably participates in the same mechanism as was just described: the organization and subordination of the perceptual field. It is in fact *the* theory of this subordination and supervision. The challenge to philosophy is to keep these two kinds of activity apart, at least in appearance.

These, then, are the terms within which can be traced the movement of the philosophical signifier in Aristotle: from philosophy as a self-constituting act of denomination (of its own proper domain and focus) to philosophy as a theory of domination; from philosophy as a theoretical act of vision to philosophy as a theory of supervision. The coordination of metaphysical and political terms, terms that otherwise tend to be kept neatly held apart, is anything but fortuitous. Their union in Aristotle reflects what might be called a universal metaphysico-political discourse, or else simply philosophical discourse prior to its division into philosophical discourses and domains.

Consider the first words of Aristotle's *Politics*, already in the form of a conclusion as the work commences: "Since we see that every state is some kind of association and that every association is organized for the sake of some good ..., it is clear that all associations are directed toward some good, and that most of all that association which is the highest of all, and which embraces all the others [the political association called the *polis*], is directed at the highest good."[4] This statement gives the skeleton of Aristotle's argument in the *Politics* as a whole. Any detailed analysis of the passage would want to inspect the *subordination* enacted by the since-clause, that is, the act of seeing, "since we see," on three levels: grammatically (in the syntactic subordination), logically (in the figure of logic that grounds the inference captured by the verb "we see"), and rhetorically (in the predication and anticipation of the whole of the *Politics* by this preamble to the work). The since-clause clearly serves as the grounds for its sequel; it invokes a logical structure with the force of a premise, out of which the conclusion flows smoothly and limpidly: "it is clear."

In a grounding act, Aristotle is thus operating a figure of logic that he himself invented and perfected into a frictionless mechanism. But this grounding act is not self-grounding. The logical structure must find itself reflected in some other structure: that invoked by the clause beginning with "we see that ...," which, through a doubly embedded but self-erasing grammatical subordination ("Since (we see that)"), invokes a truth-bearing syntax that subordinates every statement within the field of its articulations. Implied in the words "we see" is an entire domain of empirical knowledge (such as Aristotle would have acquired in his compilation and analyses of political constitutions), as well as a field of speculative knowledge (the theoretical elaboration of the first domain). The subject of (in this case) political philosophy and its logical grounds are thus inscribed within a field of perceived objects, a field of vision. The things viewed are invoked as a substantiating proof in a logical chain, as a virtual *semeion* or evidentiary sign. (Cf. *Pol.* 2.8 1268b38–39, and compare the identical procedure in *Metaphysics* 1.1 980a1.)

Let us simply note the curious interplay between, on the one hand, the initial grounding of the *Politics* in the empirical, and on the other, the speculative conclusion that follows from it. At work in the passage is a subtle betokening of the visual, which in turn permits itself to be confiscated by a logic of truth, one that the simple act of observation itself seems to have generated. Truth appears to be caught in its own reflection, in a specular play between the visible, the logical, and the speculative: between observation, language, and philosophy. For Aristotle, on the other hand, this interplay is unproblematical. It always results in clarity (*delon*, "it is clear").

The sequel will bear out this specular clarity, which, it needs to be stressed, is not quite the sort of clarity that issues from a privileging of the visual, a phenomenon frequently isolated, and discredited, under the label of ocularcentrism. It is not my intention here to accuse Aristotle of this visualist bias but only to visit the specular regimes of knowledge and power that he erects, so to speak, in the very shadow of the visual.[5] Specular regimes, I wish to argue, are constituted less by an appeal to vision per se than by an appeal to what lies beyond it, beyond the registers of the visible and the invisible, beyond even the projective imagination.[6]

James I. Porter

Of interest in this connection is not the centrality of the visual but, on the contrary, the power of *self*-evidence and the *non*-evidence—the nonappearance—of power, which is to say the construction of an *asymptomatic* locus of power.

One way to bring out the difference I am alluding to is to think of power in its classical and postmodern forms, for which a whole series of contrasts is available: power as frontal and spectacular as opposed to power as oblique and relational; display versus panoptic (but nonetheless blind) surveillance; the eye versus the gaze; the Imaginary versus the Real; the copy versus the simulacrum; coercion and subjection versus fascination, complicity, and subjectivation; and so on. Both modalities of power are present in Aristotle (as they are today), and they are mutually collaborative. There is, however, a way in which it is the postvisual, postmodern theory of power that discloses the rationale of visual hegemony—the fetishism of the eye—that is actually and effectively at work in ocularcentrism. Visuality is compensatory in nature: it exists to put a face on power, to compensate for power's eccentric (structurally decentered) dimension. Visuality is thus one of the *disguises* of power, not its source and not even its true form, but simply its screen. The true form of power, on the contrary, is its own apparent absence—an absence that always elicits the supplemental interpretive gestures of a (fascinated) subject.

Visuality exists for a subject who seeks assurances and meaning, not least of all the assurance of a meaningfulness to power. Assurances of this kind are evoked *by* a visual apparatus *for* a subject who identifies herself in the act of identifying elements in a visual field. Visuality, then, is a supplement in this precise sense. It is a stopgap and a sign of (forfended) desperation. Power as effective and binding, by contrast, is the threat of nonmeaning, of nonsense, of the realization that power is, in essence, nonsensical. So intertwined are these two modalities of power that detatching them from each other may prove possible only in theory. Their more or less successful detachment in a passage from the *Politics* to be discussed below points to the risks of such a conceptual possibility. But that is getting ahead of ourselves.

Having shown what clearly is the case, Aristotle next runs through some of the received opinions (*endoxa*) concerning what the civic state (*polis*) and in effect the art of politics (*politike*) are supposed by some to be (Plato and Socrates are the likely targets here). But these suppositions, Aristotle tells us, are poorly articulated (*Pol.* 1.1 1252a9), that is, not true (1252a16). If the endoxic beliefs are untrue, this is because they are unsystematic, unmethodic, unrigorous. The remedy Aristotle proposes is the opposite: system, method, rigor. It is only natural, then, that Aristotle should conclude his prelude with an invitation to the philosophical method: "And this will become *clear* to anyone who *inspects* what has been stated, using the customary method" (1252a17–18).[7] Aristotle's hope is to refine the *endoxa* into a technically and scientifically acceptable form (*ti technikon*, 1252a22), and then to absorb them into his inquiry.

I simply wish to indicate, for the moment, Aristotle's investment in a method for knowing truth (cf. *methodos kai techne*, *Nichomachean Ethics* 1.1 1094al), which is a technique of seeing— and not just a piece of philosophical technology, as any brief perusal of the first pages of his *Metaphysics* will decide beyond question. The passage from empirical knowledge of the particular to epistemic knowledge of the universal is a well-charted course familiar from the opening paragraphs of the *Metaphysics*. There, philosophy (*theoria*) is defined as the culmination and *telos* of that passage. But in the *Metaphysics*, Aristotle cannot separate theory from technique, nor does he try to. It is the technical or, in his own language, "architectural" component, Aristotle claims, that defines genuine knowledge.

II

Some of the greatest moralists ... have already recognized and antici- pated the truth ..., namely that one can achieve *the domination of virtue only by the same means* as those by which one can achieve domination of any kind, in any case not *by means of* virtue.

—Nietzsche, *Kritische Studien Ausgabe. Werke* (*The Will to Power*)

James I. Porter

The first paragraph of the *Metaphysics* reads as follows:

All men by nature desire to know. An indication (*semeion*) of this is the delight we take in our senses; for even apart from their usefulness they are loved for themselves; and above all others the sense of sight. For not only with a view to action, but even when we are not going to do anything, we prefer seeing (one might say) to everything else, but even when we have no action in mind. The reason is that this, most of all the senses, makes us know and brings to light many differences between things.[8]

We can follow Aristotle's train of thought in what follows. The steps from sight to insight (knowledge) form a ladder, from direct or immediate experience (*empeiria*) to memory, the retention and collation of experiences (*mneme*), to knowledge or science (*episteme*). Put differently, the progression is from the knowledge of the particular to knowledge of the universal, of "first things and causes."

Once in the realm of science we are also in the synonymous realm of technique;[9] and, optimally, not that of mere manual technicians (*cheirotechnoi*, artisans) but the kind possessed by master architects, or "architechnicians" (*architektones*). The difference between the two kinds of technique is put forth in a blunt analogy at *Metaphysics* (1.1 981b2–5): "We think the manual workers are like certain lifeless things (*apsuchoi*) which act indeed, but act without knowing what they do, *as fire burns*."[10] Architechnicians, in contrast, are in possession of a technique for knowing. Their conception of fire is not just of that which burns and produces heat; it is the concept of an intelligible fire that has knowable causes. And while the senses yield knowledge of particulars, knowledge-*that* (e.g., of fire, "*that* fire is hot"), technique yields a technical knowledge, it sees reasons (e.g., "*why* fire is hot"; ibid., 981b11–13). It is this technical component that defines genuine *episteme*.

By way of illustration, Aristotle presents a model of evolution in science, from its crude origins to the current state of the art: "Probably at first he who invented any art whatever and went beyond the common perceptions of man was naturally admired by men, not only because there was something useful in the inventions, but because he was thought wise and superior to the rest" (981b13–17). In this genealogy of art and technique (*techne*), future inventions grew in sophistication (981b18–19) as they shed their constraints of utility and pleasure and approached an abstract purity (for example, the mathematical arts [*technai*]) that could be conducted in leisure (as *theoria*, 982a1). The culmination of this sequence represents a conquest over experience, over time, and over necessity. Aristotle will later resort to political and ideological categories to describe this kind of epistemological breakthrough, or rather liberation: love of knowledge for its own sake and not for some ulterior need is like a free man who exists for his own sake and not for another's. Indeed, philosophical knowledge is "as it were the only free denizen in the domain of knowledges" (982b25–28; cf. *Pol.* 1.7). This liberation of knowledge, which is both a technical advance and an achievement for humanity, represents a subordination of competing techniques and knowledges, in addition to a subordination of the perceptual field through a reconstitution of the objects of knowledge. The philosophical technician (*technites*) outstrips the experienced eye of the common, experienced person (*empeiron*) by refining the objects of sight, purifying them, restoring them to knowledge through discipline, to discipline, to the love of knowledge for its own sake (*philosophia*).

When we combine these perspectives, a new perception of key concepts in Aristotle suggests itself: if knowledge reveals itself to be a technique, theory emerges as a special kind of praxis. Philosophy in general is now best viewed as a discipline and method for organizing the perceptual field (for reconstituting the objects within any domain controlled from the commanding perspective of the discipline that oversees it), while the *Politics*, in particular, emerges as *the* theory of this subordination and supervision of competing knowledges, techniques, and discourses (Aristotle calls it, for this reason, "the architectural science" within the practical domain, while rationality [*logos*] is in its own way an architect too [*Pol.* 1.13 1260a18–19]). More insidiously, perhaps, value-free speculations in the *Metaphysics* about the ground of being betray ideological and rhetorical biases that are somewhat less innocently articulated in Aristotle's theory of political power in the *Politics*. That theory, in turn, proves to be an elaboration of a theatrical metaphor that throws light on Aristotle's methodological conduct elsewhere in his corpus. I mention these alternative descriptions of Aristotle's theories primarily to loosen the received categories of reading that control our current picture of him. What ultimately is needed is a more adequate reformulation of the nexus that can only be suggested here: a more adequate study, in other words, of the metaphysics of politics and the politics of metaphysics. In what follows, I will take up a more modestly defined but not divorced set of issues: the theatrical relation between power and ethics; that is, the problem of knowledge, technique, and perception, and specifically their troubling synthesis as it emerges in a curious passage in the *Politics*.

III

Moralists need the *gestures of virtue*, also the gestures of truth; their error begins only when they *yield* to virtue, when they lose their domination over virtue, when they themselves become *moral*, become *true*. A great moralist is, among other things, necessarily a great actor; his danger is that his dissimulation may unintentionally become nature, while it is his ideal to keep his *esse* [sc., what he is] and his *operari* [sc., what he does] in a divine way apart; everything he does must be done *sub specie boni* [with the appearance of goodness]—a high, remote, exciting ideal!
—Nietzsche, *Kritische Studien Ausgabe. Werke* (*The Will to Power*)

We should first recall Aristotle's characterization of the political science that the *Politics* exemplifies. In the first book of the *Nichomachean Ethics*, Aristotle prepares the ground for a new knowledge (*gnosis*, 1.2 1094a22–23) and technique for managing *hai praktikai*, that ensemble of knowledges whose explicit aim is not knowledge per se, but its application in life, *praxis* (ibid., 1.3 1095a5 f.). This aggregate body of practical knowledges is subject to supervision from above. The specialized branches of warfare, household management, rhetoric, and so forth (1.2 1094b3–5) must be harnessed by the supreme practical science that subsumes beneath itself all inferior practical knowledges and capacities or powers. The highest and most authoritative of these, the master discipline (the *architechne*), is the political form of art (*politike*, 1.2 1094a26–28), whose object is the *telos* at which all the practical activities aim, and whose content Aristotle proceeds to fill in, in the work devoted to this topic, the *Politics*.

Our attention in what follows will be drawn to a curious and revealing passage from the fifth book of the *Politics*, one that, in ways no more than typical of Aristotelian political theory and the sweeping perspectives it affords, in other ways represents a peculiar distillation of that project. The stated purpose of Book 5, as it is announced in the first eight lines, is to give a theory of the metabolic transformations of states—their morphology—by way of an analysis of the causes of their degeneration and of their modes of possible salvation: "Next we should scrutinize the causes of revolutions in states (lit., "from what [causes] constitutions undergo change [from one constitution to another: *metaballousin*], their scope and nature, and what, for each of the constitutions, are the degenerative factors [the *phthorai*, the corruptions, i.e., the causes leading to their inexistence] and from what [form] to what they most often transform; and then what are the kinds of salvation (*soteria*), both generally and in each particular case; and then how each of the constitutions might best be saved" (*Pol.* 5.1 1301a19–25). Physics and politics, presiding over equally unstable realms, are both sciences of motion (*kinesis*) and change (*metabole*).[11]

Aristotle carries out his program with a remarkably unprejudiced objectivity, devoting equal attention to the vicissitudes of the monarchic, aristocratic, and mixed regimes and to their perverted counterparts (*parekbaseis*), the tyrannical, oligarchic, and democratic regimes (cf. 3.7 1279b4–6), and even more surprisingly, to the best means of their respective salvation. In many ways, his most striking analysis will be the one that occupies us here: not that concerning the degenerative causes of the positively evaluated regimes but the analysis of the maintenance and salvation of the stigmatized regimes, and in particular tyranny, defined by Aristotle as that form of government founded on deception (*apate*) and naked force (*bia*) (5.10 1313a9). The central paradox of this section of his treatise (Bk. 5 ch. 11) is that Aristotle, in the course of his dispassionate analysis, lays out lines of defense for the very regimes that on all other grounds—and not least on moral grounds—he judges to be indefensible. His defense of this defense reveals paradoxes of its own.

Two paths are available to anyone whose concern it is to prolong the life of his tyranny. The first (5.11 1313a35–1314a29) involves open repression and is reducible to a set of rules and rationales:

• Hamstring the prominent members of the community.

• Extirpate high spirits.

• Ban eating clubs and political associations; prohibit lectures and learned converse.

• Alienate the citizenry from themselves: take every measure to ensure that a mutual lack of acquaintance among citizens will prevail.

• Compel citizens to be conspicuous (*phaneroi*) at all times, to spend their hours at the public gates (for in this way their doings will not escape the tyrant).

• Keep a vigilant watch over the words and actions of subjects, using spies (*kataskopoi*), like the "female detectives" at Syracuse, and the eavesdroppers whom Hiero, the tyrant of that city, used to send to any place of resort or meeting.

• Set them at variance with one another and bring them into collision. Friends should be embroiled in conflicts with friends, the lower class with the notables, the rich with their own class.

• Impoverish subjects with public works projects (paradigmatic examples of this technique are the Egyptian pyramids, the Cypselid temple offerings,[12] the construction by the Pesistratidae of the temple of Olympian Zeus at Athens, and the colossal Polycratean monuments at Samos).

• Multiply taxes, after the manner of Dionysius, tyrant of Syracuse, who contrived that in the space of five years his subjects should bring into the treasury their whole property.

• Be fond of war, which creates a dependency on leadership.

• Distrust friends, on the assumption that everybody has the will to overthrow a tyranny, and most of all those who have the power to do so, namely, one's own friends.

Before moving on to the second method of repression, we should pause to take stock. What is Aristotle in fact recommending, with this proto-Machiavellian posture that he is adopting, as it were, for the sake of the argument? Beyond the fact that subjects of tyranny are to be deprived of external goods and the license and means to organize their internal affairs, to organize, in other words, the surface patterns of life—the autonomous disposition of wealth, of time, and of the self—there is an even deeper lesson in repression to be learned: subjects of tyranny must be banned from every private sphere, from every sanctuary and interior. The civic body of private subjects must be reconstituted into an aggregate of atomic, public objects, with no recourse to obscurity, no flight to invisibility. The tyrannical policy wipes out every interior dimension by extroverting them, objectifying them, submitting them to the blinding glare of public light. The natural cohesion of individuals (with themselves, with others) is shattered, or rather substituted by a principle: the logic of self-organization is replaced by a logic of external organization, and the political space is transformed into a perceptual field, externally dominated by an inescapable presence.

All of this is accomplished not by force or deception alone but through their elusive exchange and interlacing. Consider again the measures being recommended: destroy pride, which is to say, independence of mind (*phronemata*); create ignorance, which is to say separate and alienate subjects (for acquaintance [*gnosis*] creates bonds of trust [*pistis*]); reduce thought to humility; diminish, lower, enslave; destabilize, spy, create the spectre of fear, "for in fear of such spies, subjects are less likely to exercise *parrhesia* (frank and open expression); and if they should persist in such free expression, they will escape notice less often," which is to say not at all, given the hyperbolic implementation of this technique.

The repression is complete, because it is an inversion of every value that Aristotle was at pains to establish in his ethics. Tyranny here is a technique consciously aimed at violating the individual at the very core of her ethical being, in her psyche.[13] The extroversion of the psyche is simultaneously its evacuation. Projected to the limit, the technical perfection of psychological terror entails its own obsolescence. With the equation (or rather, leveling) of inside and outside complete, there is nothing left to fear from the parrhesiastic discourse of subjugated subjects (whom Aristotle labels *antitechnoi* or "rivals in art" [1311a17]). There is literally nothing left to express. Thus does tyranny on the first model appear to run aground on itself, in this final evacuation of its subjects and of the system of visibility that embraces them, by condemning both, effectively, to irreality.

So much for the first policy, or *epimeleia* (the standard term for cultivation of any sort, especially—here, ironically—of the self [1314a32]), or rather, this first technique that is designed to eliminate all *antitechnoi*. We now turn to the second, which Aristotle describes as "the approximation of a king's rule"; it is literally a power play, for power must, he says, be preserved as a *hypothesis*:

This method can be deduced from a comparison with the seeds of destruction of kings. For, just as one way for a kingdom to fall is through its approximation to a tyranny, so is the salvation of a tyranny achievable through an approximation to a king's rule, provided one thing and one thing alone is safe-guarded: power, so that the tyrant's rule extends over both willing and unwilling subjects; for if he once gives this up, he gives up his tyranny. This thing (power) must be preserved as a *hypothesis*; but in all other respects the tyrant should either do those things a king does or appear to do them, by playing the part (*hypokrinomenos*) of a king and playing it well. (1314a32–40).

Here, then, is the alternative, or rather antithesis to the first course of action. Of the two, it is clearly the more insidious and more subversive technique of control. It rests on a decidedly nonclassical view of power, unlike the first, and is even uncannily like power under a postmodern description. Both techniques are ways of organizing and controlling a perceptual field. But whereas the first was a technique for bringing the civic body into focus as an object for supervision, and then of refracting and dispersing the source of the gaze beyond detection and verification, the second technique is the reverse of the first. The aim here is to constitute the civic body as the subject of the gaze, and then to disperse its focus, by training it on a dissimulated object. This reversed imaging creates a set of relations that might be termed a theatricality of power, as Aristotle's use of the term *hypothesis* suggests. A richly coded word, it means "policy," "assumption," "premise," and "foundation," but also the paraphrase of the action of a play, a summary of its "plot."

The two strategies or techniques are neatly, even dialectically, contrasted. The foundation of power on the second scenario resides in the manipulation of appearances, as opposed to the prior technique's erection of a manifest appearance of manipulation. To paraphrase Aristotle: "Appear (*dokein*) to be mindful of the commonweal, appear to be respectful and not harsh, create a climate not of fear but of respect, hide behind the machinery of justice, delegate its execution to others, be paternalistic, a guardian of the people; *practice* virtue, by concealing your vices, or by *actually performing virtuous actions*" (1314a40–1315b10). In almost perfect antithesis to the first set of instructions, the new list of imperatives reads:

In the first place [the tyrant] should pretend a care of the public revenues and not waste money [in lavish expenditures].... He should give an account of what he receives and what he spends.... In the second place he should be seen to collect taxes and to require public services only for state purposes ... and he ought to make himself the guardian and treasurer of them, as if they belonged, not to him, but to the public.... Neither he or any of his associates should ever appear guilty of the least offense against the young of either sex who are his subjects, and the women of his family should observe a like self-control toward other women.... He should observe moderation, shy from extravagance.... He ought to adorn and improve his city.... He should honor men of merit.... He should abstain from all outrage.... [And so] his power will be most lasting. (1314a40–1315b8)[14]

I have reproduced the positive injunctions only, deleting the sotto voce admonitions to "appear" that occur in most but not all of them, in order to extrapolate a logic that is inherent in Aristotle's account anyway: Aristotle seems to become mesmerized by the ethical import of what he is constructing, in the course of which the critical word *appear* elliptically drops out, like the mark of difference that a tyrant eliminates from his regime.

Such a logic, taken to the extreme, necessarily leads to a vicious paradox: when power constitutes itself in spectacle and theatricality, in the mimetic exchange of one form of rule for another, such that the exchange is complete and seamless, the author of the exchange becomes indistinguishable from his projected image. The differences between, say, the vicious man and the virtuous man he theatrically approximates to appear to extinguish themselves one by one with every act the vicious man undertakes. It is as if each virtuous act suffices to annul its own vicious premise. That this vicious-virtuous man has entered into a kind of ethical gray zone is apparent in the confused equivocation with which Aristotle pronounces his discussion of the issue closed: "And so, his disposition will be virtuous, or at least half-virtuous; and he will be not wicked, but half-wicked" (1315b8–10). Here it is not just a system of power that renders itself strangely inoperable, in a way that recalls the earlier account of tyrannical technique. Aristotle has landed himself in a bit of trouble, as his precarious distinctions indicate by themselves.

The terms "half-virtuous" (*hemichreston*) and "half-vicious" (*hemiponeron*) are unusual, to say the least. "Half-wicked" appears again only once elsewhere in Aristotle's corpus (*Nichomachean Ethics* 7.10 1152a17, in a discussion of moral weakness [*akrasia*]) and the two terms never reappear in any other Greek writer, with the exception of a commentator on the passage from the *Ethics*.[15] It is not hard to see why these words should be so rarely attested: the circumstances that require them are nothing short of remarkable. And yet it is odd that their use in the passage from the *Politics* should have drawn so little critical notice.[16] Has Aristotle forgotten the disguised "hypothesis" of theatrical power? Or has he rather fallen victim, like the tyrant's subjects, to the snares of this illusory construct, which eliminates, by assimilating to itself, all legible differences from virtue? Bending the light toward himself, the tyrant becomes the focal point of all antinomies as he completely assimilates and internalizes them in his person: a reflex image of the polity he governs, such a tyrant effectively destroys all oppositions, and hence all opposition. A literal monstrosity, he defies analysis.[17]

But the doubt runs deeper still: is it possible that this hypothetical construction, bursting as it does the seams of Aristotle's ethical theory, gives the lie to all his political and ethical theory? If a tyranny can pass for a kingship and ultimately evade cogent moral analysis, where does the contagion end?[18] Morality, the summum bonum, the end of politics: is all this perhaps the supple theatrical hypothesis which, in the course of long and conscientious habituation (rehearsing), has been forgotten and codified into philosophical truth—a truth that must be maintained at all costs, along with the constitutional form that is the social and political incorporation of its essence? If so, maintenance or salvation (*soteria*) must be understood in the full pregnancy of its implications: what must be preserved is not the structure but the facade, not the organization but its appearances, the surface of relations on which a state (or condition) constitutes itself and onto which it projects its regime, which is to say, its semiotic regimentation. The convergence of a theory with a politics, in a specular regime of knowledge and power, is striking.

Consider Aristotle's general prefatory remarks on the maintenance of states: "Constitutions can be preserved not only by maintaining a distance from corruptive influences, but sometimes by establishing a *proximity* [to them]" (*Pol.* 5.8 1308a24–26). Preservation thus consists in "making the distant near" (1308a30). This feat of reduction, which is sophistic in spirit, of eliminating distance and depth in an act of suppression, and of gathering all oppositions into immediate proximity and onto a surface plane, is a technical feat of physics and optics. It is a powerful kind of magnification, which enhances and thereby magnifies power itself.[19] The principle is, moreover, a vital requirement that holds generally for all forms of government: surveillance, the erection of a governmental organ—an eye—

designed specifically to monitor the movements on this surface, is Aristotle's recommendation to all forms of government: "It is necessary to establish a magistracy that might keep an eye (*archen epopsomenen*) on those whose life is not in harmony with the government" (5.8 1308b20–24). The subjects described are like objects formally ranged on a visual plane, stripped of all dimension and depth, save one. They are no longer citizens (*politai*), but *hoi zontes*, the biological constituents of the body politic. Technique is always a matter of matter.[20]

IV

Aristotle's theory in *Politics* Book 5 seems to be in flagrant contradiction with the opening thesis of Jürgen Habermas's *Theory and Praxis*: "Ancient political teaching was geared exclusively to *praxis*, in the narrow Greek sense. It had nothing in common with *techne*, the skillful production of artifacts and the mastery of objective tasks. The art of politics was ultimately aimed at the improvement of character; its method was pedagogical, not technical."[21] The decisive break with the classical notion of *praxis*, as Habermas understands it, occurred in the seventeenth century, when a confluence of physical mechanics and a rigorous, abstract methodology came about, these things lending themselves for the first time to an application in the sphere of political theory. Thomas Hobbes was perfectly situated to benefit from this historical accident. "For Hobbes, on the other hand, the maxim formulated by Bacon is already a commonplace: *scientia propter potentiam* (knowledge is for the sake of power). Mankind owes its greatest advances to technology, and above all to the political technology concerned with the proper management of the state."[22]

The passage Habermas selects to illustrate the essentials of Hobbes's modern sophistication is taken from the beginning of chapter 29 of *Leviathan*, entitled "Those Things That Weaken or Tend to the Destruction of a Commonwealth": "Though nothing can be immortal, which mortals make: yet, if men had the use of reason they pretend to, their Commonwealths might be secured, at least, from perishing by internal diseases.... Therefore when they come to be dissolved, not by external violence, but intestine disorder, the fault is not in men, as they are the *Matter*, but as they are the *Makers* and orderers of them." Habermas isolates in this citation three "moments" that mark an advance over the classical view: (1) Hobbes's analysis seeks, independent of place, time, or circumstances, to determine how the life span of a commonwealth might be extended; (2) the application and transfer of knowledge is a technical problem based on rules not of conduct but of relations and apparatuses (the general, scientific nature of these considerations obviates an application of the classical model of prudential virtue [*phronesis*]); (3) Hobbes's social engineer, calibrators in hand, can accordingly dispense with ethical categories and approach his problem as though it were a natural object. Man becomes material for organization. No longer considered an ethical being, he is a social being caught in a network of social relations.

There are, of necessity, huge differences between two political theories separated by two millennia. But at the same time there are two issues that ought to be kept distinct. The first is the relation between moral and political theory in a classical Aristotle and a modern-age Hobbes; the second is the question of theory and practice: of a mode of praxis that evidently is not guided by an objectifying theory in the case of Aristotle; of a schema and its application or technical implementation in the case of Hobbes. And although a revolutionary change did in all likelihood occur with regard to the first point (political theory is, ideally, an ethical theory for Aristotle), there is no compelling reason to concede the claims made with regard to the second point as a consequence of the first. Moral pedagogy plainly does not rule out technique; in fact, it demands it. But is Aristotelian political theory captured by so innocent a term as *pedagogy*?[23] Moreover, if ethical theory implies political theory for Aristotle, the opposite is not obviously the case: the sophistic elements—or is it just realism?—that Aristotle assimilates in his thinking generally lead him to a reassessment of the kinds of claims that ethical thinking can make on political theory, that is, to a more pragmatic and functionalist analysis: the virtue of a good citizen and that of a good man do not always coincide; in fact, they rarely do, except in the case of "complete" or "perfect" virtue, which we find realized in the ideal state, a limiting case.[24]

A reading of Aristotle more sensitive to the implications of politics (*politike*) as a theory of technique (*techne*) would provide a more nuanced, and more realistic, view of the *Politics*. (This would be to bring out the recessed nuance of the term itself: in Greek, "politics" is an ellipsis for "the *techne* of politics.") It would also help account for what would otherwise persist as an insoluble puzzle: How can Aristotle's theory of political organization produce a theory of power in which power is to be viewed as a theatrical technique? What are the genetic links between the analysis of the norm and the unanalyzable aberration? And finally, how could Aristotle, within the closed framework of his theory, produce the concept of a technique for ordering the perceptual field, the technology for which would be brought frighteningly close to perfection only in our own day? And why has this profound discovery by Aristotle of a political potentiality been overlooked? These are questions that an investigation into normative purity will never be able to pose.

There may be no clear answer to these questions, but this should not be counted a loss. It is hoped that the specific analysis of the visual syntagm (it is surely more than a trope) in Aristotle has thrown not just some light, but some obscurity, on our understanding of the workings of his philosophical method and discourse, with implications for other theaters of philosophical discourse. The visual and the discursive do intersect, possibly more often than we might wish to acknowledge, though when they do, their result is anything but the kind of clarity one is accustomed to find in the context of the visual. Clarity is a desideratum that had been manipulated by philosophers long before René Descartes's own demands for thinking *clare et distincte*. As Theodor Adorno reminds us in a brilliant essay on G. W. F. Hegel's style, clarity is a demand that no language and no thinking can possibly or validly fulfill.[25] One could say that clarity is a metaphor or else just an ideal. I would prefer to say that clarity is an effect of discourse, and so too a reflection of any given discourse's self-imposed shadows.

Acknowledgments

This chapter is a slightly revised version of a paper presented at a seminar on *parrhesia* taught by Michel Foucault at the University of California at Berkeley in 1983. I wish to dedicate it to his memory. A shorter version was read at the Philological Association of the Pacific Coast in 1985 (and, in a different form, at the Ninth Triennial Meeting of the American Comparative Literature Association at the University of Michigan in 1986), and subsequently appeared in *Pacific Coast Philology* 21, nos. 1–2 (1986):20–24. I thank the following for their comments at the time: Daniel Brewer, Alina Clej, Eric Downing, Michel Foucault, Dalia Judovitz, G. E. R. Lloyd, and Thomas Rosenmeyer. Thanks also go to David Levin for expressing an interest in exhuming the paper for this book and for his encouragement along the way toward its publication.

Notes

1. Paul de Man, "The Epistemology of Metaphor," *Critical Inquiry* 5, no. 1 (1978):11.

2. See further J. I. Porter, *Nietzsche's Atoms* (Stanford: Stanford University Press, forthcoming). For the view that rhetoricity is primarily a function of discursive strategies and of voice in the classical sense, rather than a formal property of language, see "Nietzsche's Rhetoric: Theory and Strategy," *Philosophy and Rhetoric* 27, no. 3 (1994):218–244.

3. See G. E. R. Lloyd *Demystifying Mentalities* (Cambridge: Cambridge University Press, 1990), on the notion of styles of competing inquiry in classical antiquity, conceived by way of a view about the sociology of knowledge (esp. chap. 1, and, e.g. p. 59 on Aristotle); and compare Nietzsche, "Homers Wettkampf" (Homer's Contest), in *Friedrich Nietzsche: Kritische Studienausgabe*, ed. G. Colli and M. Montinari, (Berlin and New York: Walter de Gruyter, 1988) 1:783–792. Criteria of self-evidence as (frequently transparent) markers of competing discourses deserve to be considered in this connection.

4. Henceforth to be cited as *Pol.* Translations of this work are mine, unless otherwise indicated.

5. For a nearly exhaustive survey of ocularcentrism and its enemies, see Martin Jay, *Downcast Eyes: The Denigration of Vision in Twentieth-Century French Thought* (Berkeley and Los Angeles: University of California Press, 1993). On Aristotle's place in the Greek ocularcentric tradition, see e.g., ibid., p. 28. Establishing ocularcentrism in any given case is a relatively (and possibly all too) easy matter; assessing its implications, or its various decenterings, is not.

6. Neither Aristotelian *phantasia* nor our own, more restricted concept of imagination (for this contrast, see Malcolm Schofield, "Aristotle on the Imagination," in G. E. R. Lloyd and G. E. L. Owen, eds., *Aristotle on Mind and the Senses,*

James I. Porter

Proceedings of the Seventh Symposium Aristotelicum [Cambridge: Cambridge University Press, 1978] pp. 99–140) corresponds to the psychoanalytic concept of the imaginary, which would be the more useful notion to invoke in the discussion to follow (though I have not chosen to do so myself, except in passing or by implication).

7. The proposed method is one of analysis, of breaking wholes down into their constituent parts: "And if we *inspect* the parts from which the *polis* is composed we shall *see* all the more [clearly], in this case, how states differ from one another" (ibid., 1252a20–23). Remarkably, within the first twenty-six lines of the *Politics* alone, Aristotle deploys six different verbs of seeing.

8. *The Basic Works of Aristotle*, ed. Richard McKeon (New York: Random House, 1941), p. 689 (here, the translation by W. D. Ross). Translations from the *Metaphysics* are from this source.

9. Cf. H. Bonitz, *Index Aristotelicus*, 2d ed. (Graz: Akademische Druck u. Verlagsanstalt, 1955), s.v. *episteme*: "*epistime et techne quomodo et distinguantur et inter se confundantur.*"

10. Cf. also Plato, *Statesman* 259e–60e, for the architect as a metaphor and model of theoretical competence in charge of less knowledgeable subordinates; and Aristotle, *Metaphysics* 1.1 982b25–28 (to be quoted below).

11. Cf. Aristotle, *Physics* 3.1.

12. The reference is to Cypselus and his son Periander, tyrants of Corinth in the late seventh to early sixth centuries.

13. Cf. the paramount value attached to *megalopsychia* in the *Nichomachean Ethics* (4.3). In contemporary Greek thought, psychic impairment is abhorred as a vital diminishment of individual capacity (cf. Plato, *Laws* 832C).

14. Trans. Benjamin Jowett in *Basic Works of Aristotle*, pp. 1259–1262.

15. The anonymous commentator on Aristotle's *Nichomachean Ethics* cites only the term that appears in the *Ethics*. Plato uses *hemimoctheros* ("half-wicked") as a contrast to *pamponeros* ("wholly wicked") in Book 1 of the *Republic* (352c). *Hemimoctheros* enjoys an afterlife only among late antique authors.

16. For example, the passage receives passing, untroubled comment from Sir Ernest Barker, *The Politics of Aristotle* (Oxford: Clarendon Press, 1948) p. 247n1: "In the following sections Aristotle anticipates the character of Machiavelli, and gives 'politic' advice to a 'new prince' in a realistic way. But his advice is fundamentally different from that of Machiavelli. He bids the new prince abjure 'reason of State,' and play the king—and the man." Much as one might wish to be able to save Aristotle from himself here, he has created something of a moral puzzle. When virtue is performed with vicious intent, how do we characterize the agent of the performance? Aristotle's equivocal response points to the insolubility of the dilemma. I doubt, moreover, that he can be saved even if the moral or objective of his theoretical fiction is heightened vigilance on the part of suspecting citizens. So great is the degree of deception involved on Aristotle's con-

struction that the increase in vigilance required could only lead to a state of paranoia.

17. This paradox is far more pernicious than the problem of discovering criteria for evaluating moral conduct in the absence of any privileged access to intentional states, a difficulty Aristotle recognized, to be sure. Cf. *Eudemian Ethics* 2.11 1228a15–17: "Since it is no simple thing to see [an agent's mental act as he makes] a choice and of what sort it is, we are constrained to judge the quality of the agent from his deeds"; ibid., 1228a13–14: "even though the doing is preferable to (the possession of) virtue." Greek ethical thinking was aware of the efficacy, and risks, of the mere semblance of virtue long before Aristotle (Democritus fr. 39 Diels-Kranz: "one should either be virtuous, or simulate it"; Plato, *Sophist* 267c). But to my knowledge, the logic of ethical appearances is nowhere more consequentially and spectrally drawn than in the present passage from Aristotle.

18. That it could spread to democracy is confirmed by Plato's condemnation of the manipulation of public opinion and the fashioning of political images, as in *Gorgias* 517a–19d.

19. A similar tendency is exhibited in the *Rhetoric*, where Aristotle instructs aspiring orators in the art of dissembling their characters (1.9, 1366a23–32, and 2.1, 1377b20–1378a5). The art of making far things appear nearer than they are and other forms of optical illusion resemble a characteristically sophistic trick. Cf. Plato, *Phaedrus* 267a, *Sophist* 235e–36b; Aristotle, *Rhetoric* 3.12 1414a8; *Dissoi Logoi* D.-K. 90.3; ps.-Longinus, *On the Sublime* 17.3. In *Metaphysics* 1.2, Aristotle states that the universal is "the farthest from the senses" (982a25): metaphysics, too, consists in making the far appear near.

20. We are also now better equipped to understand Aristotle's famous caveat about looking for exactitude in the human sciences: "Things moral and just, which are the purview of the art of politics, are susceptible of so much variety and flux that these things appear entirely a matter of human convention and law, but not of nature" (*Nichomachean Ethics* 1.3 1094b14–16). It is precisely this imprecision, this hazardous elusiveness, that we are concerned with, the migration of moral terms, their malleability: "half-good," "half-evil": *beltion to kinein*, "motion is better" (*Pol.* 2.8 1268b33–34, with reference to constitutional changes).

21. Jürgen Habermas, *Theory and Praxis*, trans. John Viertel (Boston: Beacon Press, 1973), p. 42; trans. modified.

22. Ibid.

23. Hobbes's focus on "commonwealth," "security," and "perishing" or "destruction," and his view of the "architect" of the state, the framer of laws and orderer of polities, suggests that he may have had more than a casual familiarity with Aristotle's own work on politics.

24. Cf. *Nicomachean Ethics* 10.8 1178a34–b32; *Eudemean Ethics* 2.11 1228a12–17; *Rhetoric* 1.13 1374b13–14.

25. Theodor Adorno, "Skoteinos or How to Read Hegel," in *Hegel: Three Studies*, trans. Shierry Weber Nicholsen (Cambridge: MIT Press, 1993), pp. 89–148.

3

Discourses of Vision in Seventeenth-Century Metaphysics

Catherine Wilson

In Nicole Malebranche's *Dialogues on Metaphysics* of 1688, Malebranche's spokesman, Theodore, draws his interlocutor, Aristes, into his cabinet or closet in order to retreat from "those enchanted places which beguile our senses and which are too distracting in their variety."[1] They pull the curtains after them to dim the light; but after some discussion, Theodore decides against closing up the little room altogether and sitting in pitch blackness, for this maneuver would not produce the state of indifference to the sensory environment they are seeking but anxiety: "some disquiet or slight alarm in our senses."[2] The condition of philosophical reflection is a place in which the two men are neither subject to the solicitations of the illuminated world, in which objects appear in all their distracting variety, nor plunged into the night world of unseen dangers. Inner illumination demands a dimming but not an extinguishing of the ambient light.

Malebranche's philosophical works are replete with references to optics and the physiology of vision, to eyes, mirrors, and magnifying lenses, to illusions and visual deceptions. The dominance of the theory of vision in seventeenth-century epistemology has often been remarked on and associated with the new technologies and practices of observation, especially those involving the telescope and the microscope. René Descartes studied the anatomy of the eye and wrote essays on light, geometrical optics, and the design and fabrication of optical instruments. Malebranche continued work on optical theory and the psychology of vision; Spinoza, as everyone knows, ground lenses; and Leibniz poured praise on the microscope and its revelation of the ubiquity of living forms and said that the real basic constituents of the world were not inanimate particles but "living mirrors," which collected images from every part of the universe. It is in the so-called rationalist philosophers that we find the fullest exploitation of empirical theories of vision, an awareness of the curious effects of perspective, and the ubiquity of illusion, and the most strenuous use of illuminationist metaphors for the acquisition of knowledge. Across the channel, early modern empiricists like John Locke, contrary to what one might expect, have as little use for the puzzles and problems of the appearance-reality distinction that optics generates as they do for the notion of an "inner light," so determined are they to make experience, and experience alone, the source of our knowledge. Empiricism treats vision in a welcoming but on the whole rather uncritical and even unempirical spirit. The contrasting richness of rationalist discourses of vision is a function of the essentially redemptive aspirations of metaphysics, which is dedicated to showing the miraculous under the ordinary, the whole in place of its fragments.

The "oculocentrism" of the period has thus deservedly attracted attention. Yet caution is called for in positing anything like a "scopic regime," a particular coercive discourse of visuality in the seventeenth century, for within the rationalist text itself there are retreats and rebellions, exceptions and redescriptions, which threaten what has been termed "Cartesian perspectivalism."[3] I first describe three received theses about visual experience and its meaning in seventeenth-century metaphysics and then go on to evaluate them. These theses concern the *logic*, the *morality*, and the politics of *vision*:

Thesis 1: *The Logic of Vision*
The camera obscura provided a fundamentally misleading model for vision, in which the mind served as a private, inner theater

into which copies of the external scene were projected. As a result, philosophers have tended since the seventeenth century to conceive knowledge erroneously as the inner screening of reality-matching representations.

Thesis 2: *The Morality of Vision*
Seventeenth-century rationalist discourse is marked by a Platonic-Augustinian effort to transcend and repudiate embodiment, first by privileging the sense of sight over that of the senses that depend on immediate contact, second by privileging intellectual vision over corporeal vision.

Thesis 3: *The Politics of Vision*
The attempt by metaphysicians to describe God's surveillance of the world or the world itself *sub specie aeternitatis* models the absolute state that possesses all information and is therefore capable of exercising all power through well-organized, bureaucratic modes of terror rather than arbitrary feudal terror.

The seventeenth century's engagement with visuality is thus regarded not only as having produced scientifically important discoveries in optics and the theory of light, the anatomy and psychology of vision, and as having exploited its discoveries to gain new knowledge of the microworld and the distant cosmos. It is suspected of having given philosophical and scientific authority to erroneous and coercive epistemologies and encouraging the development of the injustices and malaises of modernity, from the bourgeois cult of inwardness and domestic repression, to totalitarian politics. In what follows, I discuss these prefigurings but also show how they are threatened from within the texts in which they occur by second thoughts and counterproposals. Discourses that contradict and compensate for one another, now valorizing desire and visual engagement, now evincing a kind of Augustinian disgust, play through the pages of a single text. Insofar as they are conceived as determining or validating, the three theses stated above represent a selection from the available metaphors and models suggested by rationalist theory of vision, a selection dictated both by intervening needs or apparent needs, and by contemporary unrests and dissatisfactions that arise in reflecting on those needs.

The Logic of Vision

The medieval theory of species posited the emission of immaterial visual forms or "species" from material objects that were transmitted to the subject and "received" by the eye and finally the *sensus communis.* This metaphysical theory coexisted with an optical theory with which it was not integrated (thanks to the scholastic doctrine of the separate sciences, which took mathematical representation to have no necessary connection with physical or metaphysical reality). The optical theory made use of a visual pyramid with its apex at the eye and posited the extromission of light from it, spreading out to form a cone of the visible. With Johannes Kepler's reanalysis in the *Paralipomena* of 1604, this scheme is inverted. The apex of a pyramid is now situated at every point on a visual object: light rays are reflected off each point at angles corresponding to the angle of incidence, and the array is then focused by the lens of the eye.[4] The subject does not generate visibility by opening and turning his eyes; his consciousness brings a visible world into being by interrupting, as it were, the passage of light waves reflected off surfaces that themselves are invisible. In Kepler's scheme, light and dark are associated with action and passion: light arrives from outside and "paints" on the retina, ray by ray, as on a wall or screen, a picture of the external scene.

Anatomy and mathematics were first conjoined in this account. And in the wake of Kepler's discoveries, it is a subject of controversy how far the camera obscura, which projects just such an image on a dark wall or curtain behind a small hole, furnished and continues to furnish a model for vision. Richard Rorty in particular has argued that seventeenth-century epistemology is based on the mistaken idea that the true image of the world is a perfect copy of it, received into the subject's mind or inner *camera.*[5] This copy theory is not only philosophically confused, leading us to suppose that there can be a match between a theory—a collection of statements—and some segment of the world, but morally pernicious in its sanctification of "truth" and its rejection of the possibility of multiple rival accounts. Locke is certainly compelled by the analogy when he says, "The understanding is not much unlike a closet wholly shut up from light, with some little openings left, to let in external visible images."[6] And Leibniz, in his *New Essays*, generally endorses this description while suggesting that the "screen" at the back is not flat, taut, and uniform but "diversified by folds representing innate knowledge" and, under tension, with "a kind of elasticity or active force."[7] Now Kepler himself denies that the processes of projection are similar (as the camera obscura uses a pinhole, the eye a lens), while allowing nevertheless that an inverted image is projected onto the back of the eye, and Descartes says clearly that image is not what we see. There are no species flitting through the air, and the "picture" on the retina is not an intermediate object of vision but formed adventitiously. The mind constructs what we call a visual image from pressures and motions in the brain. Seeing is not seeing but a kind of touch.[8]

Yet the metaphor has its power and its uses. Fascinated by his own image of the tense, gently oscillating folds of the mind's curtain, even Leibniz is willing to tolerate talk of species.[9] And by meditating on the cameral aspect of the camera obscura model, rather than thinking of the eye as the inlet for light and the means by which we remain in contact with the world, one can generate the Cartesian subject's privacy and interiority—and catch a glimpse, on the temporal horizon, of the snugness of the bourgeois domestic interior with its confinements and family secrets and its strict separation of private and public life. The camera obscura, says Jonathan Crary, "is a figure for the observer who is nominally a free sovereign individual but who is also a privatized isolated subject enclosed in a quasi-domestic space separated from a public exterior world.... The monadic viewpoint of the individual is legitimized by the *camera obscura*, but his or her sensory experience is subordinated to an external and pre-given world of objective truth."[10]

On the horizon as well is aestheticism, with its professed lack of interest in screening a copy of the world, for the notion of the mind as an inner theater also emphasizes the roles of fancy and imagination—the freedom to inscene and enact in the inner theater what one wishes. And the attraction to the new space of possibilities and gratifications opened up by the camera metaphor remains in fundamental contradiction to the official teaching. Both Descartes and the Locke, along with Malebranche, Leibniz, and a host of others, believe that the sensory world we experience is wholly different from the material world that gives rise to it, our perceptions do not mirror nature at all. The visual mechanisms, processes, and results are explicitly held by seventeenth-century theorists of the visual who reject visual species theory to be disanalogous to this kind of copying from exterior to interior. But it is not until the mature physiology of the nineteenth century that the "internal" place of the mind is finally collapsed, that "inside the head" is finally dissociated from "inside the mind," and it comes to seem conceivable that the human brain might be removed from its enclosure and rolled out as flat as a pancake and still perceive, dream, fantasize, and think. As Crary notes, "The body which had been a neutral or invisible term in vision now was the thickness from which knowledge of vision was derived."[11]

The Morality of Seeing

"Bodies are not strictly speaking," says Descartes, denying what everyone appreciates to be the case to speak in the higher language of philosophy, "perceived by the senses at all, but only by the intellect."[12] What is the significance of this avoidance or denial, this splitting in rationalist visual discourse? Is it not the case that metaphysics, especially rationalist metaphysics, is informed through and through by a Platonist-Augustinian *horror materialis*, which translates into a *horror naturae* or even a *horror feminae*, that its accomplishment is the escapist one of constructing, in the isolation of a darkened closet, an orderly substitute for our disorderly world, an imaginary universe in which intellectual values reign supreme and the objects that form the focus of our desires in the material world are illusions and nonbeing?[13] This antimaterialist, immortalist motive is arguably that behind rationalist metaphysics: to make matter unreal is one of Leibniz's principal aims in his early as well as his late writings. For if matter is allowed to exist in the very obviousness of existing, why do we not, with the same obviousness, go out of existence like every other individual thing, going up in smoke, or getting crushed to powder, or just slowly disintegrating into atoms? Such projects never come to completion. As Friedrich von Schiller says, when a philosophical system is trying to exclude something essential, that thing will keep breaking in on it, ruining the effort and creating problems and inconsistencies.

One manifestation of this anxiety about matter and mortalism and its confusing consequences is the pervasive indecision in seventeenth-century metaphysics about whether one could have visual experiences without having a body and whether a separated soul would feel and experience as we do. This problem is brought to a focus by the Cartesian meditative exercise, which seems to reveal that all my experiences might be exactly as they are now even if I did not possess a body and sensory organs, and even if there were no physical interaction between my body and a world of external objects independent of me. Descartes establishes that this is so in his *First Meditation,* in which it is pointed out that the hallucinated world produced by an omnipotent genius is an exact experiential replica of the visual world produced by interaction with physical objects and that sensory experience neither presupposes nor provides any direct evidence for the existence of a human body or any other bodies around it.[14] But Descartes also enunciates two propositions seemingly incompatible with the thesis that sensory experience does not imply or provide evidence for the existence of a body: that "feeling" depends on the body[15] and that "the human mind separated from the body does not have sensation strictly so called."[16] Now one might resolve this conflict by saying that, given that a nondeceiving God exists and that I know him to exist, sensory experience does in fact imply and provide evidence

Catherine Wilson

of a body (mine) and bodies (causally interacting with mine). But if sensory experience implies that I have an actual body, not merely the sensory experience *of* a body, what of the famous claim for the separability and immortality of the soul? Descartes, who perhaps is a mortalist and whose interest in this problem is accordingly far from genuine, leans toward the doctrine that in the afterlife I will indulge only in pure thought without having sensory experience, whose purpose after all is only to preserve the body during its earthly existence.[17] Then an omnipotent God could give my disembodied soul sensory experiences and refrains or would refrain from doing so in the afterlife only insofar as he does not wish to deceive me, and the inference from my experiences, feelings, and sensations to the existence of my body and other bodies does not involve the logic of those concepts alone. Descartes's conclusion at the end of his *Meditations* is that he has established the logical independence of the soul and body and, thanks to God, their empirical dependence, their intimate union.

It is not often remarked that Descartes's hyperbolic doubt, leading to the conclusion that mind and body are essentially distinct, rests on the possibility of visual illusion, dreaming, and hallucination, cases in which I seem to see—a man, in a dressing gown, seated by a fire, holding a paper—but no such thing is causing my perception. "The visions which comes to us in sleep are like paintings."[18] By contrast, Descartes is thoroughly "somatic" in his last work, *The Passions of the Soul*, intended to show the union of the soul and body, a union that, Descartes explained to Princess Elizabeth, could be shown only experientially and not metaphysically.[19] Now, logically, there is no reason that Descartes's skeptical arguments, which lead to the absolute distinction of soul and body, should not be framed in terms of nonvisual sensory modes, by reference to the possibility of aural and tactile hallucinations. Yet as a highly visual species, we have dreams that are predominantly visual; our visual sense is so differentiated and our aesthetic impulses are so keyed to the production of visual replicas that the possibility of exact sensory replication turns quite naturally on the sense of sight. And what Crary calls the "opacity or carnal density" of the visual observer was only partially internalized into seventeenth-century knowledge.

We should expect, accordingly, that philosophers who took exception to the soul-body dualism of Descartes's *Meditations*, would, like the later Descartes himself, turn their attention away from the visual sense in order to express beliefs about the unity of soul and body. This is the case with Leibniz, who rejects Cartesian dualism, maintaining that all souls, with the single exception of God's, are embodied at every stage of this life and beyond, and who rejects Descartes's withholding of sensory experience from animals and "lower" beings in general. The Leibnizian text is replete with references to somatic perception: dizziness, unease, pleasure, sleepiness. His attention is particularly held by a category of experiences, which he calls *petites perceptions*, which, he says explicitly, "come from the body."[20] These perceptions, predictably again, are construed in the first instance as tactual, not as visual:

There are hundreds of indications leading us to conclude that at every moment there is in us an infinity of perceptions unaccompanied by awareness or reflection ... of which we are unaware because these impressions are either too minute and too numerous, or else too unvarying, so that they are not sufficiently distinctive on their own....

These minute perceptions ... are more effective in their results than has been recognized. They constitute that *je ne sais quoi*, those flavours, those images of sensible qualities, vivid in the aggregate but confused in the parts; those impressions which are made on us by the bodies around us which involve the infinite; that connection each being has with the rest of the universe.[21]

The world has accordingly a two-tiered structure in which the clarity of the qualities we experience (green, crash) is the result of the confusion and multiplicity of the singly undetectable. The Cartesian project of making the maximum number of distinctions is thus frustrated, for there are some qualities that cannot be grasped both clearly and distinctly, and to comprehend the sensory phenomenon intellectually is to lose it from view. Qualities emerge as the summation of their forebears reaches a certain threshold at which point sensory novelty enters the world.

The Leibnizian soul is never without sensation "for it always expresses its body, and this body is always affected in infinitely many ways by surrounding things, though often they provide only a confused impression."[22] Note here the repeated avoidance of the optical: the unconscious is not a repository of faint images but of tiny somatic inclinations and repulsions. As Deleuze expresses it, the world is "a lapping of waves, a rumour, a fog, or a mass of dancing particles of dust. It is a state of death or catalepsy, of sleep, drowsiness or numbness."[23]

But to what extent does the rationalist text accept embodiment and materiality, let alone endorse it? "I find everything I see in this sensible material world distasteful now that I have heard you," says Aristes to Theodore in Malebranche's *Dialogues*, evoking the Augustinian disgust of the *Confessions*, Book 10. Sensory experience is only "for the sinner to preserve for a while his wretched life and perpetuate the human species until the accomplishment of the work which posterity is to enter into."[24] Here sensory experience appears in its morally problematic linkage with desire, both assigned, rather resignedly, a function, if not a value. Yet the system must move around and adapt. The withdrawal into the philosopher's cabinet turns out to be not only an act of repulsion and retreat into intellection but a generous outpouring of sanctification toward the visible and tangible. For first Theodore "proves"—we are dealing here with another central text of rationalist philosophy—in the course of a few pages that the room the speakers are in is not "strictly speaking" visible and that it is not really the room they see when they look at it (since God could have destroyed the room without altering what was seen). Having made this absurdity—the visible is actually invisible!—convincing, Theodore proceeds to rehabilitate sight. "The beauties we see," he explains, "are not material beauties but intelligible beauties rendered sensible."[25] From the initial position and its allied recommendations—shut the doors and windows, flee sensory experience, engage in thought-experiment—the dialectic inverts the old order of values by revealing what we admire and love to be intelligible beauty. What we look at is variable and corruptible, but what we see is immutable, eternal, necessary.[26] Where the static, irresolvable-except-through-faith Augustinian ambivalence ends in despair, disgust, and conversion—but also in reminiscence, and the substitution of the description, the written word of the confession, for the thing itself—we have here a surprise ending, an idea elegantly converted into its opposite. This ploy reaches parodic heights in the *Fourth Dialogue*, in which at first the pleasure in describing is perfectly balanced against the "official" value assigned to that described. "How unworthy sensible goods are! How powerless bodies appear to me to be! No, this sun, brilliant as it appears to my eyes, does not possess nor spread the light which enlightens me. The colours which beguile me in their variety and vivacity, the beauties which charm me when I turn my eyes on what surrounds me, all of this belongs to me."[27]

But now the solution to the problem of visual beguilement is given in philosophical terms. The solution consists in denying that it is something other that exerts this power over me: it is I myself. And the troubling solicitations of the visual can be further redeemed by physico-theology. "What excuse can I make for myself," Augustine asks, "when often, as I sit at home, I cannot turn my eyes from the sight of a lizard catching flies or a spider entangling them as they fly into her web?"[28] Augustine's own answer is that there is no excuse; the irresistible desire to recount and therefore to relive the experience is corrected by the frame of regret and remorse of the confessional mode. Another solution is to recount an entirely different story, to go into a dark room, polemicize against the superficial and confused knowledge of the senses, to realize your blindness,[29] to make yourself blind.[30] But there is no lack of encouragement in continental metaphysics to go through the world with open eyes, drinking everything in, so long as it is stated that it is we who produce these splendors and that we are seeing God everywhere. "As for the magnificence of his work," says Theodore in the *Tenth Dialogue*, "it bursts out in every way. From whatever side we cast our eyes on the Universe, we see a profusion of prodigies in it.... What animals, what birds, what insects, what plants, what flowers, and what fruit!"[31] In place of a general hostility to the concupiscent gaze in the rationalist tradition, a hostility with implications for the problems of alienation and distance of the modern, we have an attempt, appropriate in a new scientific age, to break free of Augustinian inhibition. Malebranche's dimmed cabinet, like Descartes's hyperbolic doubt, is a temporary, though always available, retreat.

The forgetting, erasure, or exclusion of the physical body in the rationalist text is thus balanced by awareness and acknowledgment of the physicality of perception and experience. I shall illustrate this by another example. The Cartesian method of analysis can be seen in the procedure by which the celebrated conceptual distinction between mind and body is arrived at. By attentively considering what belongs to the concept of mind, one discovers that it is conceptually distinct from the body. The mental representation of one need not include the other. An intellectual, sense-abstracted process is performed that gives, as its self-reinforcing result, the absolute distinctness of mind and body. Some commentators are quick to see here not any kind of discovery but merely the playing out of a repetitive stipulation against the involvement of the body in knowledge, a performance that reveals the essential circularity and futility of metaphysics. But this is an incorrect interpretation, for the discourse of perceptual and conceptual "distinctness" crisscrosses constantly. There is no consistent appeal to a pure intellectualism that forgets the physical nature of seeing and distinguishing. For first, the seeing and distinguishing of visual objects is the ultimate aim of a priori reflection. Cartesian method and mathematics are implicated in the development of theoretical optics, the purpose of which is ultimately, as the later sections of his *Optics* make clear, to construct magnifying equipment for resolving and observing the smaller parts of animals, for use in furthering empirical science. Conversely, Descartes can recommend physical practice as training for intellectual tasks: "Craftsmen who engage in delicate operations, and are used to fixing their eyes on a single point, acquire through practice the ability to make perfect distinctions between things, however minute and delicate."[32] He even recommends illiberal handicrafts like rug-making and embroidery, "the occupations of women," and puzzles as preparation for mental work. Thus the discourse of pure intellectuality is implicated in various ways as well as opposed to the discourse of embodiment and tactual manipulation, in which even the feminine is accorded respect.

The Politics of Seeing

I have mentioned the influential analysis of visual processes given by Johannes Kepler. One accompaniment of this portrayal of perception as a passive rather than an active process is that, in epistemological discourse, an active mind or intellectual faculty takes up many of the metaphors with which vision was formerly dressed. The mind rather than the eye is portrayed as a searchlight, a source of illumination, which can be turned and held steadily on material, which is thereby made perspicuous. The discussion of "mental vision," which he construes as a trainable faculty, in Descartes's *Rules for the Direction of the Mind* contrasts with the analysis of vision as a process of passive imprinting in which an impression is made like that of a seal in wax.[33] But if the vision of the eye is passive, that of the mind is active. "The whole method consists entirely in ordering and arranging the objects on which we must concentrate our mind's eye if we are to discover some truth."[34] Inference is a movement from the beginning of a proof to the end, which relies on the clear perception of each segment, for "our eyes cannot distinguish at one glance all the links in a very long chain, but, if we have seen the connections between each link and its neighbor, this enables us to say that we have seen how the last link is connected with the first."[35] The metaphor of the active and radiant intellectual eye is developed in various ways. Human wisdom is said to be like the sunlight;[36] we bear within us a "spark" of the divine.[37]

This irradiating intellect is not particularly new. "The understanding is the candle of the Lord" as the Bible has it, or, as Ralph Culverwell glosses it in his *Spiritual Opticks*, "God hath set up a distinct Lamp in every soul, that men might make use of their own light."[38] The problem of the origins of this "light"

Catherine Wilson

and its relation to the divine understanding are discussed in the theological literature, in which the feeble light of nature in us and the powerful light of grace that reaches us from outside are contrasted, or in which the light of nature, reinterpreted as reason, is held sufficient for both religious and secular purposes, or in which the experience of inner illumination is castigated as hallucinatory and dangerous.[39] This occurs in an age in which the physical properties of light—its speed, for example, its behavior at the interface of various media, its wave-nature—are rapidly becoming understood. Now it might be said that the same scientific confidence that produces and reacts to its own production of the analysis of light and vision as produced by *invisibilia* acting by physical pressure must find old metaphors to describe its experience of itself; that the rejection of authority associated with these new analyses of vision and new technologies of vision (e.g., the Galilean telescope) demands a new epistemology based on individual capacity; and, finally, that when an intuitively satisfying phenomenologically based account of experience, like the doctrine of visual rays and the visual power of the eye, is shown to be "incorrect" through its replacement with a scientific account, one expects to find the beloved metaphor of the active subject transferred to a realm safe from the incursions of science: metaphysics.

The visual sweep and the stare come into play in the mathematical and observational sciences, respectively. Descartes says that we confirm a lengthy deduction by seeing the relationship of each step to that next to it and then taking in the whole at a glance. Lacking a formal notion of proof, Descartes treats validity as a matter of visual order tied to subjective certitude.[40] Or—another moment in the evolution of modern science—the observer stares fixedly at a thing that has been brought into focus with a telescope or a microscope. If the notion of intellectual mastery was taken by the older historiography of science at face value, with newly acquired methodological and factual competence conceived as setting in order or suppressing the confusion and error of Renaissance superstition, it has taken on, in a postcolonial era, additional connotations. Visual ordering has more recently been interpreted—thanks to the work of Michel Foucault—as an expression of political will, which reveals itself in the modern trend toward definition, containment, separation, policing, and the distancing of self from other.[41] The marshaling and classification of ideas and their presentation in tables, the sorting out of erroneous from true representations, the policing of opinions through the development of formal scientific protocols, the segregation and surveillance of the sick, the bad, the deviant, have been regarded as a sort of colonialism whose aims are no more rational and ultimately as arbitrary as every other form of conquest and domination. Thus the visual metaphors in seventeenth-century epistemology can be seen in two complementary ways: as part of the construction of the new "private" or cameral subject, defined as one possessing moral and epistemological autonomy and deserving of political self-determination, and as part of the construction of a repressive absolute state, with its categories and coercions, rising up, as it were, as a rational creation of this new subject and meeting and enclosing him.

Nowhere else is the optical-hierarchical model of surveillance more exactly portrayed than in Leibniz's description of the monadological kingdom of spirits. Other metaphysicians of the period make the basic furniture of the world inanimate particles, atoms or corpuscles, and separate and separable minds: Leibniz makes them living, perceptive, striving "monads," which exist in a well-regulated, hierarchically organized, deterministic society. I next consider the puzzling occurrence in Leibniz of two discourses of perceptual experience. We have already noted the empirical-psychological discourse of the unintegrated somatic subject with its inner regions and zones of permanent unclarity and obscurity, who experiences the world "confusedly" in various senses. The other Leibnizian subject is the immaterial subject of a metaphysical theory, formal-geometrical perspectivalism. These discourses are related only through the doctrine of "confused omniscience" and the insistence that perception is always situational.

"*Monads*," Leibniz says, speaking in the second mode, "having no parts, can neither be formed nor unmade.... They cannot have shapes, for then they would have parts. It follows that one monad by itself and at a single moment cannot be distinguished from another except by its internal qualities and actions, and these can only be its *perceptions* ... and its appetitions; and these modifications must consist of the variety of relations of correspondence which the subject has with things outside. In the same way there may be found, in one *center* or point, though it is perfectly simple, an infinity of angles formed by the lines which meet in it."[42]

Monadic subjects have each a nonspatial site, which determines their perceptual experience location, and a ranking, which determines the quality or clarity of their perceptions. First imagine a set of points randomly distributed on plane surface; next imagine the view that each of those points would have if it were a consciousness; then imagine that the points are filled in to become infinitely dense; then imagine that we remove space from the picture so that there are neither distances nor directions, neither right nor left. And finally imagine that the monads, who are "windowless," cannot in fact "see" each other across an expanse of visual space, but that each generates a predetermined sequence of experiences for itself that bears a determinate relation to the experiences of all the rest. As God, if he were looking down at the original map, could see on the plane surface all the monads at once and know what their subjective perceptions were, so God can intuit all their experiences—not by looking, for God has no eyes and no body, but on analogy with looking. Because the experiences of the monads occur as though they saw each other across spaces and as though they saw nearer monads better and more distinctly than those far from their own site, they retain this capacity when despatialized. Each perceives the entire universe, though "remote" sectors are perceived confusedly, or, perhaps, what is perceived confusedly is what we think of as remote. The differential clarity and fineness of the monads' experience is in some way the "ground" of our perception of a spatial world with nearer and farther objects.[43]

God cannot intervene in the course of their experiences, but he has surveillance of the whole system; he has the dossier, as it were, on each. And each individual monad has the dossier on all the rest, but this knowledge is mostly confused and is anyway unusable; nothing can be changed. As God differs from the absolute monarch in being unable to intervene in his kingdom, which would be to act against the perfect order he has established, this community differs from a city of informants in being able to derive no benefit from their confused omniscience. The scheme is absolutist in positing a divine perspective on the part of one who is "outside" the system depicted and, at the same time, relativistic. Each monad has a unique series of representations that is neither correct nor incorrect but simply a function of its *situs*, for even two monads of high degree will have compatible but not superimposable experiences, and no created monad has experiences superimposable on God's.

Leibniz's interest in multiple perspectives, which he compares to varying architectural elevations or "scenographies," by contrast with the bird's-eye view of the subject, borrows equally from his interest in varying frames of reference for considering motion and from certain practices of multiple representation, especially observed in engravings of cities.[44] Now it is sometimes said that the discovery of perspectival schemes includes a movement not only toward a morally neutral objectivity in representation but toward an inappropriate and nonreciprocal form of objectification.[45] Nowhere does Leibniz say that God—a member of the system of monads who sees into every monad—is in turn an object of perception for them. Leibniz's universe has a colonial structure insofar as its subordinate entities are looked at and theorized by the dominant power, without being given the privilege of looking back. If we theorize God, it is not because we perceive him. But, of course, even the colony of monads experiences only an artificial reciprocity as subjects all of one another's hallucinations. For all their numerousness, they cannot touch or crowd, so it is natural to think of them as spread out like individual stars in the sky.

What then is the significance of the conjunction of these two paradigms: one a view *sub specie aeternitatis*, in which every trace of embodied experience—materiality, causal interaction, spatiality, temporality—save only force and action is eliminated or redescribed; one a view from within the embodied subject, in which there is no escape from corporeality and confusion? Philosophers studying the internal motivations for the construction of each picture trace them to specific puzzles about causation and individuality. And there has been no lack of efforts to prove that these two pictures are fully compatible, via a conception of matter as a "well-founded phenomenon." But we may also ask, To what impetuses, to what projects or programs, do the parts of this split scheme correspond? And if these impetuses are the urgings of a divided self, should we expect their realizations to be consistent rather than mutually compensatory? Now insofar as the philosopher proposes and invites his philosophical audience to contemplate the formal-geometrical monadic scheme, he is moving the object of the discourse—the subject with its merely relativized, confused knowledge—to the position of the absolute subject, God, who sees in a nonperspectival way that embraces all perspectives. Metaphysical discourse makes a distinction between the world as experienced and the world as known, a distinction that disappears only for God. To participate as reader or writer in a metaphysics like that of the *Monadology* is to lose one's relational and embodied view, though in fact one can participate in this structure only by retaining one's physical intuitions, as the explication of the monadology showed. But metaphysicians want to become not only higher but deeper. And correspondingly, by moving into the interior of the subject, into zones of indistinctness and confused representation, the philosopher nestles into the luxurious and secret world of pleasures that Leibniz describes for us in the *New Essays*: the world of heady swoons, delicate inclinations, vague unrests, and the fascinating and strange "mixtures" of psychology, such as the one we experience when, during the deepest sorrow or sharpest anguish, we find pleasure in drink or music.[46] Yet this too is a world of epiphanies and revelations, in which the "living fires or flashes of light hidden inside us but made visible by the stimulation of the senses, as sparks can be struck from steel" alert us to our own episodic brilliance.[47]

The monads are each locked in their individual dream worlds. They generate within themselves their experience like tiny living factories of images. This duplicative faculty is particularly amazing. As Leibniz says, "There is one very remarkable thing in dreams, for which I believe no one can give a reason. It is the formation of visions by a spontaneous organization carried out in a moment." We can dream what we could not even imagine;[48] we can imagine what we could not draw.[49] And yet there are people who can draw what we imagine and dream, and the pictorial imagination and capacity of the baroque with its sudden flooding of the world with pictures, copies, and images perhaps accounts for the fascination with and the exploitation of the Cartesian theme of visual doubling, which is at the center of every rationalist analysis of the relation of the sense of vision to the external world.

In a chapter from the *New Essays* on signification, Leibniz meditates in a less than wholly serious vein on the ancestry of the word *oeil.* He begins by linking it to the sound *Ah,* the first letter of the alphabet and produced by mild aspiration, so that *aer, atmos, haleine,* and *aqua* are all signifiers of movement and flow. Now water frequently floods pastures, and the German word *Auge* refers to a flooded pasture or an island, or a blob of oil on water; *ach* (as in the Frankish place names *Biberach* or *Anspach*) is a suffix meaning "water." The eye, then, the *oculus, oeil,* or *Auge,* is like a pond "a brilliant isolated hole" in the face.[50] The eye does not only flash and radiate from its reflecting surface, but swallows up images into its dark depths.

The rationalist philosophers move between a conception of vision that they construct as a phenomenon of embodiment, explained, conditioned, and sometimes degraded by its involvement with the material and the corporeally dense, and a conception of vision they construct as an intellective act, implicating geometrical principles, as a way of having while keeping one's distance, as a satisfaction—but of a thirst for light and knowledge. From this melange, it is no surprise that we can extract what prefigurations we like: community or terror; embodiment or transcendence; engagement or dissociation; the active gaze of Augustinian concupiscence; or the retreat into the shadows of philosophy and the colorless, formless world of midcentury ontology. The ocular emphasis of seventeenth-century metaphysics supplied not only the richness of positive science in optics, microscopy, and telescopy, the anatomy of the visual system and the psychology of vision, but a multitude of compelling and misleading visual metaphors.

Notes

1. Nicole Malebranche, *Dialogues on Metaphysics*, trans. Willis Doney (New York, Abaris, 1980), p. 23.

2. Ibid., p. 25.

3. The phrase is that of Martin Jay, "Scopic Regimes of Modernity," in *Vision and Visuality*, ed. H. Foster (Seattle: Bay Press, 1988), p. 3. Jay, drawing on the study of Dutch painting by Svetlana Alpers, *The Art of Describing* (Chicago: University of Chicago Press, 1983), calls attention to the plurality of such regimes.

4. Johannes Kepler, *Paralipomena in Vitellionem*, in *Gesammelte Werke*, ed. F. Hammer (Munich, 1939), vol. 2: *Astronomiae pars Optica*, chap. 5, sec. 2, pp. 151 ff.

5. Richard Rorty, *Philosophy and the Mirror of Nature* (Princeton: Princeton University Press, 1979), pp. 49 ff. See, on the prevalence of the model and the notion that we bear within us a "microcosm" or little world that duplicates the outer world, John Yolton, "Perceptual Optics," in *Perceptual Acquaintance from Descartes to Reid* (Minneapolis: University of Minnesota Press, 1984), pp. 124 ff.

6. John Locke, *An Essay Concerning Human* Understanding, ed. P. H. Nidditch (Oxford: Clarendon Press, 1975), 2:11–17.

7. Leibniz, *New Essays*, trans. Peter Remnant and Jonathan Bennet (Cambridge: Cambridge University Press, 1981), pp. 144 f.

8. René Descartes, *Optics*, Discourse 6 in *The Philosophical Writings of Descartes*, ed. and trans. John Cottingham, Robert Stoothoff, and Dugald Murdoch (Cambridge: Cambridge University Press, 1985), 2:167 ff. See also Yolton's comprehensive treatment of these issues in *Perceptual Aquaintance*, chap. 7 et passim.

9. Leibniz, *New Essays*, p. 144; cf. p. 343.

10. Jonathan Crary, "Modernizing Vision," in Foster, *Vision and Visuality*, p. 33.

11. Ibid., p. 43.

12. Descartes, *Replies to Objections II*, in *Philosophical Writings*, 2:95.

13. See, for example, Susan Bordo, *The Flight to Objectivity: Essays on Cartesianism and Culture* (Albany: State University of New York Press, 1987).

14. Descartes, *Meditation I*, in *Philosophical Writings*, 2:13–15.

Discourses of Vision in Seventeenth-Century Metaphysics

15. Descartes, *Meditation II*, in *Philosophical Writings*, 2:18.

16. Letter to Henry More, August 1649, in Anthony Kenny, trans. and ed., *Descartes: Philosophical Letters* (Oxford: Clarendon Press, 1970), p. 256.

17. Descartes, *Principles of Philosophy*, 2:3, in *Philosophical Writings*, 2:224.

18. Descartes, *Meditations I*, 2:13.

19. Letter to Elizabeth, June 28, 1643, in Kenny, *Descartes*, pp. 141–142.

20. Leibniz, *New Essays*, p. 195.

21. Ibid., preface, p. 55.

22. Ibid., p. 117; cf. pp. 221, 307.

23. Gilles Deleuze, *The Fold: Leibniz and the Baroque*, trans. T. Conley (Minneapolis: University of Minnesota, 1993), p. 86.

24. Malebranche, *Dialogues on Metaphysics*, p. 97.

25. Ibid., p. 31.

26. Ibid., p. 33.

27. Ibid., p. 82.

28. St. Augustine, *Confessions*, trans. R. S. Pine-Coffin (Harmondsworth, Penguin, 1961), p. 243.

29. "Your modalities are total darkness, remember ...," says Theodore. "Silence your senses, your imagination, and your passions.... The more lively our sensations are, the more darkness they spread." *Dialogues*, p. 61.

30. Descartes begins his *Third Meditation* with the words, "I will shut my eyes, stop my ears, and withdraw all my senses. I will eliminate from my thoughts all images of bodily things, or rather, since this is hardly possible, I will regard all such images as vacuous, false, and worthless." *Philosophical Writings*, 2:24.

31. Malebranche, *Dialogues*, p. 227.

32. Descartes, *Rules for the Direction of the Mind*, in *Philosophical Writings*, 1:33.

33. Ibid., p. 40.

34. Ibid., p. 20.

35. Ibid., p. 26.

36. Ibid., p. 9.

37. Ibid., p. 17.

38. Culverwell, *Spiritual Opticks*, in *An Elegant and Learned Discourse on the Light of Nature* (London, 1652), p. 155.

39. See Rosalie L. Cole, *Light and Enlightenment* (Cambridge: Cambridge University Press, 1957).

40. See Ian Hacking, "Leibniz and Descartes: Proofs and Eternal Truths," in S. Gaukroger, ed., *Descartes: Philosophy, Mathematics, and Physics* (Brighton, Sussex: Harvester, 1980), pp. 169–180.

41. Especially in *Surveiller et punir* (Paris: Gallimard, 1975).

42. Leibniz, *The Monadology*, in L. Loemker, ed. and trans., *Leibniz: Philosophical Papers and Letters*, 2d ed. (Dordrecht: D. Reidel, 1969), p. 636.

43. Leibniz, letter to Arnauld, October 6/9, 1687, in ibid., p. 339. On space as a "well-founded phenomenon," see letter to Des Bosses, June 16, 1712, in ibid., p. 604.

44. "The plan of a city, looked down at from the top of a great tower placed upright in its midst .... differs from the almost infinite horizontal perspectives with which it delights the eye of travellers who approach it from one direction or another." Leibniz, "An Example of Demonstrations about the Nature of Corporeal Things," in Leroy Loemker, *Philosophical Papers and Letters*, 2d ed. (Dordrecht: D. Reidel, 1969), p. 142.

45. See Jay, "Scopic Regimes," p. 8. Cf. Normal Bryson: 'The gaze of the painter arrests the flux of phenomena, contemplates the visual field from a vantage point outside the mobility of duration, in an eternal moment of disclosed presence; while in the moment of viewing, the viewing subject unites his gaze with the Founding Perception in a moment of perfect recreation of that first epiphany." *Vision and Painting: The Logic of the Gaze* (New Haven: Yale University Press, 1983), p. 94, quoted in Jay, "Scopic Regimes," in Foster, ed. *Vision and Visuality*, p. 7.

46. Leibniz, *New Essays*, p. 166.

47. Ibid., preface, p. 49.

48. Leibniz, *De somnio et vigilia*, in Loemker, *Philosophical Papers and Letters*, p. 115.

49. Leibniz, *Theodicy*, trans. E. M. Huggard (La Salle, Ill.: Open Court, 1985), p. 403.

50. Leibniz, *New Essays*, pp. 284–285. Recall Rimbaud's "Jouet de cet oeil d'eau morne" in the last verse of his poem *Mémoire*.

4

How to Write the History of Vision: Understanding the Relationship between Berkeley and Descartes

Margaret Atherton

In any account of the history of vision, René Descartes's name quite appropriately looms large. Descartes is the author of a treatise of vision, the *Dioptrics*, which puts forward an important account of how perceivers see, an account that encapsulates and rests on principles of geometric optics. But Descartes sometimes takes on a larger-than-life role, a role of mythic proportions, in which his views are made to stand for the thought of an age. This is illustrated, for example, in Martin Jay's decision to characterize that "scopic regime," which he says is usually identified with "the modern scopic regime per se" as "Cartesian perspectivalism." Jay writes: "As has often been remarked, Descartes was a quintessentially visual philosopher, who tacitly adopted the position of a perspectivalist painter using a camera obscura to reproduce the observed world. "Cartesian perspectivalism," in fact, may nicely serve as a shorthand way to characterize the dominant scopic regime of the modern era."[1] In support of this nomenclature, Jay cites Richard Rorty, who also makes Descartes emblematic of an age that assimilates knowing to seeing, so that knowing is described as gazing with the mind's eye on mental representations that mirror the exterior world.[2]

I have some doubts about the usefulness of this mythic Descartes, for I think this tendency to use Descartes as the leading character in an account of intellectual events in the seventeenth and eighteenth centuries often results in a dual oversimplification: it reduces the highly complex thought of Descartes to a caricature, and it removes attention from events that do not fit neatly into the Cartesian mold.[3] In discussions of vision, what can often get ignored is the alternative account of George Berkeley. Such an oversight is strongly detrimental to an adequate understanding of the history of vision since it is Berkeley's theory that virtually replaced Descartes's as the prevailing account of the nature of vision.

In order to illustrate the dangers of overlooking Berkeley, I examine some arguments made by Jonathan Crary in *Techniques of the Observer: On Vision and Modernity in the Nineteenth Century.*[4] Crary is not writing a history of vision. He is an art historian, whose actual project is to encourage a rethinking of the history of modernity. The way he conceptualizes his project and the very careful way in which he carries it out, however, provides an excellent example for me of what can happen when Descartes's thought is overgeneralized to stand for the thought of an entire period.

Crary's central claim I want to investigate is that the concept of an observer should be understood as a historicized notion and one that, moreover, exhibited very significant shifts at the beginning of the nineteenth century. "It is a shift," he writes, "signalled by the passage from the geometrical optics of the seventeenth and eighteenth centuries to physiological optics, which dominated both scientific and philosophical discussion of vision in the nineteenth century" (*TO*, p. 16). Geometric optics, for Crary, is to be understood as represented by the figure of the camera obscura, a device he tells us achieved popularity in this period. The camera obscura is an object, of varying sizes, that was designed to take advantage of the fact that if light passes through a small hole into a darkened box, then an inverted image of the scene in front of the hole will appear inside at the back wall of the box. "Historically speaking," Crary says, "we must recognize how for nearly two hundred years, from the late 1500s to the end of the 1700s, the structure and optical principles of the camera obscura coalesced into a dominant paradigm through which was described the status and possibilities of an observer.... During the seventeenth and eighteenth centuries the camera obscura was without question the most widely used model for explaining human vision" (p. 27).

Crary explains that it was thought that we could understand how it is that a human observer sees the world outside, when we discover that light, entering through the pupil, causes an inverted representation of the exterior scene to be projected on the retina, inside the observer. The human eye is a camera obscura. Following Rorty, moreover, Crary wants to take the image of the camera obscura as more than a way of representing in the large the geometric relations of light rays to the retina. He also takes the camera obscura as a model for how the observer knows. Crary stresses that, according to Descartes, what the observer contemplates are disembodied images, but since these images, like the images of the camera obscura, reproduce the world outside the camera, this model allows us to see how the observer is able to make "truthful inferences about the world" (*TO*, p. 29). Vision, for Crary, according to the camera obscura model, is both disembodied and veridical.

Crary's view, in an approach that exhibits the influence of Michel Foucault, is that the early nineteenth century witnessed a rupture and a new beginning to the way in which vision was conceptualized. What for Crary forms the basis of this new beginning was the sudden importance of physiology to the study of vision. "Physiology at this moment of the nineteenth century is one of those sciences that stand for the rupture that Foucault poses between the eighteenth and nineteenth centuries, in which man emerges as a being in whom the transcendent is mapped onto the empirical. It was the discovery that knowledge was conditioned by the physical and anatomical functioning of the body, and in particular of the eyes" (*TO*, p. 79). According to Crary, the study of vision in the early nineteenth century is now firmly located within the body of the observer. Seeing is no longer to be understood as a transaction between an observer and an external

Margaret Atherton

world but is the product of an autonomous, organic system. This way of thinking about vision, Crary tells us, reaches its culmination in Johannes Mueller's theory of specific nerve endings:

The theory was based on the discovery that the nerves of the different senses were physiologically distinct, that is, capable of one determinant kind of sensation only, and not of those proper to other organs of sense. It asserted quite simply—and this is what marks its epistemological scandal—that a uniform cause (for example, electricity) generates utterly different sensations from one kind of nerve to another. Electricity applied to the optic nerve produces the experience of light, applied to the skin the sensation of touch. Conversely, Mueller showed that a variety of different causes will produce the *same* sensation in a given sensory nerve. In other words, he is describing a fundamentally arbitrary relation between stimulus and sensation. It is an account of a body with an innate capacity, one might even say a transcendental faculty, to *misperceive*—of an eye that renders differences equivalent. (*TO*, pp. 89–90)

Nineteenth-century vision, as firmly located in the body of the observer, is fundamentally subjective. As such, vision is no longer the source of veridical representations of the world. It does not receive copies of what is out there; instead, it independently generates illusion.

Crary wants to draw a number of interesting conclusions from this account, which it is not my purpose to go into here.[5] My concern is the historical account he gives and the historiographical principles on which it is based. Crary's telling of the history of vision from the seventeenth to the early nineteenth centuries is flawed for two important reasons. He provides a vastly oversimplified account of Descartes's optics and of the epistemology relating to it, which seriously underplays the importance of physiology in Descartes's own theory. Second, he ignores a very important chapter in the history of vision: Berkeley's successful challenge to Descartes's geometric optics at the beginning of the eighteenth century. The result is that many of the features Crary takes to characterize a rupture in the understanding of the nature of vision occurring in the early nineteenth century are actually features of theories of vision that had come to the fore a century earlier. Instead of consisting of a series of disconnected models of vision, the theory of vision presents a relatively smooth development.

Crary's account sees Descartes as using a single model, one that emphasizes geometry. This model is based on an account of vision and is then assumed by analogy to provide an account of knowing. According to Crary, knowing for Descartes is a kind of seeing, which is itself a geometrically described, disembodied, and veridical event. But this account is achieved by reading back some of what Descartes says about knowledge into his account of vision. In fact, it is safe to say that Descartes did not have a single descriptive model for vision. At best, it is possible to find at least three different lines of thought in his account of vision, not all of which mesh very successfully together. Therefore, it is not obvious what sense can be made of Descartes's visual language in his description of knowing.[6]

What causes problems for Descartes is that seeing is for him an embodied but mental event. In humans, seeing takes place as a result of what he calls the union of mind of body. Descartes's handling of the mind-body union has never been regarded as fully satisfactory, but what is crucial to recognize about his account of vision is that he was struggling to deal with a phenomenon he conceived as both mental and physical. It is not then true to say that Descartes's account of vision was without a physiological component, which plays an important role in the way he thinks of vision. At least a part of Descartes's account of vision is in terms that he considered appropriate for discussing bodily states and events, that is, mechanical terms.

Descartes's first approach to vision describes the way light rays affect the retina. He is quite clear there is no vision unless it rests on the appropriate corporeal event. Descartes provided a number of images to show how it is that vision should be understood in terms of light rays that strike the retina according to mechanical laws, of which the most telling is that of the blind man with a stick.[7] Just as the blind man can become aware of different pressures on his stick, so the eye can become aware of all the qualities it sees as a result of the impact of light reflected off bodies onto the retina. The result of such a mechanical account allows

Margaret Atherton

Descartes to conclude that what we see, so far from being a picture copying an exterior world, in fact bears no resemblance to that world at all. He writes:

And first of all, regarding light and color, which alone properly belong to the sense of sight, it is necessary to think that the nature of our mind is such that the force of the movements in the areas of the brain where the small fibers of the optic nerves originate cause it to perceive light; and the character of these movements cause it to have the perception of color; just as the movements of the nerves which respond to the ears cause it to hear sounds, and those of the nerves of the tongue cause it to taste flavors, and, generally, those of the nerves of the entire body cause it to feel some tickling, when they are moderate, and when they are too violent, some pain; yet in all this, there need be no resemblance between the ideas that the mind conceives and the movements which cause these ideas. You will readily believe this if you note that it seems to those who receive some injury in the eye that they see an infinity of fireworks and lightning flashes before them, even though they shut their eyes or else are in a very dark place; so that this sensation can be attributed only to the force of the blow which moves the small fibers of the optic nerve, as a strong light would do. And if this same force touched the ears, it could cause some sound to be heard; and if it touched the body in other parts, could cause it to feel some pain.[8]

A major goal of Descartes's writing on optics was to argue against those who believed that we saw by means of little images, "intentional species," in their terminology, that resemble the objects in the world to be seen. As the quotation makes clear, he seeks to refute this theory by means of a physiological theory that is not unlike the one Crary attributes to Mueller. From his physiological theory, Descartes wants to draw the same sort of epistemological conclusion that Crary highlighted: that since our sensations are generated within our various sense faculties, what we have are faculties that enable us to misperceive the world. So at least one important way in which Descartes talks about vision stresses its physiological nature and reveals the extent to which vision is nonveridical.

No matter how much Descartes wanted to disabuse his readers of any belief in "all those small images flitting through the air, called *intentional species*" (*O*, p. 68), he still could not rid himself entirely of the grip of the "picture model" of vision, and this shows up most clearly in his discussion of the pictures on the back of the retina. These are among the passages Crary discusses in order to indicate the importance of the camera obscura model for Descartes. While I do not think these passages show the hold the model had on Descartes was quite as tight as Crary suggests, nevertheless, I do find that he did not entirely escape its seductions. Descartes first raises the issue of the images on the retina in a way that shows he understands that his own account of vision, in terms of the impact of light rays on nerve endings, precludes any significant roles for images on the retina. He says: "Thus you can clearly see that in order to perceive, the mind need not contemplate any images resembling the things that it senses. But this makes it no less true that the objects we look at do imprint very perfect images on the back of the eye" (*O*, p. 91). Before he says anything at all about the images on the retina, Descartes moves to point out that we do not see by looking at pictures on the retina. He proceeds by invoking a description of a camera obscura, which he then compares to what can be seen at the back of the eye, most conveniently, he suggests, an ox eye. Crary refers to this eye as disembodied, and of course it is, in the sense that it has been removed from the body of the ox, but it is not disembodied in the sense important to Descartes. The ox eye is a body, and Descartes is using it as an example to discuss the way in which the corporeal nature of a particular kind of body, the eye, affects what is imprinted on the retina, so as to affect what we see. For example, the shape of the eye means that only what falls into the center of the retina is in focus. Therefore, that our visual field is blurry at the edges can be understood through an examination of the anatomy of the eye. In general, what Descartes's use of the camera obscura model allows him to do is to discuss the way in which the body records a distorted image of an exterior scene. So far from imagining that the eye's resemblance to a camera obscura shows that we are designed to see a faithfully recorded replica of a visual scene, Descartes actually uses it to reinforce the opposite conclusion.

It is only in his discussion of our perception of position or situation that Descartes traps himself into the view that what is on our retina is operative as a picture of what is to be seen. The problem is to explain the mechanism whereby we see the position of objects with respect to us, whether they are up or down, for example, and the reason that Descartes takes this to be a problem is that the image on the retina, like the image in the camera obscura, is upside down. Descartes's solution is to reinvoke the image of the blind man with the stick. This time the blind man is perceiving the location of objects by means of crossed sticks held in each hand, and we are to imagine that we can similarly perceive the location of objects by tracing back crossed light rays: "So that you must not be surprised that the objects can be seen in their true position, even though the picture they imprint upon the eye is inverted: for this is just like our blind man's being able to sense the object B, which is to his right, by means of his left hand, and the object D, which is to his left, by means of his right hand at one and the same time" (O, p. 105).

Descartes's solution is ingenious, but on his own terms he should not have thought there was a problem at all, since the picture on the back of the retina does not function in his own account of vision as a picture to be seen at all. It is merely one of a series of mechanical steps through the optic system. So in this one instance Descartes does not seem to have rid himself of the picture theory that the camera obscura model supports. But this aspect of the camera obscura model is far from being a dominant theme in his thinking about vision, and in particular, he nowhere uses this model in order to claim that our visual perception is veridical.

What is perhaps more significant about the disembodied eye of the ox is that it is also disem*mind*ed, and this, at least as far as humans are concerned, is, for Descartes, a highly significant omission. In a famous phrase, he says, "It is the mind, which sees, not the eye" (O, p. 108). The mind sees by virtue of, among other things, the retina, but it does not see by looking at the retina. The camera obscura model can never tell the whole story of vision for Descartes, for the camera obscura model explains only what is imprinted on the retina, and we do not see what is on the retina. In fact there are significant differences between what is imprinted on the retina and what we experience ourselves as seeing. The example of situation perception is one case in point, since what we experience ourselves as seeing is actually in a different spatial orientation from what is on the retina, but there are many others as well. For example, two objects may project images that are the same size on the retina, but the child who is close to me will be experienced as smaller than the adult who is farther away. In order to deal with cases like these, Descartes makes use of an intellectualist way of talking about vision, in which the mind introduces geometrical properties into the visual array by means of calculations that correct what is on the retina. The mind is imagined to reason back from the inverted image to the actual position of the object, and to, as it were, reinvert the image that is seen. Or, it reasons back, using geometrical principles, to calculate the actual size of the object at the distance at which it is located, so that the child is seen as smaller than the adult.

In this way of talking, Descartes comes closest to suggesting that, in vision, the mind constructs a picture that is geometrically isomorphic to the world the picture represents. Even in this case, however, the result is not a veridical picture of the external world: "In judging of distance by size, or shape, or color, or light, pictures in perspective sufficiently demonstrate to us how easy it is to be mistaken. For often because the things which are pictured there are smaller than we imagine that they should be, and because their outlines are less distinct, and their colors darker or more feeble, they appear to us to be farther away than they are in actuality" (O, pp. 112–113). Even in these intellectually guided cases, the effect of the corporeal nature of vision is to produce a visual array that is an inaccurate representation of the geometric properties of the world, which is its ultimate cause. In general, while Descartes's account of vision does make use of some pictorial features such as are suggested by a camera obscura model, he is far from suggesting that seeing is a matter of gazing at an inner pictorial representation. Seeing is mediated by both physical and mental processes so as to result in an inaccurate portrayal of the world to be known.

Descartes's theory of optics is not, as the camera obscura model put forward by Crary would suggest, a straightforward transference of a visual metaphor for knowledge onto the visual realm itself. Instead, in addition to using the camera obscura as a way of explaining something about the anatomy and the optics of the visual system, he also used two other models, a mechanical model and an intellectualist, and these two do not have exactly the same consequences. Thanks to the mechanical properties of our bodies and of the bodies that surround us, we see certain pictorial properties, colors, and these colors we perceive, mediated through our bodies, do not resemble their causes in the external world. Thanks to these same mechanical principles, we also see these color patches as spatially organized, and here the situation is more complicated.[9] The spatial organization we see is not a copy of the organization of items in the world, such that we could read off the spatial properties of the world from the properties of what we see. Nevertheless, the visual world we see is not a direct reflection of what is registered on the retina either but involves some kind of correction in favor of the geometrical properties of the actual world, properties, moreover, we are intellectually equipped to grasp, even if we cannot read them off our visual sensations. The tensions embodied in Descartes's account make it unlikely that it could serve for long as a dominant version of what vision is like. In fact, the Cartesian theory of vision was successfully challenged by Berkeley early in the eighteenth century.

For all Descartes's praise of vision of the beginning of the *Optics*, what he produced was an account that encouraged a distrust of vision. This attitude of distrust was in fact picked up and extended by later Cartesians, such as Malebranche. What we see on the Cartesian account is a misleading, and in fact, false representation of the world. The exterior world was not supposed to be colored, as is the world we see, nor does the world being represented even have the same geometric properties as does the visual representation. Berkeley's effort can be seen as one of restoring vision to an honorable place, by showing that, when its nature is properly understood, vision can be seen to work. What this requires is to give up the presupposition on which Descartes's account rests that, in vision, what we see is a picture misrepresenting a nonpictorial world, in favor of a different model entirely. It is Berkeley's contention that we will understand vision to work if we take it to represent as if it were a language, in which visual cues serve as signs for meanings that, like the meanings our words stand for, do not resemble the cues themselves.

I have argued that Descartes's discussion of vision was an amalgam of mechanical, pictorial, and intellectual talk. A part of what Berkeley did was to straighten out the sources of these various vocabularies. In *The Theory of Vision Vindicated*, he is careful to establish exactly what portion of the prevailing theories he was taking issue with:[10]

To explain how the mind or soul of man simply sees is one thing, and belongs to philosophy. To consider particles as moving in certain lines, rays of light as refracted or reflected, or crossing, or including angles, is quite another thing, and appertaineth to geometry. To account for the sense of vision by the mechanism of the eye is a third thing, which appertaineth to anatomy and experiments. The two latter speculations are of use in practice, to assist the defects and remedy the distempers of sight, agreeably to the natural laws obtaining in this mundane system. But the former theory is that which makes us understand the true nature of vision, considered as a faculty of the soul. (*TVV*, 43)

Berkeley did not intend his account to subvert in any way the optics, the geometry, on which Descartes's theory relies, or his anatomy, his physiology. Berkeley's account, like Descartes's, is physiologically based. It assumes we can see only what our corporeal, visual organs can register. He takes issue just with Descartes's account of how the mind or soul sees. Berkeley's language theory is going to replace Descartes's intellectualist account, in which the mind is supposed to be constructing a pictorial representation by geometrical reasoning.

Berkeley's project, therefore, is to provide a theory, superior to Descartes's, of the way in which we visually perceive the spatial properties of distance, size, and situation. I need to stress, since this is something frequently overlooked, that this means that the nature of Berkeley's project is essentially positive: he is assuming we do perceive distance, size, and situation by sight, and he is going to explain how we do so. This is something that Crary, for example, gets badly wrong about Berkeley. Crary claims that "for Berkeley there is no such thing as visual perception of depth," and he assimilates Berkeley to other seventeenth- and eighteenth-century writers who have what he calls "an anti-optical notion of sight" (*TO*, p. 62). This is in fact quite the reverse of Berkeley's actual procedure. He thinks and seeks to show that we do perceive spatial properties by sight, and he thinks we can understand how this is possible only if we remove from our notion of vision everything that is not genuinely optical in nature.

While Berkeley's theory is most often discussed in terms of his account of distance perception, and indeed it is sometimes discussed as if distance were the only phenomenon under discussion, this is not an aspect of his theory by which Berkeley himself sets most store. In the *Theory of Vision Vindicated*, he singles out aspects of his account of situation perception as being of primary importance: "The solution of this knot about inverted images seems the principal point in the whole optic theory, the most difficult perhaps to comprehend, but the most deserving of our attention, and, when rightly understood, the surest way to lead the mind into a thorough knowledge of the true nature of vision" (*TVV*, 52). In his discussion of situation perception, the problem of how we are able to see where to reach for, and the attendant knot about inverted images, the puzzle that what appears on the retina is inverted with respect to what we see, Berkeley attacks Descartes's theory at its weakest point. More important, he gives an account that undercuts a description of vision that sees its primary purpose as the deliverance of "pictures," as in the camera obscura model, which then may or may not resemble what they represent. I believe that the best way to see how it is that Berkeley's theory contrasts with that of Descartes is to concentrate on the example of situation perception.

In order to develop his account of our perception of the spatial organization and orientation of what we see, Berkeley needs to identify what it is we learn about in seeing, what it is in our perception of situation that is purely optical in nature, and he needs to discriminate this purely optical element from what we learn about through other sense modalities. This distinction forms the bedrock of his theory of space perception and is the principal way in which he distinguishes himself from his predecessors. In Berkeley's terminology, he needs a distinction between the proper and immediate objects of each sense modality and the mediate objects that do not belong to each sense but are rather suggested to it by the imagination. The idea is that for each sense organ, there is a range of sensations we become aware of by virtue of possessing that sense organ. Because we have a visual system, we sense light and colors; because we have an auditory system, we sense sounds; and so forth. Berkeley's idea is to get us to strip down our understanding of each sensory system to just what that system is physiologically equipped to provide. What our eyes can do is register light and colors, and this is all we can learn about strictly through seeing. Whatever else we become aware of in seeing, as the distance objects are from us, we do not strictly speaking see; rather, distance is suggested to us by what we see. Berkeley's theory presupposes the physiology of the eye and of our various sense organs.

In introducing the distinction between immediate and mediate objects of sense in *Theory of Vision Vindicated*, Berkeley makes use of the analogy with language:

Things properly perceived by sight are immediately perceived. Besides things properly and immediately perceived by any sense, there may be also other things suggested to the mind by means of those proper and immediate objects. Which things so suggested are not objects of that sense, being in truth only objects of the imagination and originally belonging to some other sense or faculty. Thus, sounds are the proper object of hearing, being properly and immediately perceived by that, and by no other sense. But, by the mediation of sounds or words, all other things may be suggested to the mind, and yet things so suggested are not thought the object of hearing. (*TVV*, 9)

Just as, strictly speaking, what we hear by having ears are sounds and not meanings, so what we see are no more than light and color patches. Berkeley's theory is predicated on an idea Crary reserves for the nineteenth century: the notion of the innocent eye. In introducing this idea, Crary quotes John Ruskin as follows: "The whole technical power of painting depends on our recovery of what may be called the *innocence of the eye;* that is to say, of a sort of childish perception of these flat stains of colour, merely as such, without consciousness of what they signify,—as a blind man would see them if suddenly gifted with sight."[11] The device of the blind man made to see is used by Berkeley throughout his account of vision in order to help the reader to become restored to a sense of visual innocence. It is a central element of his work.

Although the innocent eye, the eye that sees color patches, may be the eye we are born with, it is not the eye we see with. Berkeley enters into the same problematic as Descartes: the way in which we are physiologically equipped to see does not account for what we end up seeing. There must be some enrichment of what is registered on the retina. Descartes had offered a whole slew of ways in which retinal information is enriched, some of which, those that fit into his intellectualist account, imagine that in seeing, we construct a visual picture by reasoning from the information contained on the retina. Descartes's account of situation perception is like this. The visual system is assumed to be working out the orientation of the objects it sees by tracing them back from the images that appear upside down on the retina.

Berkeley's main criticism of this account is that it assumes that the mind has at its disposal information about lines and angles for which there is no mental representation, and it assumes that it makes sense to attribute to a mind calculations that mind has no consciousness of having performed. Instead, Berkeley points out, there is an easier theory available, which relies on mechanisms Descartes is prepared to admit. Berkeley observes that not all the cues that Descartes mentions can be treated as elements in a reasoning process that relies on necessary connections between the retinal information and the constructed visual field. When Descartes observes that we take something small and faint as a sign for distance, however, then he cannot suppose we can calculate a distance based on smallness or faintness. The connection between smallness and faintness and distance is habitual and customary: "They have none of them in their own nature, any relation or connection with it."[12] These arbitrary connections, Berkeley points out, are just like the ones that exist between words in a language and what they signify. We have to learn the meaning of words.

Berkeley proposes to take cases like these as a model for how the visual system works. We learn to see distance by associating our kinesthetic sense of distance with small and faint color blobs, because we have learned that when we see something small and faint, it will take a good time to get there. But a man born blind, if made to see, would not similarly suppose small and faint color patches to be at a great distance. He would have no reason to associate what he is seeing with any distance at all. Berkeley's theory presupposes that vision is the product of an independent visual system, a view that Crary reserves for nineteenth-century theories of vision.

The effect of isolating the visual system means that Berkeley is looking at an entirely different way in which visual ideas represent than was understood by Descartes's account. Because visual ideas are completely independent of any of our other ideas, then visual ideas cannot be assumed to represent a nonvisual world through resemblance, as a picture copies an original. Nor are visual ideas a pictorial version of something nonpictorial to which we can reason. This is the thrust of what lies behind Berkeley's claim that vision is best regarded as a language:

Upon the whole, I think we may fairly conclude that the proper objects of vision constitute an universal language of the Author of nature, whereby we are instructed how to regulate our actions in order to attain those things that are necessary to the preservation and well-being of our bodies, as also to avoid whatever may be hurtful and destructive of them. It is by their information that we are principally guided in all the transactions and concerns of life. And the manner wherein they signify and mark unto us the objects which are at a distance is the same with that of languages and signs of human appointment, which do not suggest the things signified by any likeness or identity of nature, but only by an habitual connexion that experience has made us to observe between them. (NTV, 147)

If vision is a language, then seeing is something we had to learn how to do. We had to learn to associate the light and colors which are all that properly speaking we see with ideas derived from other sense modalities. It is this approach, that takes seeing as something that requires learning through arbitrary associations, that had a tremendous impact on subsequent theories of vision.

The idea that nature is a book that can be read is not a new one, but Berkeley is introducing some new twists. In arguing that nature is a language that can be read, he is denying that natural signs represent by means of resemblance, in the way in which it was sometimes thought that the medical qualities of plants could be recognized because the plants looked like the organs for whose disorders they provided a cure. For Berkeley, the important property of a language is that words do not resemble what they represent, so that it is only through experience that the various arbitrary sounds and shapes come to suggest to us what they signify. It was also important to Berkeley that languages have speakers, so that when he came to publish *Alciphron*, his most theologically oriented work, he reprinted *The New Theory of Vision* along with it, because of the way in which the view that vision is a language provided a new and, Berkeley thought, convincing proof for the existence of God as speaker of the language of vision. But interestingly, the *New Theory* itself is almost completely free from theological references, and this is not the lesson that subsequent readers took from the language analogy. While they found the claim that seeing is an acquired skill to be totally convincing, they were far more likely to take what they were inclined to see as the skeptical tendencies of Berkeley's later works to be a threat to traditional causal proofs for the existence of God. So Berkeley's language theory of vision, as it survives in the nineteenth century, is entirely secular in form.

If we think of vision as a language, in which visual ideas derive their meaning predominantly by suggesting to us ideas of touch, then the problem of situation perception—of how we perceive the position of things, as Descartes calls it—is going to be conceived in a different manner from the way Descartes did.

Descartes's account presupposes that seeing is a matter of constructing a visual display that itself has positions like up or down, that can be correlated with and can represent corresponding positions of up or down in the external causes of the visual array. But for Berkeley, it becomes relevant to ask, Is situation properly perceived by sight or by some other means? and his answer is that situation is the proper object of touch. We learn whether something is up or down, erect or inverted by touch. Up is reaching away from gravitational pull, and down is reaching toward it. If this is the primary sense of words like *up* and *down*, then they can have no application to the light and colors of the visual array per se. A blind man made to see would not have any sense of how to reach out and touch the confusion of light and colors he now sees and so would not be able to locate what he sees as up or down or erect or inverted. Such terms become applicable only when he learns to "read" his visual ideas by correlating them with his tangible ideas. We learn that we must reach up to touch something we see by raising our eyes up. We come to see the figure of a man as erect when we come to correlate an array of colors with those tactile qualities of the man's head that are felt as farthest from the earth. Until we have learned to make such associations, Berkeley claims, we would have no way of recognizing something visual as erect.

In seeking to meet what seems like an obvious objection to his claim that the man born blind would not be able to apply terms like *erect* or *inverted* to what he initially sees, Berkeley reveals the radical nature of his theory. The objection he considers runs as follows:

It will, perhaps, be objected to our opinion that a man, for instance, being thought erect when his feet are next the earth, and inverted when his head is next the earth, it doth hence follow that by the meer act of vision, without any experience or altering the situation of the eye, we should have determined whether he were erect or inverted: For both the earth it self, and the limbs of the man who stand thereon, being equally perceived by sight, one cannot choose seeing what part of the man is nearest the earth, and what part farthest from it, *i.e.* whether he be erect or inverted. (*NTV*, 101)

The objection assumes that a man born blind when made to see would be looking at something like a picture, of a person, say, and so could identify the erectness of the person pictured in his visual field. Berkeley's response is to point out that what such a person would be seeing would not be in the least like a picture (although it would be exactly what all sighted persons see by virtue of having eyes). He would be seeing visual qualities, light and colors, but since these visual qualities have no connection with the tangible qualities with which he is familiar, he would have no grounds for parceling out what he is seeing into a person with a head and feet. Until the man born blind has learned to associate what he is now seeing with the tangible qualities with which he is familiar, the colors he sees would not represent anything to him. He would not be so much as able to tell that he was seeing one head and two feet, because he would not be able to sort out the colors into a head blob and feet blobs until he could associate the colors with tangible qualities. The structural organization of the visual field is created only when the visual qualities are associated with tangible and other qualities.

Berkeley's account is very different from that presupposed by the camera obscura model, because, according to Berkeley, we do not see anything like a picture. The job of the visual system is to register light and colors, and this is all that it does. These lights and colors are not in themselves supposed to be structurally like anything else or to be resemblances of anything else. They acquire a representational function when they are combined into collections by the mind. At that point they may be said to represent the collections of which they form a part. But the idea is that things have visual qualities and these we see with our eyes, and they have other kinds of qualities too, which we become aware of through other means. Our visual experiences become meaningful when they suggest to us these other qualities that have become associated with the visual. I argued earlier that the camera obscura model does not adequately capture Descartes's theory of vision, because of the various ways in which Descartes conceived the spectator as involved both corporeally and intellectually in the act of seeing. But it should be clear that it has even less to do with Berkeley's theory. Berkeley is trying to show that the picture, at which the spectator is assumed to be gazing in the camera obscura model, does not even exist until after that spectator has become thoroughly engaged tactilely and kinesthetically.

With this account in hand, Berkeley is able to dispel the problem of the inverted image on the retina, the problem embedded in a camera obscura model of vision. The problem comes about because the image of the man imprinted on the retina is upside down. The eye is supposed to be puzzled because what it immediately sees is inverted and to have a reason for wanting to work out the correct orientation of what it sees. But according to Berkeley, an eye has no information about the tangible orientation and so never has a reason for trying to invert what it sees. The eye registers a visual array in which, as Berkeley says, the head is farthest from the earth. Alternatively, we could imagine that we are looking at a retina at the back of an eye, with a picture appearing on it, like Descartes's ox eye. But in this case, the head is still farthest from the earth, and so there is still no problem. It is only when we imagine ourselves comparing the two, that is, a visual scene and the scene of a retina looking at that scene, that we think there is a problem, but this is a problem not for the visual system but only for someone else who is looking at both the retina and the visual scene. What the little picture that is being experienced on the retina copies is another visual experience, that of looking at the world. What is experienced on the retina is not a copy of a nonvisual or tangible world, and what is actually on the retina is itself tangible; it is the impact of light rays. For this reason, Berkeley exposes a place where Descartes has become confused by the camera obscura model. For, of course, Descartes himself did not hold that a visual array could copy a mind-independent world.

I have tried to show that Crary's account of the nature of vision in the seventeenth and eighteenth centuries, as dominated by a single model, the camera obscura model, goes badly wrong for a couple of reasons. The first is that this model is too simplistic to capture the complexity of thought even of that thinker it was most designed to fit, René Descartes. Most especially, by ignoring the fact that Descartes's account of vision describes a process that was corporeal in nature, Crary misses an important element in Descartes's theory: that our visual representations misrepresent the world. The second way in which Crary's use of the camera obscura model leads him astray lies in the way in which it papers over the vast difference between Descartes and Berkeley. In particular, Berkeley's account of vision in terms of language is specifically intended to provide an alternative account to Descartes, one in which vision does not misrepresent. Berkeley thought we would cease to take vision to be a faulty way of knowing when we understand that each of our sense organs presents us with an independent set of qualities. These qualities are not a misleading version of something else, which they imperfectly represent. Instead, some qualities, such as visual qualities, come to represent other qualities, such as tangible qualities, when they have been observed to go together. What Crary misses is the presence in the early eighteenth century of a way of thinking about vision that is not only other than but contrary to the camera obscura model.

The upshot is that there is no justification for Crary's claim that the early nineteenth century witnessed a rupture in the way the observer was conceived. For one thing, many of the features Crary cites as unique to the nineteenth-century conception of vision, such as the importance of physiology, were in fact present in accounts of vision throughout the period under discussion. I am not, of course, maintaining that there were no advances in understanding of physiology from the seventeenth to the nineteenth centuries—this is certainly not the case—merely that it is not true to say there was a shift from a view of vision as disembodied to one in which it was rooted in the body. Second, to the extent that the theory of vision took a turn away from a geometric account, it did so not at the beginning of the nineteenth century but at the beginning of the eighteenth, with the work of

Berkeley. Other elements Crary cites as important to the nineteenth century, such as the notion of the "innocent eye," were key to Berkeley's work. And the presence of these elements is not surprising, since in fact, the paradigm Berkeley established for work in vision was still proving fruitful well into the nineteenth century. But finally, it would be a mistake to characterize the transition from Descartes's geometric optics to Berkeley's linguistic optics as a rupture in any case. It makes far too much sense to see Berkeley not merely as incorporating elements of Descartes's theory into his own, but as developing his alternative account in response to difficulties perceived in Descartes's theory.

There are several different responses that Crary might be presumed to want to make to the way in which I have been trying to warn him off his use of the texts I have been discussing. The first would be to say that my account of Berkeley's theory should not actually serve to interrupt the grand narrative he is telling because he is perfectly prepared to agree that there are oppositional moments to the general thematic account he is giving.[13] But my point is that Berkeley's rejection of geometric optics does not constitute an oppositional moment to an otherwise dominant theme, but instead served to shift decisively the way vision was described. Almost midway through the nineteenth century, John Stuart Mill said of Berkeley's theory that it "had remained, almost from its first promulgation, one of the least disputed doctrines in the most disputed and most disputable of all sciences, the Science of Man."[14] What Mill is reporting is that it is in fact Berkeley's associationistic, language-based model that provided the dominant account of vision throughout the eighteenth and well into the nineteenth centuries. In fact, it did not begin to loosen its grip until the middle of the twentieth century, with the rise of alternative theories, such as David Marr's, and even with these new rivals, it still remains influential.

The second kind of response Crary seems likely to make is to say there are many different paths to be followed through the history of vision, and that his is as available as any other. What Crary says is this:

It should not be necessary to point out that there are no such things as continuities and discontinuities in history, only in historical explanation. So my broad temporalizing is not in the interest of a "true history", or of restoring to the record "what actually happened." The stakes are quite different: how one periodizes and where one locates ruptures or denies them are all political choices that determine the construction of the present. Whether one excludes or foregrounds certain events and processes at the expense of others affects the intelligibility of the contemporary functioning of power in which we ourselves are enmeshed. Such choices affect whether the shape of the present seems "natural" or whether its historically fabricated and densely sedimented makeup is made evident. (*TO*, p. 7)

But I am not myself so readily inclined as is Crary to reject out of hand the value of restoring to the record "what really happened." The relativism behind his approach comes up against the reality of Descartes's and Berkeley's texts themselves, which, for me, provide a fact of the matter that cannot be gainsaid. These texts Crary discusses cannot be made to fit the mold he tries to fit over them; there are far too many occasions on which Crary makes claims about the texts that are simply false.

In order to support his claim, for example, that Berkeley's theory of the dissimilarity of sight and touch is different from the nineteenth-century autonomy of the senses, Crary describes Berkeley as "not alone in the eighteenth century in his concern with achieving a fundamental harmonization of the senses, in which a key model for visual perception is the sense of touch (*TO*, p. 58). But this seems an extremely unlikely way to characterize the thought of someone whose theory was predicated on the claim that the deliverances of sight and touch were thoroughly unlike each other and connected only arbitrarily. Or again, Crary supports his rather surprising claim that Berkeley's theory was in the camera obscura tradition by referring to a passage in the *Theory of Vision Vindicated* where Berkeley asks us to imagine ourselves as looking through a grid. But Berkeley was not by means of this device suggesting that our visual field is a projection in perspective of the world it represents. Quite the contrary, he is using the device of the grid to help us divorce ourselves from the represented world and to recapture the innocent eye. Crary cites but misses the importance of Berkeley's claim that the grid through which we imagine ourselves to be looking is really tactual. A tactual grid does have spatial organization, but Berkeley in fact wants to deny this of a visual array. It is therefore quite false to read this passage as providing a reason to suppose that Berkeley thought that "the observer is still one who observes a projection onto a field exterior to himself" (*TO*, p. 55). As I hope my discussion of Berkeley's account of situation perception has made clear, this is exactly the opposite of what Berkeley intended. So whether or not Crary's decision to divide the history of vision into a seventeenth- and eighteenth-century geometric period to be followed by a nineteenth-century physiological period was influenced by Crary's politics, his treatment of Berkeley shows that this periodization cannot be made to fit the facts.

Whatever else is true of Crary's account, it is not a story about what actually happened. Does this matter? Crary tells his story in order to get us to rethink our allegiance to a different story, a story about visual representation. He is suggesting that the rupture between perspectivalism and impressionism should be located not as events in the history of visual representation itself suggest, in the 1870s and 1880s, but rather should be seen as part of a wider rupture, taking place earlier in the century. To the extent that I have not challenged his account of optics in the nineteenth century, I have not said anything to discourage Crary's attempt to place our understanding of visual representation in a wider framework. But I have challenged his account of this rupture, and this in the end casts doubt on his enterprise. I have suggested that close attention to the texts of Descartes and Berkeley not only suggest that what dramatic changes occurred in the understanding of the nature of vision took place in the eighteenth and not in the nineteenth century, they also suggest that they took place as the result of a dialogue. The story these texts tell is not one of rupture, of a break in the pattern. Instead, we trace an ongoing conversation. And this suggests to me that any patterns that emerge are going to be limited to the subject of the conversation, to concern, in this case, the history of vision, and will intersect only in very complex ways, with other conversations.

Crary himself explicitly disagrees with any attempt to see the history of vision as displaying developmental continuities. He writes: "It would be completely misleading to pose the camera obscura as an early stage in an ongoing autonomization and specialization of vision that continues into the nineteenth and twentieth centuries. Vision can be privileged at different historical moments in ways that simply are not continuous with one another" (*TO*, p. 57). I have tried to show that the appearance of a lack of continuity is an artifact of Crary's method of privileging a single paradigm, the camera obscura, as capturing the thought of an age. The camera obscura does provide a fitting metaphor for both an epistemological and an optical theory in which the knower or perceiver is provided with an optical truth. Crary, in common with numerous others, tends to identify this theory as Descartes's. Unfortunately, this image is not a very accurate portrayal of either Descartes's epistemology or his theory of vision. It provides an easy way of reading Descartes, one that sees him as upholding a naive faith in vision, itself a view with which many readers feel comfortable. More accurate readings of Descartes are harder to sustain because they portray Descartes as struggling with issues that actually tend to undermine our faith in vision. Such more accurate, richly textured readings are in the end, however, more worthwhile when it comes to challenging those views that in the present seem natural to us.

Crary has, I think, adopted a certain ethos that recommends that the right way to understand some event or phenomenon, such as the emergence of modern art, is to place it against a historical background. And it is hard to quarrel with a well-intentioned program such as is implied by this method. But perhaps in the long run, history is hard enough to do properly that it ought to be left to the historians. What I think in the end is not appropriate is to expect to be able to read off the answer to a contemporary problem via a quick dive back into the past. I have tried to suggest that when the past is approached on its own terms, it yields a richness that can be obscured when we look at prior events simply in order to "understand" how we got from there to here. Such an approach can create the caricature of Descartes, who turns out, more often than not, simply to be represented as "not us," whomever we happen to be.

Finally, to treat Descartes as the spokesperson for an age entirely obscures the actual function he tended to provide for the thinkers immediately following him. While there may be a sense in which Descartes articulated the vision of an age, if matters are looked at in a more fine grained way, it becomes clear that his actual role was to provoke dispute and controversy, as in one way or another people struggled to move beyond the problems and inconsistencies his thought so amply demonstrated. Berkeley's work on vision shows how it is possible to draw on Descartes in order to refute him. A method such as Crary's, which papers over the way thinkers at one time disagree with each other in order to highlight discontinuities between one period and another, makes it harder to observe the actual connections and the nature of the connections as they exist between one period and the next. It is in fact in the end such close attention to detail that reveals the artificial nature of any particular system of periodization.

There is a way in which Descartes dominates the history of philosophy, but it is from the vantage point of the present. Descartes has come to stand for a certain model of rationality and clarity that, for better or worse, is now identified with the nature of philosophy. But we get a different view of Descartes if we look more closely at what he had to say about specific issues that engaged him, and we tell a different story when we start with Descartes and move forward. As far as the history of vision is concerned, when we tell such a story that starts with Descartes and moves forward, then Berkeley eclipses Descartes. But if we tell a story that embodies our current pictures of these two men, then Descartes certainly outshines Berkeley—quite hides him, in fact, by his own brightness.

Margaret Atherton

Acknowledgments

Work on this chapter was in part supported by a grant from the Institute for the Humanities at the University of Wisconsin, Madison. I thank the Fellows of the institute for conversations that were very useful in helping me frame the issues discussed here. I am also grateful to Robert Schwartz and David Michael Levin for helpful suggestions to improve this chapter.

Notes

1. Martin Jay *Downcast Eyes: The Denigration of Vision in Twentieth Century French Thought* (Berkeley: University of California Press, 1993), p. 69. See also "Scopic Regimes of Modernity" in *Vision and Visuality*, ed. Hal Foster (Seattle: Bay Press, 1988).

2. Richard Rorty, *Philosophy and the Mirror of Nature* (Princeton: Princeton University Press, 1979).

3. I have written about a similar manifestation of the phenomenon among some recent feminist theorists in "Cartesian Reason and Gendered Reason," in *A Mind of One's Own: Feminist Essays on Reason and Objectivity*, ed. Louise M. Antony and Charlotte Witt (Boulder, Colo.: Westview Press, 1993).

4. Jonathan Crary, *Techniques of the Observer: On Vision and Modernity in the Nineteenth Century* (Cambridge: MIT Press, 1990). Further references to this book will occur within the body of the text, abbreviated as *TO.*

5. Further discussion of Crary's work can be found in W. J. T. Mitchell, "The Pictorial Turn," *ArtForum* (March 1992):89–94.

6. For some further accounts that recognize the complexity of Descartes's work on vision, see Dalia Judowitz, "Vision, Representation and Technology in Descartes" (pp. 63–86), and Stephen Houlgate, "Vision, Reflection and Openness" (pp. 87–123), both in *Modernity and the Hegemony of Vision*, ed. David Michael Levin (Berkeley: University of California Press, 1993). Houlgate also very interestingly discusses the relationship between Descartes and Berkeley on vision.

7. Judowitz has a very nice discussion of the role of this image in Descartes's account of vision in "Vision, Representation and Technology."

8. René Descartes, *Discourse on Method, Optics, Geometry and Meteorology* trans. Paul Olscamp (Indianapolis: Bobbs-Merrill, 1961), pp. 101–102. Further references to this work will be in the text as *O* and page number.

9. For further discussion of the issues involved, see Margaret Wilson, "Descartes on the Perception of Primary Qualities," in *Essays on the Philosophy and Science of René Descartes*, ed. Stephen Voss (New York: Oxford University Press, 1993), pp. 162–176.

10. *The Works of George Berkeley Bishop of Cloyne,* ed. A. A. Luce and T. E. Jessop (London: Thomas Nelson and Sons, 1948), vol. 1. All references to this work will be in the text as *TVV*, with the section number.

11. *TO*, p. 95, quoting *The Works of John Ruskin,* 15:27.

12. *Essay towards a New Theory of Vision,* 28, *Works,* vol. 1. All further references will be in the text as *NTV* and section number.

13. Crary writes: "What is *not* addressed in this study are the marginal and local forms by which dominant practices of vision were resisted, deflected, or imperfectly constituted. The history of such oppositional moments needs to be written, but it only becomes legible against the more hegemonic set of discourses and practices in which vision took shape" (*TO*, p. 7).

14. J. S. Mill, "Bailey on Berkeley's Theory of Vision" in *Dissertations and Discussions* (New York, 1973), p. 84.

5

Embodying the Eye of Humanism:
Giambattista Vico and the Eye of *Ingenium*

Sandra Rudnick Luft

In response to the question asked him by Jean Beaufret, "How can we restore meaning to the word 'humanism'?" Martin Heidegger lays bare an original complicity between humanism and the metaphysical determination of human essence. Humanism is metaphysical, and metaphysics determines the essence of *humanitas* without asking the truth of Being. That essence was fixed for the West in the Roman mistranslation of *zōon logon echon* as *animal rationale*, the positing of *animalitas* as *anima* (soul), and *anima* as *animus sive mens* (spirit and mind), and ultimately as subject, person, or spirit (*Geist*).[1] In the context of that metaphysical formulation, epistemic concerns came to the fore in the tradition. With René Descartes's secularization of the soul as *res cogitans*, humans became epistemological subjects, knowers, and Descartes's age the "age of the world picture."

Heidegger insists that the moderns' objectification, representation, and systematization of an object of knowledge for that subject was already implicit in Greek metaphysics. It was Plato who identified Being as the unchanging, characterized the unchanging as *eidos* and *eidos* as the rational and intelligible, and attributed the possibility of knowledge of the intelligible to a *homoiosis* between *eidos* and what was essential to humans, which he identified as soul. The soul's "likeness" to being—its nature as self-moved and therefore immortal and ontologically distinct from the physical body—ensured the possibility of knowledge as

a contemplative activity of the soul. From the earliest Greek philosophers, contemplation was characterized in the language of
vision. Knowledge grounded on the *homoiosis* of soul and the
intelligible was *theoria*, an immediate contemplation of the eternal, unchanging, and necessary by what was "like." *Theoria* was
an "active viewing which enabled us to assimilate to the divine,"
producing in the soul a sublime state of wonder or rapture.[2] The
conception of knowledge as ocularcentric, an active seeing of
what is, persisted into the modern period, despite the fact that
the object of knowledge was no longer presumed to be either
ontologically given or divine, and the viewing was no longer
contemplative. In the context of the metaphysically overdeter-
mined nature of the activity of knowing, all other activities and
forms of mediation with the world were devalued. Doing (*praxis*)
and making (*poiēsis*), and whatever mediatory role language
played, for example, were devalued when measured against the
immediacy and clarity of specularity.

Heidegger's critique of modernism as the age in which representation came to the fore and the world became a "structured
image that is the creature of man's producing which represents
and sets before," is a condemnation of the enframing tendencies
of that ocularcentric epistemology.[3] Humanism, "that philosophical interpretation of man which explains and evaluates whatever
is, in its entirety, from the standpoint of man and in relation to
man," is for him the source of the nihilism Nietzsche claimed to
be the *telos* of the entire tradition.[4] "In the planetary imperialism
of technologically organized man ... subjectivism ... attains its
acme, from which point it will descend to the level of organized
uniformity and there firmly establish itself. This uniformity becomes the surest instrument of total, i.e., technological, rule over
the earth."[5] Immediately after this apocalyptic pronouncement,
however, and his acknowledgment that "man cannot, of himself,
abandon this destining of his modern essence or abolish it by
fiat," Heidegger says, "but man can, as he thinks ahead, ponder
this: Being subject as humanity has not always been the sole possibility belonging to the essence of historical man, which is always
beginning in a primal way, nor will it always be. A fleeting cloud

shadow over a concealed land, such is the darkening which that truth as the certainty of subjectivity ... lays over a disclosing event [*Ereignis*] that it remains denied to subjectivity itself to experience."[6]

Heidegger's critique of modernism's enframing of the world as picture at the twilight of the age is matched by one that foresaw the dangers inherent in the objectifying eye of intellect at its dawning. Giambattista Vico was among the first to sound the alarm against the totalizing tendencies of system inherent in Cartesian philosophy, against that "unlimited power for the calculating, planning, and molding of all things" that Descartes's optical conception of philosophic method ensured. Vico did this in the name of humanism, and in his early writings his humanism was that of the philosophic and the Latin rhetorical traditions that the age had cast aside in its desire for the certainty of objective knowledge. Although Vico's humanism would remain anthropocentric, by the third edition of the *New Science*, his last work, his emerging understanding of the existential condition of being-human freed him from precisely that subjectivist assumption that Heidegger thought determinate of Western humanism. The understanding of being-human that he finally achieved was his way of saying to his age that "Being subject as humanity has not always been the sole possibility belonging to the essence of historical man."

Vico had grasped the meaning of what he called the master key of the *New Science*, that the "first gentile peoples" were " 'poets,' which is Greek for 'creators.' " He claimed it had cost him "the persistent research of almost all our literary life, because with our civilized natures we [moderns] cannot at all imagine, and can understand only by great toil, the poetic nature of those first men."[7] He had come to understand a way of being in the world that was wholly "indefinite," wholly embedded in the world, wholly open to what showed up. *Humanitas* was not given but made. His "poets" were not themselves humans but makers of the human, and making (*poiēsis*) was the activity not of subjects or of subjectivity but of language. Language was eventful: it had the power to make what did not exist in nature or thought, the power of setting up a world. *Poiēsis* was a way of seeing as well, but its vision was not that of the eye of soul or rational intellect. It was the imaginative, inventive (*ingenium* in Latin, *ingegno* in Italian) vision of corporeal beings. The eye of *ingenium* did not represent or enframe what it saw. Its way of seeing was itself originary and ontological—the making of a real, though fictive, world within which the poets lived human, that is, social lives.[8]

Vico's contemporaries, caught by the power of intellectual sight, could not understand the poetic vision he attributed to humans. Ironically, however, even those who have read him appreciatively since the eighteenth century have not understood just how innovative Vico's understanding of *humanitas* had become. They themselves succumbed to what Vico called the "common property of the human mind," that of judging the unknown by what is familiar and at hand.[9] Nothing was more "familiar" to Vico's tradition than the identification of *humanitas* with soul or subjectivity, the priority of epistemic concerns, and the privileging of an objectifying gaze. Thus, despite their awareness of Vico's "strangeness," his readers have always interpreted him in the context of epistemological concerns. His principle, *verum et factum convertuntur*, the convertibility of the true and the made, was understood as an epistemological principle delimiting knowledge to that which the knower has made, thus providing a theoretical justification for the historical knowledge Descartes did not think possible. The making of the philosopher-historian was understood as an intellectual activity and the made in some sense a conceptual product of thought. Neoplatonic interpreters of Vico, for example, "remake" in their own minds the *storia ideale eterna* of divine providence, while historicists derive an empathic understanding of the primitive "minds" of the makers of history and the knower using recollective imagination (*fantasia*) "correctly orders [historical] events" of the original imaginative process.[10] Each of these interpretations, and in effect almost all interpretations of the *New Science,* make the assumption that though Vico countered the Cartesian conception of knowledge, he retained the view of humans as subjective beings. This makes it possible to read him in a way that ultimately legitimates the epistemic concerns of the philosopher-historian. His accomplishment, it is claimed, was a justification of humanist and historical knowledge against the claims of rationalist and scientific method. Vico is credited with the humanist response to Cartesian epistemology that led to historicism and the development of the human sciences in the nineteenth century. By placing Vico within the epistemological project of modernity, however, this interpretation takes for granted his position within the Cartesianism he struggled to reject.

This view of Vico is so pervasive that despite acknowledgment of the uniqueness of his thought, there have been no sustained challenges to the notion that Vico's philosophical concerns were epistemological and that he agreed with his contemporaries in conceiving of humans as subjective beings. To this day, his identification with the dominant assumptions of Western humanism remains widely unquestioned. Yet such a "rethinking" is as important today as it was when Pietro Piovani questioned the "presumed affinities" between Vico and Hegelian idealism, arguing that since "in the context of contemporary philosophy" it has become possible to "discern the multiplicity of the forms of historicism, and to combat the monopolistic claims of one form ... over the others, doubt concerning the essential affinity ... [between] Vico and Hegel acquires particular value."[11] A similar situation exists today in the context of postmodern critiques of the presumption of subjectivity in Western humanism and the hegemony of epistemology that presumption enables. As Piovani's doubts led to richer, more diverse readings of Vico, so too can doubts concerning the presumed role of subjectivity in his conception of human nature lead to an appreciation of the more original, alien, and tragic humanism taking shape in Vico's writings. I am not suggesting yet another anachronistic reading of Vico as historical or theoretical precursor to postmodern writers. Rather, insofar as recent critiques of traditional and modernist views denaturalize the presumption of humans as subjective beings and contextualize the historical and cultural origins of that presumption, they serve to correct the co-optation of Vico's writings for epistemological concerns. It is that co-optation that may itself be anachronistic.

Because of his critique of rationalism and its method and his relation to the rhetorical tradition, Vico seemingly escaped the ocularcentrism of the tradition. As one commentator, reemphasizing Vico's ties to the rhetorical tradition, says, "Vico operated with an oral analogue for intellect, which he inherited from classical and humanist rhetoric, rather than with the visual analogue for intellect developed by Descartes with sources in Plato."[12] I agree with this claim as far as it goes. Vico was, however, more than an inheritor of the past: he was a highly original thinker— so original that his thinking was ultimately alien to his tradition. His struggles to understand an original condition of human existence took him beyond that tradition, beyond the mere revaluing of the rhetorical over the philosophic or the substitution of an imaginative for an intellectual subjectivity, to an understanding of a different way of being in the world. Vico did draw on an oral analogue, but orality became for him a new and alien—a poetic—way of seeing. By reading the *New Science* as Vico's realization of that poetic way of seeing, I argue for an appreciation of his "unfamiliarity," an appreciation of that new and uncanny "poetic" humanism emerging in his writings.

Vico signaled the turn from one kind of vision to another in his explanation of the frontispiece in the *New Science,* when he identified the "luminous triangle with the seeing eye" at the upper left corner as God with the aspect of providence. Lady metaphysic, standing on the globe of the world in "ecstasy contemplates [in] Him ... the world of human minds ... in order to show His providence in the ... world of nations." The "ray of divine providence illuminate[s] a convex jewel" on the breast of metaphysics and is reflected from there to the statue of Homer, the first gentile author. This indicates "that the knowledge of God does not have its end in metaphysic taking private illumination from intellectual institutions ... as hitherto the philosophers have done ... but ... [in metaphysic] enabl[ing] us finally to descend into the crude minds of the first founders of the gentile nations, all robust sense and vast imagination ... [and thence] to poetic wisdom ... the first wisdom of the world."[13] In this imagistic way, Vico announced a different conception of metaphysic, a metaphysic of poetic wisdom, and a way of seeing that differed from the vision of the philosophers in not presupposing subjectivity.

The persistent research that brought Vico to his master key—that the first men were poets—began in his early commitment to the more traditional humanisms of Platonism and the Latin rhetorical tradition. He drew on those traditions when he returned to Naples after an absence of nine years, "a stranger in his own land," to find that "the physics of René Descartes has eclipsed all preceding systems."[14] He was critical of the primacy Cartesian philosophy gave to method and warned of the pernicious effects of method on pedagogy—the impoverishment of the ability to think imaginatively and inventively—and indeed on social existence in general.

Most threatening in the priority that the moderns gave to geometric method was the elimination of concern for the probable. The moderns distinguished between the arts of discovery and of judgment, and they identified philosophy entirely with the latter. For Vico, however, criticism and judgment must be preceded by the art of discovery, which he attributed to invention (*ingenium*). For the rhetorical tradition, *ingenium* was that part of imagination that "connects disparate and diverse things."[15] "Disparate and diverse" things are accumulated inductively by perception and organized by verisimilitude into topics. Topical thinking was the source of eloquence and the common sense of social beings, which made men "apt in the affairs of civil life."[16]

In an early work, *De antiquissima Italorum sapientia*, Vico characterized the rhetorical faculty of *ingenium*, so fundamental to his pedagogy, as an essential faculty of the soul. His materialist conception of the soul as air and motion (*conatus*) was closer to that of Epicurus than to Plato.[17] More specifically the soul was "a faculty of making ... the word *facultas* ... signif[ying] an unhindered and ready disposition for making (*facere*). Hence, faculty is the ability to turn power into action. The soul is power, sight an activity, and the sense of sight a faculty." Making begins, he thought, in the corporeal senses: there was, indeed, "no sect of gentile philosophy that recognized that the human mind was free from all corporeity. Hence they thought every work of the mind was sense." This truth of the corporeality of "mind" (he continued to use the language of subjectivity throughout his life) Vico distinguished from the truths of revealed religion. "But our religion teaches that the mind is quite incorporeal."[18] He identified the corporeal skills that were the sources of making as perception, memory (in which perceptions were stored), and, since memory "also signified the faculty that fashions images," imagination.

Ingenium, which, Vico said, was one and the same as *natura*, was the inventive capacity of imagination. Its ability to "connect disparate and diverse things" was first used in geometry, from which the term derived its original meaning, "acute."[19] Because "an acute wit penetrates more quickly and unites diverse things," it was considered an art of discovery, a means of "finding something new."[20] Where method "inhibits intuitive wit while aiding facility, [and] dissolves curiosity while providing for truth," "creative *ingenium*" is a synthetic process in which "we do not just discover the truth but make it." A synthetic method of composition, Vico said, would "strengthen the imagination, which is the eye of *ingenium*, just as judgment is the eye of intellect."[21] The eye of *ingenium*, here presented as the source of the intellectual process of making the conceptual truths of mathematics, would later, in the *New Science*, become a poetic way of seeing and making concrete "truths," the social customs and institutions of the real, historical world.

In the *De antiquissima* Vico made use of a little-known scholastic principle to delimit knowing to the activity of making: "*Verum esse ipsum factum*, the true is precisely what is made."[22] Despite his conception of the corporeal nature of the soul in this early work, Vico described making as an intellectual activity, the construction of mathematical truths.[23] It was only through his reading of Grotius in 1717 that Vico came to realize that a more significant *factum* of human making was the making of positive law, and indeed, of all the social institutions of the historical world. He had transformed a logical relation between the true and the made into, first, a historical, then a genetic process. The *factum* of making was recovered from the *certum* of history: the certain his age desired would be found not in rational concepts but in history.

The unquestioned interpretation of Vico's *verum/factum* as an epistemological principle is based on its explicit formulation in the *De antiquissima*. To be sure, Vico continued to use the epistemological language of his tradition—the language of mind and mental activity, of ideas and truth—in his later works. He called his final work a "new science" in the sense that "science" meant the knowledge of causes. "In reasoning of the origins of institutions in the gentile world, we reach those first beginnings beyond which it is vain curiosity to demand others earlier; and this is the divining character of [first] principles. We explain the particular ways in which they came into being, that is to say, their nature, the explanation of which is the distinctive mark of science."[24] Since the causes studied in the *New Science* were historical, philosophers were to give "certainty to their reasoning by appealing to the authority of the philologians" and philologists to "give their authority sanction by truth."[25]

Despite these apparently epistemological characterizations of his work, it must be granted that by the time he wrote the *New Science*, Vico had grasped his master key: that causes in the human world are not only historical but also poetic. Though he stressed the great toil on his part to comprehend the "wild and savage natures" of the poets, even he may not have realized what a radical break with the traditional conception of knowledge and science that master key brought about. It meant, as he stated in an axiom, that "the nature of institutions is nothing but their coming into being at certain times and in certain guises."[26] Knowledge was as subject to this genetic principle as were all other institutions. As a *factum* of making, knowledge was itself conditioned by the process of its making. The knowing that originated in *poiēsis* and was genetically descended from it was not a conceptual activity—not even an activity of subjective thought that was imaginative rather than rational. Rather, it was a way of being in the world. "Knowing" for Vico was an activity of making social customs and institutions in the concrete historical world—what I am calling an ontological process—an activity inseparable from the "knowing" which was, in effect, a hermeneutic understanding by the "knower" that he or she was genetically descended from the original makers of the made and of the truths this process yielded.

Though the poets had neither noncorporeal soul nor rational eye, *ingenium* as a power of the soul to make and know poetically was a way of seeing as well. By the last edition of the *New Science*, Vico had come to understand the poetic way of seeing of the eye of *ingenium* as radically different from that of intellectual sight. He was able to get beyond the Western determination of humans as subjective beings—whether as *animal rationale* or as *imago Dei*—by constructing a different myth of origins than the one in Genesis to which his tradition appealed. His gentiles were not simply fallen. Like Epicurus and Lucretius, Vico went back to a pre-human condition, to the beasts of the forests.[27] In this primitive condition the first men had lost the ability to reason or think, lost language, sociality, and even, eventually, their human bodies. They were sons of the earth (autochthones).[28]

These *giganti* were the tabula rasa on which Vico wrote his own narrative of origins: it is "from these first men, stupid, insensate and horrible beasts, all the philosophers and philologians should have begun their investigations of the wisdom of the ancient gentiles."[29] In the poverty of their condition they had only the corporeal skills of perception, memory, and imagination. Sensations occurred to them as discrete, random, fleeting, retained in memory as randomly as they had been felt until brought together in some way. Imagination was nothing other than the activity of bringing sensations together, while invention made something new out of them. Vico used the word *ingenium*, whose etymology and history he had traced to the ancients, for that activity; but in the *New Science*, *ingenium* became a radically different way of making from that conceived within the tradition. As an activity of making similarities out of differences, of making relations with an "acute" vision, *ingenium* was essentially a metaphoric activity. Metaphor was in fact the mode of "discovery" for the ancients, and the dominant conception was Aristotle's, for whom metaphor "consists in giving the thing a name that belongs to something else ... on [the] grounds of analogy.... A good metaphor implies an intuitive perception of the similarity in dissimilarities."[30] The ancient philosophers could conceive of nothing more originary than that essentially mimetic process. The only model of a radically creative activity Vico's tradition offered was the creation *ex nihilo* of the Old Testament.[31] In the context of what Hans Blumenberg calls their "presumption of order," the ancients had no need—or any cosmological or logical place—for the radically new.

The poetic vision of *ingenium*, which transformed the bestial existence of the poets into a human one, could not, however, have been one of seeing similarities, since even an imaginative activity understood as the "recognition of similarities" presupposes some form of mediation—some process of determining common features, some process of "measuring" newly perceived particulars against the standard of the common. If philosophers had begun their investigations with the *grossi bestioni* as Vico had done, they would have realized, as he had, that the original existential condition of the first men made necessary a more radical way of seeing than the inventive seeing of the ancients. Vico went beyond concern for a formative process within human history to raise more radical questions about the very setting up of that historical world. Seeing had to be both originary and ontological. It had to be originary in seeing what did not already exist in nature or in reason, originary in making fictive images. But it also had to be ontological, in that those fictive images, the only images the poetic eye could see, would constitute the real world for the seers—the only world they could inhabit.

Originary and ontological vision, a way of seeing that is at one and the same time a corporeal, imagistic, linguistic making, is a metaphoric vision. However, in the pages of the *New Science*, metaphor became something other than the purely figurative and mimetic rhetorical activity it had been for Aristotle. The

metaphoric seeing and making that Vico attributed to the poets
was an event in the world, an act of violence that forced together
sensations that did not belong together under the impetus of
violent passions, fixed the identity of dissimilar sensations with
the dissimilarity of language, and fixed as the real and the true
what did not exist in nature or thought.[32] His metaphorical seeing was thus a "disclosing event" in which a world was set up—an
event of ontological import.

In Vico's account of this metaphorical seeing, one can distinguish but not separate two aspects of the "disclosing event": the
making of images that Vico claimed constituted the metaphysics
of the poets, their "forms of being"—and the process of signifying those "forms of being," thus fixing their identity and
meaning. The necessity for poetic imaging and signifying was
due to the poverty of corporeal nature: while individual senses
took in sensations, the *giganti* could not make sense out of them.
By itself, seeing was a kaleidoscope of fleeting, random, disparate
sensations. The poets could make sense of these sensations only
by making them into images and fixing those images with language. Vico gave a vivid account of that poetic imaging in the
narrative of Jove, the first, most important image ever made by
the poets. I shall reproduce at length his account of that violent
conjoining of dissimilar sensations that gave rise to a "confused
idea of divinity" in creatures incapable of thought, because that
event was for Vico the exemplar of poetic vision. To heighten the
traumatic circumstances of the event, he postulated that for several hundred years after the flood, the air was not dry enough to
produce lightning, until

at last the sky fearfully rolled with thunder and flashed with lightning....
Thereupon a few giants ... were frightened and astonished by the great
effect whose cause they did not know, and raised their eyes and became
aware of the sky. And because in such a case the nature of the human
mind leads it to attribute its own nature to the effect, and because in
that state their nature was that of men all robust bodily strength, who
expressed their very violent passions by shouting and grumbling, they
pictured the sky to themselves as a great animated body, which in that
aspect they called Jove ... who meant to tell them something by the hiss
of his bolts and the clap of his thunder.... In this fashion the first

theological poets created the first divine fable, the greatest they ever created: that of Jove, king and father of men and gods, in the act of hurling the lightning bolt; an image so popular, disturbing, and instructive that its creators themselves believed in it, and feared, revered, and worshipped it in frightful religions.[33]

The Jove narrative is the heart of the *New Science*. It is the treasure uncovered by the master key it took Vico twenty years to grasp—his recovery of the poetic nature of the first men. Despite his disclaimer that it is "beyond our power" to enter into their "vast imaginations," his narrative is just that—an imaginative recreation of that originary making. Vico had gone beyond the epistemological vision of the "eye of judgment" to find in the eye of *ingenium* an ontological power of the corporeal soul to make what was not given in nature. In that poetic vision, imaging was a *metaphoric* activity. As such, the word "seeing" is itself a metaphor for all bodily sensing that made up the metaphoric image the poets "saw."

In the midst of the primordial kaleidoscope of sensations, it was not until one opened the eye of *ingenium* that sense could be made. The sensation that opened that poetic eye was that of hearing. When "at last the sky fearfully rolled with thunder and flashed with lightning as could not but follow from the bursting upon the air for the first time of an impression so violent," it was the sound of thunder that forced the poets to raise their bodily eyes and see, for the first time (since they had lived for centuries under the canopy of the trees, eyes downward, without occasion to look up), the vast emptiness of the sky.[34] They saw it with the eye of *ingenium*, an eye whose sight was inseparable from the sound of thunder that evoked it—and from the fear that the sky and the thunder occasioned in them. Their fear was incarnate in their bodily shaking, shouting, and grumbling. When thunder forced the poets to raise their bodily eyes, they projected those bodily sensations and sounds onto the sky and saw—that is, imaged—the sky as the animate body of a god.[35]

The image of the sky as the animate body of Jove is metaphoric in another sense as well, since, for Vico, inventive seeing was one and the same with the event of signification.[36] The image projected onto the sky was "fixed" as a self-identical *res* by the two poetic languages that originated in the same event that made the image: the mute language of gestures and hieroglyphs, which Vico called "divine," and the articulate, poetic language he called "heroic." (A third, vulgar language of men was created at the same time.) Mute hieroglyphic language was a writing—*in* the body and *with* the body—of the image seen with the "eye of *ingenium.*" The beasts imitated the turbulence of a stormy sky, Jove's own violent motions, in their gestures, facial expressions, shaking, pointing, running, which the sound of thunder and the sight of the sky elicited. Those agitated gestures expressed in bodily writing the terror they felt: a writing that, as the bodily imitation of a metaphoric image which in turn signified that image, was trebly metaphoric.

Mute language was accompanied by an articulate language. It began with the sound "*pa*" uttered by the beasts in their terror at the sight of the being imaged in the sky, a sound that fixed that image with the power of a name: "They pictured the sky to themselves as a great animated body, which in that aspect they called Jove." The language that began with the sound *pa* was the language of "poetic locutions of images" made necessary by the incapacity of the poets "to form intelligible class concepts of things."[37] These images were poetic characters that, though concrete and imaginative, were the "universal concepts"—*universale fantastico*—of the poets. But of all their poetic locutions (synechdoche, for example, or metonymy), it was metaphor that enabled the poets to imagine, to envision and create, images of what did not exist in nature: "metaphor ... gives sense and passion to insensate things in accordance with the metaphysics by which the first poets attributed to bodies the beings of animate substances, with capacities measured by their own, namely sense and passions, and in this way made fables of them."[38]

The fables, however, were not mere images and signs. Vico was not an idealist. For him, as for Heidegger, language arises "from the overpowering, the strange and terrible, through man's departure into being. In this departure language was being, embodied in the word: poetry. Language is the primordial poetry in which a people speaks being."[39] Vico reminded his readers that *logos*, which "meant not only word but idea" in the languages of the first men, "meant also deed to the Hebrews and thing to the Greeks."[40] In the text he made it clear that metaphoric vision, the bringing together of the radically dissimilar, is inseparable from the social customs and institutions it occasions. Accordingly, the making of the image of Jove was the origin of religion. Before the face of that image, the fathers fled to caves with the shy women with whom they would produce the first families, thus establishing the institutions of marriage and burial. Those institutions led to the labor of clearing the forests, tilling the soil, building walled cities, originating crafts, making laws and constitutions, and performing the ritual aspects of communal life.[41]

Vico gave us an ironic image of this setting up of a world, at one and the same time an activity of poetic vision and an activity of concrete physical labor, with the Cyclops. He attributed Homer's reference to giants with one eye in the middle of their forehead to the corruption of the "true heroic phase" that "every giant had his *lucus*." The word *lucus* meant both "clearing" and "eye," and the original meaning of the term referred to the first *orbes terrarum* of the poets, the lands they cleared and cultivated, which were always circular. Thus every clearing "was called a *lucus*, in the sense of an eye."[42] With a fanciful etymology Vico associated the poetic vision of the giants with the clearing of the forests and brought together the two senses—Heidegger's and Marx's—in which a clearing is the setting up of a world.

As poetic imaging and signifying were the makings of all things human, they made human ways of knowing as well. The genetic origin of knowledge was poetic wisdom, made possible by the poetic vision that imaged nature as a signifying system. "The first men ... believed that lightning bolts and thunderclaps were signs made to them by Jove ... [and that t]he science of this language ... [was] divination."[43] Thus the poets were called "sages who understood the language of the gods expressed in the auspices of Jove; and were properly called divine in the sense of diviners, from *divinari*, to divine or predict."[44] From the moment the fathers experienced nature as the language of God, they became wise men, their poetic wisdom consisting in the interpretation of that divine language. The "history of human ideas" began "with divine ideas by way of contemplation of the heavens with the bodily eyes. Thus in their science of augury the Romans used the verb *contemplari* for observing the parts of the sky whence the augures came or the auspices were taken. These religions, marked out by the augurs with their wands, were called temples of the sky, whence must have come to the Greeks their first *theōrēmata* and *mathēmata*, things divine or sublime to contemplate, which eventuated in metaphysical and mathematical abstractions."[45]

Vico found in this history of ideas "the rough origins both of the practical sciences in use among the nations and of the speculative sciences which are now cultivated by the learned," and he traced the development of human wisdom from the interpretive study of the auspices: theology, law, mathematics, astrology, astronomy, chronology, and geography.[46] Because those studies were not the contemplative activities of soul or mind, however, but a "contemplation with bodily eyes," they were practices that took place within the *sensus communis*, the world of shared social and linguistic customs. They were inseparable as well from the "mechanical arts" and from the physical labor without which that social world could not exist.

Vico traced the history of ideas that originated in poetic wisdom and divination to the making of mind, subjectivity, and abstract ideas at the end of the heroic age. At the moment when the Athenians established popular commonwealths, philosophy arose, "ordained by providence to take the place of religion in prompting virtuous actions."[47] Toward this end providence "permitted eloquence to arise" from philosophy and become impassioned for justice. The making of abstract thought also took place within the institutions of the social world, particularly in the practice of jurisprudence "in the great assemblies," where "intellect was brought into play" in the abstraction of "universal legal concepts." Thence grew up the notion of a "common rational utility," of "rights which did not attach to corporeal things," and were thus "modes of spiritual substance."[48] It was through the example of "agreement in an idea of an equal utility common to all ... that Socrates began to adumbrate intelligible genera or abstract universals by induction," and Plato, "reflecting how in public assemblies the minds of particular men, each passionately bent on his private utility, are brought together in a dispassionate idea of common utility ... raised himself to the meditation of the highest intelligible ideas."[49]

The emergence of philosophy as "eloquence" was the high point of human development, but it was not to last. It was followed by philosophic skepticism, false eloquence, civil wars and total disorder, the perfect tyranny of anarchy and "the unchecked liberty of the free peoples," which characterized the age of men.[50] At that point, for Vico as for Heidegger, "only a God can save us," but even salvation took the form of the end of days. For those "rotting in the ultimate civil disease," who had reverted to the state of wild beasts living in a "deep solitude of spirit and will," each pursuing his own interest, providence ordained an extreme remedy: "Through obstinate factions and desperate civil wars, they shall turn their cities into forests and the forests into dens and lairs of men. In this way, through long centuries of barbarism, rust will consume the misbegotten subtleties of malicious wits that have turned them into beasts made more inhuman by the barbarism of reflection than the first men had been made by the barbarism of sense."[51]

The genetic process that originated in the glorious vision of the eye of *ingenium* and led to the making of intellect in the heroic age continued in the age of men, though in that period "making" took place as the pedagogic practices of men capable of abstract thought. In this regard it is important to bear in mind that in his early writings, Vico had distinguished between two very different pedagogies: one that strengthened the "eye of judgment" and the skills of analysis, leading to such methodic philosophies as the Cartesian; and a second, which nurtured the inventive vision of imagination with the study of "eloquence," of languages, literature, jurisprudence. For Vico those practices described not merely two different pedagogies but two different ways of being in the world.

The first way of being was that of Cartesian subjects, cut off from their own imaginative natures and from the *sensus communis* of social beings. It was the existence and optics of beings incapable of civic life. Vico did not hold out much hope for preventing a fall into that barbarism of detached and disembodied reflection. In the parable in the *Autobiography* with which he narrated his own life, however, he suggested a way of retaining access to imaginative vision by means of a different pedagogy. He did so by creating a fable of himself as an outsider alienated from his contemporaries by virtue of a fall he suffered at age seven, which kept him from formal schooling and the methodic pedagogy of the day. This estrangement deepened with his nine-year absence from Naples during the very period in which Cartesian philosophy reached its ascendancy. Vico presented himself as an autodidact, pursuing the study of languages, law, history, poetry, oratory, and topics that strengthened the natural skills of perception, memory, and imagination. He claimed that those studies nurtured his imaginative eye—and the practice of eloquence that makes men "apt in social existence." Those studies enabled him, "after long labor," to discover the master key of the *New Science*.

Vico's autodidactic development had indeed enabled him to "know" in a way different from his contemporaries. The natural law theorists and Cartesian philosophers understood all human existence in accordance with their own rational nature. They had fallen into the conceit of scholars, "who will have it that what they know is as old as the world."[52] Their rationalism had forgotten its own origins. By contrast, Vico's philosopher-historian was a knower who did not forget the origins of his knowledge: Vico's new science would be a science of origins. Those origins were not only historical and genetic, however, but poetic, that is, originary. In making the *factum* of the historical world, *poiēsis* had made both the *verum* humans could know and the "knowers" capable of recovering the true. The way the true was known, however, was itself conditioned by the poetic nature of its origin and by the educational practices that enabled knowers to become philosopher-historians.

Vico's distinction between two ways of knowing—the epistemic and the poetic—and thus two kinds of science and two different pedagogies, is also a distinction between two ways of seeing: an intellectual vision proper to the disembodied, denatured eye of reason abstracted from history, culture, and life, and the originary, ontological, metaphoric vision of the "eye of *ingenium*." Intellectual vision is based on the assumptions foundational to philosophy: a *homoiosis* between knower and known and the determination of humans as souls, minds, eventually subjects. In contrast to this, the principle of the second way of seeing was *verum/factum*. Though *verum/factum* did not assume that *homoiosis* which made epistemic knowledge possible, it did contain a poetic variant of the belief that only like can know like. Knowing and making were united in the maker, since it was the activity of making that enabled the maker to be a knower.[53]

As the philosopher-historians were the genetic descendants of the poets, their way of knowing was genetically descended from the poetic way of knowing. Poetic wisdom began in divination, the interpretive "science of that language" that the poets "envisioned" in the sky. Moreover, poetic knowing was thus hermeneutic, for the language that the poets interpreted was one they themselves had written, which meant that the meaning they could find in it was only the meaning they had put there. Poetic wisdom was an artifact of poetic making.

The historical process that began in poetic making would lead, for Vico, to ways of knowing in the age of men: both the way of rationalist philosophers and the way of philosopher-historians. The philosophers, however, would not remember that humans were the makers of their ideas, nor that they did so by means of the power of language. Instead, they would attribute their ideas to the intellectual seeing with which the eye of their rational soul contemplated being. The making of knowing that took place in the methodic practices of the philosophers would culminate in the making of the rational systems of natural law theorists and Cartesian philosophers, who also forgot the linguistic and social origins of their rational way of knowing and their own rational nature.

Sandra Rudnick Luft

The second way of knowing in the age of men was the one that strengthened the imaginative skills of humans and accordingly strengthened the bonds that bring humans together in the social world. It would make possible the philosopher-historian's discovery of the master key of the *New Science*. It was a way of knowing genetically descended not only from poetic making but from the wisdom of the poets. As their poetic wisdom was a "divining" of the signs they had made with imaginative vision, so too the "knowing" of the philosopher-historian was a divining of the originary language that made the *factum* of history. The truth this second way of knowing and seeing yielded was, ultimately, the understanding that has always been at the heart of hermeneutics: the truth that what one knows one has made oneself, the understanding that truths do not have epistemic import, but that they are artifacts of linguistic and social practices. The philosopher-historians knew that, as humans, they were genetically descended from those poet-makers of the human world; and they knew that, *as knowers*, their knowing was genetically related to divination.

The philosopher-historian knew himself to be a descendant of the poets in a third sense as well: he knew that insofar as he was a descendant of the first men who were makers, he was himself a maker. As the first men had made the human world and their poetic wisdom with language, so too the philosopher-historian made a textual narrative about that originary making. The *New Science* was Vico's narrative, a narrative remaking of originary historical making—an act of making performatively telling the reader that the narrator knew himself as maker, an acting out of the truth that humans are makers who make their own human reality and their truths, and do so with language.

The sense in which the *New Science* is itself a making has not been appreciated because it has always been understood within the context of epistemology, albeit as a quirky, idiosyncratic, "humanist" variant of epistemology. If, however, the "knowledge" of the philosopher-historian is his self-understanding that he and all ways of knowing are artifacts of an originary making, then his way of knowing cannot be other than a making as well, the making of a narrative about that making. The significance of narrative in Vico's new, poetic science is missed when it is read as epistemology. In the words of one commentator, "To apprehend human nature, one must know, not an essence or definition, but a story. The narrative provided by the *New Science* is therefore the essential vehicle by which human nature comes to be recognized by human beings: narration for Vico is the means—the only means—of human self-recognition.... The presence to self achieved through the narration of the ideal eternal history is not described, but produced."[54] I agree with this interpretation, but I believe that the "recognition" that takes place in narration, the self-presentation that takes place in the production of the narrative, takes place for the self not only in the narrative but also in the very making of the narrative. The *New Science* is the vehicle of this recognition, not only in that it recounts a story in narrative form of the making of history, but in that it is a performative linguistic remaking, by the narrator, of that originary linguistic process.

Vico distinguished *his* performative narrative from rationalist epistemologies written by philosophers who had forgotten the poetic origins of their science by making his in his own metaphoric language, re-creating the metaphoric making of the first men. His first men are *giganti*, for example, and *grossi bestioni*; his heroes Cyclops; the pattern of history a *storia ideale eterna*; history itself a *corso*, then a *ricorso*. Vico's metaphors are ironic, to be sure, because, unlike the poets, he not only created his metaphors and images but knew them to be his creations. They are a way of reminding his readers that he knew his truths did not have epistemic import, that they did not reflect either actual historical events or an ideal pattern of history, but rather are made in his own ironic, poetic, textual narrative. They remind his readers that in the age of men, the only way of knowing that escapes the barbarism of reflection is the one that remembers its own origins in originary language. It is therefore doubly ironic that Vico's readers have found the *New Science* obscure precisely because it was written in metaphors, not realizing that those metaphors were a sign to them that they could not read the *New Science* as a traditional work containing truth in any epistemic sense, but must read it, rather, as an exemplary instance of the metaphoric way in which truth is made.

There is another sense in which Vico told his readers that his narrative was a performative remaking of an originary making. Vico called the *New Science* a *Rational Civil Theology of Divine Providence* because it was a "history of the institutions by which, without human discernment or counsel, and often against the designs of men, providence has ordered this great city of the human race." He was referring to the fact that, in the *New Science*, he identified as "providential" the immanent means by which the private and egocentric choices of the men of the divine and heroic ages realized social ends. Stoics, Epicureans, and natural philosophers, who found in history only fate, chance, or the "order of natural things," should "have studied [providence] in the economy of civil institutions," Vico claimed, "in keeping with the full meaning of applying to providence the term 'divinity,' [i.e., the power of divining], from *divinari*, to divine, which is to understand what is hidden *from* men—the future—or what is hidden *in* them, their consciousness."[55]

In identifying divination as a power "hidden in [men]," a power by which human choices realized social ends, Vico was claiming that the activity of finding social purpose and meaning in history is that of divination. The divination of the philosopher-historian—the study of the workings of providence in the "economy of civil institutions"—was genetically related to the divination practiced by the poets. In "divining" mind in nature, poetic vision saw the natural world as meaningful—that is, as the language of Jove—and made the human world by imitating that language. Just so, by "divining" mind in historical institutions, the philosopher-historian—Vico—made a narrative that made history meaningful. What the poets called Jove, the philosopher-historian called the providence of his narrative.[56] The image of divine providence was the greatest of the metaphors that Vico made in his narrative. It was an ironic image of that "mind" or "order" that both poets and philosopher-historians "found" in the human world. In creating that ironic metaphor, Vico expressed his understanding that mind in history was created by the poets. What was ultimately "divine" was not the *factum* "Jove" that the poets had created, or the *factum* "providence" that the narrator of the *New Science* created, but the creators—poets and philosopher-historians—themselves. When Vico claimed that the narrator of the *New Science* and his readers received a divine pleasure from the narrative, since only in God "knowing and creating are one and the same thing," he was reminding his readers of the sense in which they too were "divine." Unlike the first poets, who made without knowing, Vico and his readers knew they were the makers of their history.

I began this chapter with Heidegger's comment—as much plaint as challenge—that "being subject as humanity has not always been the sole possibility belonging to the essence of historical man." I have argued that Vico's understanding of humans as makers, and of making as the activity of being in the world, is an understanding of a way of being that does not assume subjectivity or lead to the human as subject. That way of being is *poiēsis*, the poetic making of one's human existence through language and social practices—and the physical labor without which beings embodied and embedded in the world of natural necessity could not survive. Vico's poetic anthropology is, in effect, a "new humanism," one that escapes the nihilism inherent in the determination of *humanitas* as soul, spirit, or subjectivity. It does not lead to the hegemony of epistemology, since it understands that, as humans are makers, they make their ways of knowing, and that knowledge can never be more than the hermeneutic understanding of the artifactual, fictive nature of human truths, and of knowers as the makers of those truths. Vico's own *New Science* is itself a narrative performance of that truth of the poetic nature of knowers.

There is no question that in Vico's writings one finds the concerns of a humanist of the rhetorical tradition: an appreciation of the value of communal existence and of the pedagogic and social practices that nurture it. The value of social existence was itself ungrounded and unquestioned for Vico. The belief that humans are humans only insofar as they are social beings was for him as much a metaphysical assumption as was the traditional determination of humans as soul or spirit. There was more, however, to Vico than the traditional humanist; there was also a tragic sensibility, an awareness of the darkness of the forest outside the clearing, of an abyss beyond the fragile institutions of the social world. Above all, there was the anxiety of origins. Ernesto Grassi, the only Vico scholar to explore in depth the affinity between Heidegger and Vico, says:

The essence of Vico's thought is not understood by those who limit themselves to uncovering the function of the imaginative universals as a substitution for rational concepts.... [It] emerges by recognizing— which is rarely done—that the problem of Vico is the realm within which man appears in his concrete and total realization.... Vico has recognized that it is not beings ... which are to be considered the essential subject matter of a new science. With this insight he has hit upon a completely new way of confronting traditional metaphysics.... For Vico the problem of the true is subordinate to the problem of the appearance of human reality. The bursting forth of Being in human historicity from time to time, always in new forms, realizes itself originally in the poetic, imaginative word (*parola fantastica*) in function of which the world appears in its human significance. Vico's problem is that of what opens the realm of human sociality, and he identifies this original opening with the metaphoric, mythic word.[57]

Grassi identifies what I have called the "ontological" rather than epistemological character of the *New Science.* Vico's discovery that humans are poets so incapable of seeing order and meaning in the world around them that they have to make it, took him outside the assumptions of humanism. He was raising the question humanism did not ask—the question of the possibility of human existence at all, of the nature of radical beginnings. He found those radical beginnings in the poetic vision of creatures without the power of intellectual sight.

Hayden White rejected the possibility of a relation between Vico and the "radical wing" of the human sciences in the light of Vico's belief in a philological science of history and the value Vico placed on social existence.[58] But White's conclusion does not do justice to the radical nature of Vico's thought. The genetic relation between the true and the made identified both as artifactual. Although there is no deconstructive play of language in the *New Science*, there is certainly a powerful rhetoric on behalf of the ultimate fictiveness of linguistic constructions. The realization that science, and reality itself, are both human creations, that the relation between them is a hermeneutic circle that never takes us beyond our own making, was as much the radical core of Vico's thought as it was of Nietzsche's.

While Vico believed that humane knowledge and prudential social practices are the only means by which human society could be maintained, he did not have much hope that they would prevail over the barbarism of reflection. Only the hermeneutic understanding that what we know is our own creation reminds us of the artifactuality of our humanity, and that understanding is as finite and fallible as all human artifacts. The abyss is always below the surface, and the fall into it all the more tragic for the fact that humane learning and practices might have kept us from it.[59]

I have come back to the relation between Vico and the "radical wing," and have done so in the context of the distinction between the intellectual vision of humans understood as subjects and knowers, and the poetic vision of beings as makers, which Vico had grasped in his last work. I do so in the spirit in which David Michael Levin invokes Heidegger, Michel Foucault, and Jacques Derrida, each of whom, he says, has "seen, traced and attempted to understand the advent of a distinctly modern form of ocularcentrism ... in his own way and from his own perspective. But ... each has gone beyond critique, using the textuality, the *work* of critique to articulate and practice what might be called 'countervisions': ... historically new ways of seeing, ways that model visions very different in character from the one that has become hegemonic."[60] Once Vico realized the poetic nature of the first men—the poverty of their nature, their only skill that of metaphoric making—he understood the fictive nature of all things human, even the fictive nature of his own poetic narrative of originary making. That understanding of humans as makers of their human world, of the truths of that world, was in effect a new humanism. Though I do not think his tragic

Sandra Rudnick Luft

sensibility allowed him much hope that even a poetic way of seeing could keep us from the abyss, his countervision offered the only alternative to the one that has led to what Heidegger called the "planetary imperialism of technologically organized man" and Vico the "barbarism of reflection."

Notes

1. Martin Heidegger, "Letter on Humanism," in *Basic Writings*, ed. David Farrell Krell (New York: Harper & Row, 1977), pp. 201–203.

2. I have used as references for this discussion of *theoria* Nathan Rotenstreich, *Theory and Practice: An Essay in Human Intentionalities* (The Hague: Martinus Nijhoff, 1977), pp. 3–4; Nicholas Lobkowicz, *Theory and Practice: History of a Concept from Aristotle to Marx* (Notre Dame: University of Notre Dame Press, 1967), pp. 5–8. See also Lobkowicz, "On the History of Theory and Practice," in Terence Ball, ed., *Political Theory and Practice* (Minneapolis: University of Minnesota Press, 1977), pp. 13–27.

3. Martin Heidegger, "The Age of the World Picture," in *The Question Concerning Technology and Other Essays*, trans. William Lovitt (New York: Harper & Row, 1977), p. 134.

4. Ibid., pp. 128–135.

5. Ibid., p. 152.

6. Ibid., p. 153.

7. Giambattista Vico, *The New Science*, trans. Thomas G. Bergin and Max H. Fisch (Ithaca: Cornell University Press, 1988), nos. 34, 376. See also 338, 349, 367.

8. I am not using the term *ontology* in the sense in which Heidegger used it to characterize Western metaphysics but, rather, in what he calls in *Introduction to Metaphysics* its "broadest sense ... [as] the endeavor to make being manifest itself" (p. 41). In this "broadest sense" it is distinguished from predominantly epistemological concerns.

9. Vico, *New Science*, nos. 120, 122.

10. The reference for the last example is Donald Phillip Verene, *Vico's Science of Imagination* (Ithaca: Cornell University Press, 1981), pp. 154–156.

11. Pietro Piovani, "Vico without Hegel," in Giorgio Tagliacozzo and Hayden V. White, eds., *Giambattista Vico: An International Symposium* (Baltimore: John Hopkins University Press, 1976), pp. 110–111. Interpreters who emphasized Vico's "idealism" and "proto-Hegelianism" include Croce, Quinet, Michelet, Cousin, De Sanctis, Spaveti, Gentile, Nicolini, and Berlin.

12. John D. Schaeffer, *Sensus Communis: Vico, Rhetoric, and the Limits of Relativism* (Durham, N.C.: Duke University Press, 1990), p. 3. Another work on Vico's relation to the rhetorical tradition is Michael Mooney, *Vico in the Tradition of Rhetoric* (Princeton, N.J.: Princeton University Press, 1985).

13. Vico, *New Science*, nos. 2, 5–6.

14. Giambattista Vico, *The Autobiography*, trans. Max H. Fisch and Thomas G. Bergin (Ithaca: Cornell University Press, 1963), p. 132. See pp. 128–132.

15. Giambattista Vico, *De antiquissima Italorum sapientia*, trans. L. M. Palmer as *On the Most Ancient Wisdom of the Italians* (Ithaca: Cornell University Press, 1988), pp. 96–97, 104.

16. Vico, *Autobiography*, pp. 124–125.

17. The translator of *Ancient Wisdom*, Palmer, says her translation of Vico's use of *animus* and *anima* as spirit and soul follows the practice of Max Fisch, one of the translators of the *New Science*, rather than "the obvious alternatives 'the principle of life' and 'the principle of feeling.' " (See n. 1, p. 85.)

18. Palmer, *Ancient Wisdom*, p. 93.

19. Ibid., p. 97.

20. Ibid., pp. 96–97. See also Giambattista Vico, *On the Study Methods of Our Time*, trans. Elio Gianturco (New York: Library of Liberal Arts, 1965), p. 24.

21. Ibid., pp. 96–97, 104. See also Vico, *Study Methods*, p. 24. Palmer translates *ingenium* as "mother wit," primarily, she says, because it was the customary term in the period for mental activity. (See n. 5, p. 96.) I agree with Michael Mooney, however, who points out that the term *wit*, associated with aesthetic and literary usage, has a narrower meaning than *ingenium* came to have for Vico, that is, as "mind," "human nature," the "human capacity for making." See Mooney, *Vico*, n. 84, p. 135. Unless quoting directly from Palmer's translation, I shall use the term *invention* for *ingenium*.

22. Ibid., pp. 45–47.

23. Ibid., p. 94. Vico's use of the principle in the *De antiquissima* was thus consistent with earlier scholastic uses. For a longer discussion of Vico's use of the principle, see my "Legitimacy of Hans Blumenberg's Conception of Originary Activity," *Annals of Scholarship* 5, no. 1 (Fall 1987):3–36.

24. Vico, *New Science*, no. 346.

25. Ibid., no. 140. The *verum/factum* principle is not stated explicitly in the *New Science*, but versions of it are expressed in nos. 331 and 349.

26. Ibid., no. 147.

27. Ibid., no. 369. See also nos. 169, 192, 301, 369–370, 524.

28. Ibid., nos. 13, 61, 369–373. Vico speculates that it was perhaps "in abomination of giantism that the Hebrews had so many ceremonial laws pertaining to bodily cleanliness" (no. 371).

29. Ibid., no. 374; see also no. 338.

30. Aristotle, "Poetics," in Richard McKeon, ed., *The Basic Works of Aristotle* (New York: Random House, 1941), 1457b, 1459a.

31. In other writings I have explored the thematic relation between Vico's conception of originary activity and the model of divine creativity in the Old Testament. See my "Legitimacy" and "Creative Activity in Vico and the Secularization of Providence," in Roseann Runte, ed., *Studies in Eighteenth Century Culture* (Madison: University of Wisconsin Press, 1979), 9:337–356; and "Derrida, Vico, Genesis and the Originary Power of Language," *Eighteenth Century: Theory and Interpretation* 34, no. 1 (Spring 1993):65–84.

32. In *Vico, Metaphor, and the Origin of Language*, Marcel Danesi claims Vico attributed all conceptual development to the metaphoric origins of language. Metaphor was the "bridge" between the imagistic character of audio-oral language and concept formation, thus explaining the transition from perceptual to conceptual language. I agree with him on this but differ with his assumption that that process was a mental one. He considers metaphor, *fantasia*, and *ingegno* all as mental activities and says of the metaphoric link between the perceptual and conceptual that "only a conscious mind" could make that link. Marcel Danesi, *Vico, Metaphor, and the Origin of Language* (Bloomington: Indiana University Press, 1993), p. 72; see also pp. 72–77.

33. Vico, *New Science*, nos. 377, 379.

34. Ibid., no. 377.

35. Ibid., no. 376. In stressing hearing over visual "seeing" in the Jove experience, I again differ with Danesi. He bases his argument that for Vico the "first form of consciousness was visual" on several points. First, he considers imaging a visual activity of "internal iconicity," a state of mind resulting from the formations of percepts from bodily sensations on the "deep level." He cites in support such common terms as the "mind's eye" and the "inner eye," which he seems to think universal and natural rather than cultural, an assumption—indeed, the very assumption, along with that of consciousness or subjectivity—which I believe Vico's understanding of poetic nature problematizes (see pp. 84–89). Second, Danesi argues that mute language, the language of the age of gods, was a language of gestures that assumed the priority of vision, while an articulate language did not. This argument does not take seriously Vico's claim that both languages originated together. Danesi supports his position with anthropological and archaeological evidence "that the first expressions of thought are visual, not vocal" (pp. 68, 105). My own understanding of the originary event in Vico is closer to John Schaeffer's, who overall emphasizes the power of the oral and the audio in Vico's writings. "The Jove metaphor is both auditory and visual ... but orality is primary in that it is sound that identifies the sky as alive, and it is sound that provides the opportunity for interpretation. The giants ... respond to the immediacy of sound with bodily fear, which in turn

Embodying the Eye of Humanism

provokes the metaphoric leap" (p. 91), and "In Vico's account language begins, not with men speaking, but with men listening" (p. 87).

36. Danesi seems to think that the metaphoric capacity existed before speech while I am arguing that metaphoric "vision" was as much linguistic as imagistic.

37. Ibid., no. 227.

38. Ibid., no. 205.

39. Martin Heidegger, *An Introduction to Metaphysics*, trans. Ralph Manheim (New Haven: Yale University Press, 1987), pp. 171–172.

40. Vico, *New Science*, no. 401. See no. 225.

41. Ibid., no. 217. It was this aspect of Vico that appealed to Marx. In a footnote in *Das Kapital* he wrote, "As Vico says, the essence of the distinction between human history and natural history is that the former is made by man and the latter is not." Karl Marx, *Das Kapital*, bk. I, pt. IV, chap. 13, n. 89, Quoted in Eugene Kamenka, "Vico and Marxism," in Giorgio Tagliacozzo and Hayden V. White, eds., *Giambattista Vico: An International Symposium* (Baltimore: Johns Hopkins Press, 1976), p. 139.

42. Vico, *New Science*, no. 550.

43. Ibid., no. 379.

44. Ibid., no. 381.

45. Ibid., no. 391.

46. Ibid., nos. 483–484, 490.

47. Ibid., nos. 1038–1040.

48. Ibid., no. 1038.

49. Ibid., no. 1043.

50. Ibid., nos. 1101–1102.

51. Ibid., no. 1106.

52. Ibid., nos. 120, 127.

53. Vico himself asserted the unity of knowing and creating both for the maker and reader of the *New Science*. See 349.

54. Robert P. Crease, "Vico's 'Mirror Stage': Narrative, the *Scienza Nuova*, and the Barbarism of Reflection," *Studies in Eighteenth Century Culture* 24 (1994):107–119. Crease goes on to call "self-apprehension" an ultimate epistemological triumph and to say that Vico "oddly enough precisely at this point appears indebted to the Cartesian model of knowledge." I argue that the narrative is

itself the performative act of "self-apprehension"—though I would call it "self-making"—and does not fulfill an epistemological function.

55. Vico, 342. Though Vico said "hidden in consciousness," the *New Science* was an account of the workings of a "consciousness" wholly embodied in linguistic and social practices. This is another example of Vico's use of traditional language, despite the radical implications of the text.

56. Ibid. I am not making a claim about Vico's conscious intentions or imputing to him antitheological sentiments. My interpretation is based on the implications of the text.

57. Ernesto Grassi, "Vico, Marx, and Heidegger," in Giorgio Tagliacozzo, ed., *Vico and Marx: Affinities and Contrasts* (Atlantic Highlands, N.J.: Humanities Press Inc., 1983), pp. 233–250. Also see Grassi, *Heidegger and the Question of Renaissance Humanism: Four Studies* (Binghamton, N.Y.: Center for Medieval and Renaissance Studies, 1983), and my article in *Historical Reflections* (1994 or 1995) for a comparison of Vico and Heidegger, Nietzsche and Derrida, in which I discuss Grassi's work on Heidegger and Vico.

58. Hayden V. White, "Vico and the Radical Wing of Structuralist/Post-Structuralist Thought Today," *New Vico Studies* (Atlantic Highlands, N.J.: Humanities Press, 1983), pp. 63–68.

59. For other discussions of the relation between Vico and postmodern writers, see my article mentioned above in *Historical Reflections/Reflexions Historiques*, Vol. 22, no. 3, 1996, and an article devoted to Vico and Nietzsche in *The Personalist Forum*, Vol. 10, no. 2, Fall, 1994. For a comparison of the originary understanding of metaphor in Vico and Derrida, see my "Derrida and Vico."

60. David Michael Levin, ed., *Modernity and the Hegemony of Vico* (Berkeley: University of California Press, 1993), p. 7.

6

"For Now We See Through a Glass Darkly": The Systematics of Hegel's Visual Imagery

John Russon

In absolute clearness there is seen just as much, and as little, as in absolute darkness.

—Hegel, *Science of Logic*

What we have learned in this twentieth century is to be wary of the clear-sighted ego, to distrust the ease of daytime vision, to not limit our sights to the waking reality that passes before our eyes. At the end of the century, we have grown suspicious of our easy self-awareness, and we know the need to hunt for ourselves in our dreams, in our diseases, in the darkness of our unconscious, and in the opacity of our bodies. It is the tradition of existential phenomenology that has been our guide through these subterranean grounds of meaning, and it is figures such as Friedrich Nietzsche, Martin Heidegger, Jean-Paul Sartre, and Maurice Merleau-Ponty to whom we would usually think to turn for the discovery that the inconspicuous relationship to the world in which we live and which founds the meaningfulness of the obvious and comfortable world of everyday life is the real center of the dynamism of our experience. These are the figures who have turned us to the prereflective dimensions of our experience, to the Dionysiac, to being-in-the-world, to the prethetic consciousness-(of)-self, to the lived body. It is these figures to whom we would normally turn for the critique of the primacy of the reflective ego. Yet this critique is not new with these figures.

This same turning to the subterranean, the nonreflective, the embodied, is equally at the heart of G. W. F. Hegel's dialectical philosophy, and his conceptual analysis is mirrored in his systematic use of visual imagery.

Hegel's vision-based images correspond to distinct positions and logical roles along the path of knowledge, and dealing with Hegel's use of visual images and metaphors will therefore require that Hegel's conceptual critique of the ego be developed alongside the consideration of the images. We will begin with "reflection," which is an image essentially about the alienation of viewer and viewed, the alienation of truth and its medium of manifestation, the alienation of substance and surface, and "enlightenment," which is an image of a light turned on to illuminate an already existent reality to which the light is a superfluous addition, a light that does not light itself up as the source of illumination. Ordinary consciousness presents as its truth the enlightened, reflective ego, and this ego models its life on the completeness of clear vision; the first principle of this purported truth of ordinary consciousness can thus be formulated as "I = Eye." In criticizing this self to which these images of reflection and enlightenment belong, we will be led to images of darkness, of night, of the cunning and deceptive powers that operate out of sight, behind our backs, concealing themselves from our view, creating for us the very illusion of a daylight in which there is the obviousness and clarity of a fully determinate world already given; the ease with which this reality is presented will belie the fact of its being a product of the labor of a communal subjectivity struggling to find for itself an identity. We will see this labor in the inherently idolatrous religious ritual that simultaneously provides for us the images we need for our self-understanding and fails to see its own purpose behind the images it celebrates. Religion is a system of ritualized practices that establishes for a community an immediate sensible certainty—a faith in the immediacy of one's vision—which offers both a context in which individuals can develop but also a situation that fails to see its own significance and is oppressive in its conservatism. This tension within religion will point us to the necessity for absolute knowing, and we will move, finally, from the religious imagery of light and revelation to speculation as the image for the perfected vision that apprehends the universal light of concrete reason as both the ground and the goal of even our darkest activities. Hegel's philosophy puts an end to the exotifying gaze of the I = Eye of reflective philosophy, and thereby offers us an inherently multicultural vision with which to enter the twenty-first century.

I Now It Is Day: Reflection and Enlightenment

"In ordinary consciousness," Hegel writes in his *Differenzschrift*, "the Ego occurs in opposition. Philosophy must explain this opposition to an object."[1] In ordinary consciousness, in other words, the object appears to us to be something intrinsically other than us. Perfected or absolute knowing, however, is the "pure self-recognition in absolute otherness,"[2] that is, philosophy will ultimately teach us to recognize that the apparent other is really ourselves. It is this gap between ordinary consciousness and absolute knowledge, between the experience of the other as other and the experience of the other as self, that marks out the terrain within which this study will situate Hegel's use of visual rhetoric.

The reflective ego is the self that each of us recognizes from our day-to-day conscious life. When the doorbell rings and I answer, "I'll get it," the subject—both grammatical and experiential—of my sentence is the reflective ego. The reflective ego is the human self as it posits itself—as it recognizes itself—in its explicit acts of noticing itself as a discrete subjectivity. Let us consider what happens when we so reflect. What does experience look like to the reflective ego?

When I say "me," I identify myself in contradistinction to everything else. The act of self-positing is the act of announcing the severance of my self from the world. It is thus implicitly the act of announcing the alienness of the world. The act of saying "I" is precisely the act within ordinary experience in which the opposition of self and other, of subject and object, is announced.

This portrayal of the situation of the reflective ego has its direct analog in Hegel's portrayal of the structures that characterize sight.

Hegel studies sight in the *Zusatz* of section 401 of his *Encyclopedia of the Philosophical Sciences.* His discussion makes it clear why sight is an appropriate metaphor for the rationality of the reflective ego and why the story of reason can easily be told in images of vision: "The really material aspect of corporeity ... does not as yet concern us in seeing. Therefore the objects we see can be remote from us. In seeing things we form, as it were, a merely theoretical, not as yet a practical, relationship; for in seeing things we let them continue to exist in peace and relate ourselves only to their ideal side."[3]

Like the reflective "I," the curious eye takes itself to be encountering an alien reality that is untouched by its gaze. This very alienation of vision from corporeality that gives it the power of ranging universally over a whole field is equally the ground of its inability to really appreciate the reality of its object: "On account of this independence of sight of corporeity proper, it can be called the noblest sense. On the other hand, sight is a very imperfect sense because by it the object does not present itself to us immediately as a spatial totality, not as *body*, but always only as surface."[4] Sight, in other words, is not unbiased in its portrayal of its object but implicitly makes a decision about its nature: "Sight, which is concerned with the object as predominantly self-subsistent, as persisting ideally and materially and which has only an ideal relation to it, senses only its ideal aspect, colour, by means of light, but leaves the material side of the object untouched."[5] There is thus a parallel between the logic of sight and the logic of the reflective ego in that each portrays its object as an alien and self-subsistent reality that it experiences as a surface and not as a body and that it portrays as not affected by the gaze that falls on it or the light that illuminates it.

Hegel's critique of sight as not grasping itself and its other as embodied parallels Hegel's critique of reflection, which in the end is that reflection must unearth a bodily contact that underlies reflection's apparent alienation from its other and is misrepresented in reflection's immediate apprehension of the other as alien and indifferent. If we now follow the dialectic of the reflective consciousness, we will come ultimately to see its need to look behind its back to see what unacknowledged truth its own activity is reflecting, to see what life it embodies. We will see this ultimately when we see the need for "external reflection" to recognize its truth as "determining reflection." We turn first to the ego's self-description to see how the ego's description of itself as immediately opposed to an alien other is not a merely innocent description that latches on to an already existent division within the nature of being but is in fact a performative utterance: the announcement of the separation of subject and object is equally the effecting of this very division. We can see this if we consider the experience of the world as alienated from the self.

As separated from its object, the subject can only be an observer. The key to the metaphysics of the reflective ego is precisely this: since its very definition is to be other to whatever counts as its object, the ego must be an impermeable and independent substance into which nothing alien can ever enter intrinsically (that is, its identity, its "what it is," is not affected) and which can itself never enter into a real participation in its object. The ego is always isolated, single, alien, and an unchanging onlooker; the ego faces the world like the stereotypic North American faces television.

Not only is this ego an alien onlooker; it is furthermore in charge of its own destiny, for, *qua* impermeable, it can only look to itself to account for its condition. Thus the self can only be auto-effecting, and, accordingly, it will get its knowledge of things right when it knows itself as the auto-effecting alien who cannot be a participant in any "external" world—hence the imperative of enlightenment: come to recognize your own truth, and accept the responsibility for your own situation, since you have that responsibility already. Indeed, the enlightenment's charge to the ego is like the charge the academy makes to the stereotypic North American. Advocating something that resembles the image of the light bulb coming on in the head of the inventor, the enlightenment commands the day-to-day self to look at its self: to shine a light—Descartes's "light of nature"—on itself and see what it is really doing.

So the ego on this account is auto-effecting, and therefore it can never encounter anything truly alien to itself. Whatever the ego experiences as object, then, can only ever be its own mirror, its own reflection, and this very fact is the basis of consciousness's intrinsic self-imperative to enlightenment, that is, to the self-reflective recognition of itself as something that can only ever be encountering its own self. We began with the experience of subject and object as mutually alien, and our attention to the implications of this metaphysics has led us to see that the reflective ego is never in a real position to talk about an encounter with an alien. Hence the imperative of enlightenment is the imperative for the reflective ego to acknowledge this truth about itself. And we can thus see why the very nature of our consciousness makes enlightenment seem the right stance. Enlightenment says to ordinary consciousness, "Wake up; open your eyes." Ordinary consciousness, then, naturally tends to reflection and enlightenment as to its truth.

Both reflection and enlightenment, in Hegel's discussions, are players implicated in a logic of day vision, of nonparticipant observation, in the assumed ideal of disinterested, noninvasive access to an (alien) truth that easily reflects off the surface of things. Hegel studies enlightenment as a stance, both personal and cultural, that has a systematic place in the development of the potentialities of human experience, and he studies reflection as a pivotal logical relationship for understanding selfhood and cognition.

Chapter 6 of the *Phenomenology of Spirit* is Hegel's main consideration of enlightenment, and his account is primarily devoted to studying the idea of alienated, self-reliant egohood as a cultural ideal. The world of enlightenment is the world of humanism, the world animated by the scientific revolution, by the spirit of capitalist self-advancement, by the Protestant religion, which "builds its temples and altars in the heart of the individual,"[6] by the secular love of culture as the locus and the product of human self-development. This is very much the world into which our generation has been born. It is the world that is built on the assumption that we can easily see what we ourselves are doing, the world that assumes it knows its own identity easily and immediately, the world criticized by Freud and Marx. The key to this vision of reality is the belief that "you can do it," *simpliciter.* The model for this conception of self-reliance is reason. In reasoning, we work out the answers—the truth—for ourselves, by ourselves. When I find the answer to a mathematical puzzle, I need turn to no one other than myself for confirmation that this answer is correct.[7] Similarly, in a scientific experiment, I know the truth of my results because I did the experiment myself, and, further, I know that any other subject who conducts the same experiment will get the same results. In reasoning, then, we experience ourselves as the bearers of the criterion of truth. Rather than having to look to outside authority to justify our views, we know that anyone outside, if they are to claim truth for their views, must conform to what we ourselves know. Hegel's phenomenological description of this view of the self-reliance of the rational being as it functions as a cultural ideal shows that the social institutions built around this ideal destroy themselves precisely because, by recognizing as valuable only what universally and necessarily belongs to all human beings *qua* rational, this cultural ideal negates the value of all human particularity, and thus ends up negating the very basis of our self-identity.[8] I will not trace out the cultural dialectic, but we must note the inadequacy of reflective reason's self-conception on which this cultural self-criticism turns.

In reasoning it is true that in an important sense we hold the initiative, the agency, that accomplishes truth. If someone else solves the puzzle, or if I merely repeat an answer by rote, my action was not reasoning. I am speaking accurately, in other words, when, after solving a mathematical puzzle, I say, "I did that." The crucial question, however, is, "Who is this 'I'?" Is it the same I, for example, that I identify when I say, "I like to type"? Is the ego that speaks with the authority of universal rationality simply identical with the idiosyncratic ego of my personal life?

In general, Hegel argues that reflection misdescribes its own experience, for if the ego spoke honestly, it would say that it finds its actions can harness rational ability but can never "own" it. We find ourselves as products of the synthetic activities of self-consciousness, but it is only in and as the determinate realization of these activities that we are able to identify ourselves. It is true that I am the synthetic activity of my own consciousness, but this synthesis, this power, is something I receive. I experience myself as given to myself; whatever power I have comes to me from beyond my immediate self, and thus *qua* rational my action is not a product of my empirical ego.[9] Thus the self who says, "I did that," is right, but that self has not looked carefully enough. This self does not recognize that whatever it defines as itself and its object come already given, already as products of a synthetic activity of self-consciousness that is not here one player within the system but is the ground of the whole determinate system. This self-already-in-situation does not see that the very presence to it of its self and an other already outside it marks the work of a positing power: this already determinately situated self does not see that it has already presupposed the distinction of self and other, and it, as the finite self that it takes itself (immediately) to be, cannot therefore be held up as the agent responsible for the distinction; it exists on the basis of presupposition, so it is a product, and it must look for the real truth of its experience, the real agency behind the scenes, in the power that did the preliminary "supposing," that is, the original positing power for which the distinguishing of self and other is its act. This is the determining power for which the determined elements of self and other are its determinate reflection. Hegel's critique of enlightenment thus leads us to look at Hegel's treatment of this determining power, that reflects itself in the mutual externality of self and other, each of which reflects back to the other the determinateness—the already determined-ness—of its identity. It leads us to Hegel's treatment of "External Reflection" and "Determining Reflection" in the *Science of Logic.*

"Reflection," used as an image to characterize the structure of truth, suggests that what we directly experience is an optical stand-in for the real thing; in regard to this surface show that reflects the real essence, we would ask whether the medium of the reflection plays a role, whether the posture of the viewer is relevant, whether the reflection itself has a reality beyond its role as a conveyor of the essence and its role as potential deceiver. As an epistemological structure, Hegel's "reflection" is fundamentally the relationship that characterizes the forms of the activity of the cognitive agent (whether this activity is recognized by the cognitive agent or not), and the issues Hegel's analysis raises mirror the issues raised by the image.[10]

First (in "positing reflection"), the dialectic of reflection shows that the cognitive agent can never be passive in cognition (or at least not solely passive), for any recognition of determinateness involves an act of positing; that is, recognition is itself an activity. Now the enlightened reasoner—the self who has seen the light of her auto-effection—has recognized her own power of positing and is fundamentally characterized by the second stance of reflection, which Hegel terms "external reflection." External reflection is the situation in which we recognize ourselves to be active thinkers, and we take ourselves to be performing our thinking on an already formed object that confronts us. The object is outside of us, and our task is to take what is thus given and to find out the truth about it. We take the object, in other words, to be unrecognized in its immediate state, and we see the need to recognize it as something that is showing some truth that is more than its immediate self; reflection is "the movement of the faculty of judgment that goes beyond a given immediate conception and seeks universal determinations for it or compares such determinations with it."[11] For reflection, the other is a show (*Schein*). It is on the one hand "merely" a show, for we have yet to penetrate it to the essential truth reflected in it; the immediacy of the show is the inessential, the superfluous. On the other hand the immediate is a show precisely in that it is that which shows us the truth, that without which nothing would show up; the dialectic of reflection moves to the recognition of the essentiality of the immediate show itself. For reflection in general, then, the relation to the object is a relation to a structure of show and essence, or, in more familiar terms, appearance (*Erscheinung*) and reality. External reflection, like the enlightened ego, does realize of itself that it is active, and it takes its activity to be the act of transforming the object of its consciousness from its immediate show to its truth; it knows that it seeks the essence that will explain the show it immediately encounters, where this immediacy itself is deemed superfluous.

What this project of finding the essence of a given other entails, however, is that in taking up its object, in trying to determine the essence of its show, the reflecting subject can never break out of its own self. As Hegel says, "The determinations posited by the external reflection in the immediate are to that extent [that is, to the extent that they are posited by external reflection] external to the latter."[12] The alien, given other, must remain permanently impenetrable, opaque, a thing-in-itself that defines the self-contradictory ideal of an object that is to be known (that is, to be in relation to a subject) precisely as devoid of any relations. The very activity of looking for the truth of the other is precluded from succeeding by the very fact of its being an activity; indeed, the superfluous medium that had seemed to be the residueless mediator of subject to object-as-essence becomes the very point of absolute resistance, the mark of the limit of the ability of the subject's gaze to penetrate to the truth. What we need to see to resolve the problem of external reflection is that its problems emerge from inadequate assumptions built into its original posture; this means seeing that its immediate other is not really so immediate and that its activity does not start with the operation upon this given other, but that the very givenness of the other presupposes a logically prior act of positing on the part of reflection. This is what we see in the move to determining reflection.

Hegel makes this clear in his concluding remarks about external reflection:

But if the activity of external reflection is more closely considered [*Aber das Tun der äußern Reflexion näher betrachtet*], it is secondly a positing of the immediate, which consequently becomes the negative or the determinate; but external reflection is immediately also the sublating of this its positing; for it *presupposes* the immediate; in negating, it is the negating of this its negating. But in doing so it is immediately equally a *positing*, a sublating of the immediate negatively related to it, and this immediate from which it seemed to start as from something alien, *is* only in this its beginning.[13]

Hegel's point is this: initially, external reflection appeared as a relation of self, and other in which the other-as-determined (only) reflects back the self, and the other in its immediacy becomes inaccessible; what we now realize is that this whole relation is the determinateness, the "show," which reflects the determining power of subjectivity as such, that is, the very relation, the very division of subject and object, is the way the real agency within experience shows itself. The real essence of experience is thus as much subject as object or, more precisely, the very form in which the players "subject" and "object" are defined in relation to each other is the self-expression, the determinateness, the show, of a single determining power.[14] The relation itself—the very presence to a subject of an immediately alien other—presupposes a single positing power. Hegel calls this total relation "determining reflection."

What we have seen with the observing ego is that it is right to identify the light that shines within its experience to be its self, but what reflection and enlightenment fail to see is that this, their very self, is not immediately identical with them insofar as they are alienated egos. Enlightenment suffers from a kind of blindness, much like the blindness of an eyeglass wearer to her glasses: the very power that makes a world or an object visible itself slips outside the field of vision and conceals itself as essence in its very act of showing its power in its establishment of an articulated relation of subject and object. Indeed, real insight comes when we take up the relation of subject and object as the articulate expression of this power, its self-expression, the real act of saying "I": the "I" not as alien eye, but as the total situation of embodied intentionality. Reflection needs to see itself qua totality as the real image of its identity. As Hegel implies in always insisting we "observe more closely," vision is not as simple as it "presents" itself to be, and we need to see the self-absenting of the perceptive power, the agency that does not put itself in full view in front of our eyes but works its cunning machinations behind our backs.[15]

Sight is the natural analog for the rational ego as reflection, and the inadequacy of sight that Hegel notes is that it does not experience its other bodily. We can say the same thing of the reflective ego: it only experiences its other, as Hegel would say, "ideally," which means it does not engage with it as a carnal contact. Equally, the reflective ego holds itself aloof from the object it studies, thereby failing to realize of itself that it is of the flesh and therefore vulnerable to the other. What the reflective ego needs to learn is that the situation it finds itself in is not primary but is derivative of a more fundamental dynamism, and this is the structure we have seen in determining reflection. The reflective ego participates in the embodiment of the dynamism that gives rise to both it and its other as apparently immediately alien to one another. This alienation must be overcome, and we will see this in seeing how our knowledge of the other is originally a bodily knowledge, that is, in seeing that our relation to the other begins as an immediate lived participation in a shared system of meanings that are the basis for our being able to act and are not first known by way of a process of alienated observation. It is our living relation with the other, not our looking at it, that is our fundamental reality and that upon which the reflective stance is based. Hegel remarks that we would starve if we had to first learn physiology in order to eat, or again that to learn to swim one must abandon the manuals and jump into the water; the manuals and the scientific observation can only be derivative commentaries on what is already a living bodily communion.

What we can now look for is, to continue this image, how we are already "swimming in" our object exactly when we experience it as alien: in turning to the determining reason of which our very relation to the object is the determinate, concrete expression, we turn to our real identity, which is precisely what is embodied as our relation to the other. This discovery that the immediate alienation of self and other is itself a derivative phenomenon is the thread that will allow us to trace a way back through the labyrinth, the night, of the ethical substance in which we are already embodied; we must pursue this route through Hegel's treatment of Sophocles' *Antigone* in order later to pick up this thread of immediate presence, which is here shown to be the already mediated result of an absent ground. Just as reflection must turn back to the determining power operating outside its field of awareness, we must now turn to this power, that cloaks itself in darkness in order to found our everydayness.[16] We must turn to night's children, the gods which are our earth, the Chthonian gods of *Antigone*. We, like everyday consciousness, thought we began basking in the obviousness of the daylight of enlightenment, but now it is night, and we must see how we had already begun well before daybreak.

II Now It Is Night: The Ethical Substance

Antigone does not have to find out through a process of alienated reflection whether the right thing to do is to bury her dead brother Polynices. The imperative to so act is inscribed in the very situation of his corpse lying unburied. It is as obvious as the sunshine that Creon's edict disallowing the burial is a violation of the laws governing the very nature of things. Hegel's analysis of Sophocles' *Antigone* studies this situation of Antigone as paradigmatic for the immediate form of free human social life.[17] His objective is to unearth the dynamic dimensions of our life that constitute for us this appearance of unachieved, unmediated immediacy, which achieve for us the appearance of an immediately present set of ethical values simply inherent "in the nature of things."[18]

Now Antigone can be asked, "Why is it right to bury Polynices?" and she will have an answer: "Because it is so; the gods decree it." Who are these gods? Hegel describes this power that overrides Creon's edict: "Confronting this clearly manifest ethical power [the human law] there is, however, another power, the Divine Law. For the ethical power of the state, being the movement of self-conscious action, finds its antithesis in the simple and immediate essence of the ethical sphere.... This movement

which expresses the ethical sphere in this element of immediacy
... is the Family. The Family, as the *unconscious*, still inner concept, stands opposed to its actual self-conscious existence.''[19]
Hegel further develops the portrayal of this power through reference to Sophocles' *Antigone*, and he continues to describe it
through images that show this power to be in contrast to the
ideal of the clarity and light of enlightenment reflection: "The
feminine, in the form of the sister, has the highest *intuitive*
awareness of what is ethical. She does not attain to *consciousness*
of it, or to the objective existence of it, because the law of the
Family is an implicit, inner essence which is not exposed to the
daylight of consciousness.''[20]

This divine law, "the power of the nether world (*die unterirdi-
sche Macht*)," this "power which shuns the light of day (*eine licht-
scheue Macht*)," the "hidden divine law (*das verborgene göttliche
Gesetz*)," this law that hides in the dark, is the real power that sets
for us the standards by which we see the objects of our daily life.[21]
Antigone's view that bodies should be buried is the expression of
a value—it is a product of an activity of evaluation on her part—
but she does not recognize it (posit it) as such; she sees it as a
simple fact. Antigone does not first see a corpse and only subsequently decide that it should be buried; rather, for her the very
experience of "corpse" is "to be buried." Her vision—her immediate sensing—is intelligent, is understanding, that is, her
sensing is not passive and innocent, but is decisive, already committed, already judgmental. She, however, does not see that what
she takes as a given other is really the product of a judging—a
prejudging—activity of consciousness by which objects become
possible. In this regard she is the very consciousness that will
have to follow the path to enlightenment. But she gives us a clue
to the real determining power in things, for in her we see that
behind the immediate subject there is a founding power of prejudice by which there is first allowed to be a world, by which
"there is" anything at all. It is this power that gives us the given.
For Hegel the day is the place of deceptive simplicity; the gift of
immediate presence that, in its claim to clarity and manifestness,
conceals the very giving power, conceals the very determining

foundation of, equally, the subject and the object.[22] What is this dark power that gives us the light of day? What is this force that cunningly lays out for us a world as if it were already there waiting for us?

With the daytime world of enlightenment culture, there goes a conception of self-consciously reflective, abstract reason. The opposed image of the nighttime world of ethicality equally brings with it an opposite concept of reason that is intuitive and concrete and shows forth something else while concealing itself. This reason is the *nous* to which Hegel refers in his introduction to his *Lectures on the Philosophy of History*: "Anaxagoras ... was the first to point out that *nous*, understanding in general or Reason, rules the world—but not an intelligence in the sense of an individual consciousness.... These two must be carefully distinguished. The motion of the solar system proceeds according to immutable laws; these laws are its reason. But neither the sun nor the planets, which according to these laws rotate around it, have any consciousness of it." Hegel goes on to discuss how Socrates, in Plato's *Phaedo*, embraces this idea of a governing reason that is invisible to that which it governs but is disappointed with Anaxagoras's use of it: "It is evident that the insufficiency which Socrates found in the principle of Anaxagoras has nothing to do with the principle itself, but with Anaxagoras' failure to apply it to concrete nature. Nature was not understood or comprehended through this principle; the principle remained abstract—nature was not understood as a development of Reason, as an organization brought forth by it. I wish at the very outset to draw your attention to this difference between a concept, a principle, a truth, as confined to the abstract and as determining concrete application and development. This difference is fundamental."[23] This is a *nous*—a reason—that cannot have its own identity apart from the elements it organizes, for these very elements are the substance of the *nous*'s self-expressive act: they are not instances to which reason is applied but are its embodiment.

The reason of enlightenment and external reflection is the reason that applies to an other. This is the reason for which the paradigm instances are mathematics and formal logic. The very mark of the authority of these systems of reasoning is the universality and necessity that comes from their being solely formal truths; that is, these systems of reasoning claim to tell us the truth about any situation irrespective of the content. These are truths derived solely from the notion of simple self-identity, and they therefore apply to anything *qua* self-identical. This whole conception of reasoning, then, is based on the premise of a distinction between form and content, such that formal truths are never conditioned by the content to which they apply. Such a notion of reason, however, is constitutively incapable of comprehending any identity in which form and content are not distinguishable, for the very premise of formal reasoning is the denial of the very essence of that which it would have to understand.[24] The Anaxagorean *nous*, however, is the conception of an organic reason, a reason realized through that of which it is the rationality. This concrete reason is a reason premised on a reciprocity of determination between form and content, and this reason's own identity cannot be articulated in independence of articulating that of which it is the organizing reason.[25] It is this reason for which its *explananda* are its own articulation that is the concrete, self-developing reason that grounds our everydayness.

This *nous*, then—that is, reason as concrete—is reason for which that which it explains is in fact its own self-expression. It is animative rather than applied, that is, the relations it explains are its living substance, its body, not its alien object. This reason is the determining power for which the concrete development it explains is its own reflection; thus its other—it differs from its other as *explanans* from *explandum*—is its own self-articulation, and it will adequately explain its other when it explains it as its own self-reflection. This *nous* is the determining power we sought at the end of section I and is the determining power in ethical life, and we will see that this *nous* precisely is spirit's self-recognition, and it is what is effected uncomprehendingly in and through religion (section III) and self-consciously in absolute knowing (section IV). But we have seen in Sophocles' *Antigone* that this *nous*, which organizes our world, this *nous*, which drives our history, hides itself as ground precisely in its manifestation of itself as articulation. The living reality of Antigone's *sittliche Substanz*, of her ethical world, is really the expression of such a founding rationality, and the organization of her world reflects the values that characterize this rationale, but for her, this rationality is not manifest as such. Instead, she lives an identity already attuned to a certain perception of the nature of things, already harmonized to determinate values that she experiences as fixed directly in the nature of things. She does not recognize herself and her world to be products of this founding rationality and thinks instead that she innocently reads the manifest meanings that lie open on the surface of things. This is the "cunning of reason," the reason that gets its work done through subjects who do not recognize their own complicity in passing judgment. Of this reason, Hegel says in the *Phenomenology of Spirit* that it works "behind the backs" of subjects, and it is this logical structure of unacknowledged behavioral complicity that is reflected in the image of concealment from sight. Like the gods of Antigone's netherworld, this real power in our experience works behind the scenes, out of sight and out of mind, concealing its cunning manipulation of events behind a veil of everyday obviousness.

Precisely what this cunning reason does is produce us as subjects immediately alienated from our objects, and by so producing us as observers actually effects its own project of participant self-observation. Our alienation from the object, in other words, is its self-relation. It is the coalescence of these two sides of our experience that is "absolute knowing," for absolute knowing is precisely the concrete project of recognizing that and how our apparent other is really a reflection of our own true (determining) identity, that is, absolute knowing realizes that it is only by understanding the determinate form of its own relation to its object that it will know itself.

In these first two sections, we have examined the basic logical relationships that characterize natural consciousness, enlightenment, ethicality, and absolute knowing, and we have seen that these logical relations are paralleled in Hegel's uses of visual images. Hegel uses images of a vision that takes itself to be unproblematic to characterize the epistemological and psychological stance that advocates the primacy of the independent reflective ego, and the limitations that his arguments reveal in the reflective stance are mirrored in the limitations to vision that he diagnoses in his explicit discussion of sight. In keeping with this system of images, Hegel uses images of that which is not accessible to sight to characterize the stance that advocates the concrete, embodied reason operating through individual subjects without their explicit recognition of it.

We can now consider how the theme of imagery is itself thematic in Hegel's analysis. Hegel defines religion as the system of ritualized practices that unite a community around a shared "vision," a socially endorsed system of *Vorstellungen*—images—in and as which a society portrays itself to itself. These images are precisely the expression of the concrete reason we found to be animating the member of the ethical community. In turning now to consider Hegel's philosophy of religion, we will learn both why we depend on images and how we should understand them, and we will watch the development of the image for this socially embodied reason from "light" to "revelation" (and, finally, in section IV, to "speculation"). Along the way we will be led to consider the foundations of our immediate vision itself and why this "sense-certainty" is always constructed through images. Let us turn now to the dynamics of the politico-religious vision that emerges from this rejection of the I = Eye in favor of the nocturnal reason, which uses the obviousness of daylight to veil the subtle machinations by which it enforces its vision of reality.

III   The Veil of Immediacy: The Religious Foundation of Sense-Certainty

Antigone's own actions function according to a logic she does not see: her ownmost values are not judgments to which she "owns up" (for which reason she represents a stage of consciousness that must still develop to the point of enlightenment). We have seen that her real animating value—the real core of her self-identity—is a cunning reason that operates behind her back: it is a determining power that fundamentally has its reflection in the determinate relation that it establishes between her and her surroundings, in the immediate form of the opposition of the terms *self* and *other*. Precisely what this mediating ground does is establish an immediacy, a relationship of presence, the presence of something for someone. This is the logical structure involved (a structure of determining reflection), but we have not yet seen the experiential dynamics of how this is effected.

The enlightened, externally reflecting "I" was alienated from its others and thus alienated from other egos. If *Antigone* shows us an ethical situation in which this alienation of self and other cannot be primary but where it is only this very relation that is the reflection of the real determining reason, then it must equally be only in the relation of selves that this founding power, that is the real source of the identity of these selves, is expressed. In particular, the nonalienation of the members of an ethical community is the system of recognition (*Anerkennung*) in Hegel's language, that is, the system by which there is a mutual supporting of identity: we do not hold our own identity within ourselves but require, rather, the reflections of others to tell us who we are, and Hegel understands social life essentially as this system of interpersonal communication whereby we tell each other who we are.[26]

In an ethical community, an overarching sense of the community's identity is constantly rearticulated through the practices of community life, which means that the actions of the members effect at each time—along with their manifest, particular goals—an annunciation of "we are ... "[27] Just as we earlier saw that the very relation of subject and object is the expression of the determining power, which is the real identity of both, so do we here see how social actions are precisely the point at which the particular identities that all of the members perform through their behavior equally serve to perform for each and all the expression of their shared identity as members of this "we." Thus once again, even in the determinate oppositions that make one person not another, this immediate opposition is already more fundamentally a demonstration of a shared identity. The shared identity—the universal—according to its own logic expresses itself through diverse or even opposed finite identities—the particulars—and it is the single self that performs both its particular and its universal identity in each action.

Indeed, it is the very ability of each particular self to recognize itself and the other (that is, its ability to notice the self-identity of each and the difference between them and to agree on this) that is the proof of the presence of the universal identity, for it is only because the selves operate with a shared sense of the relevant categories for evaluation of each other that they can share a sense of who they both are. It is precisely the recognizability of the world—both other selves and nonselves—that is the shared situation of the members of the ethical world, and it is in the actions in which the various agents communicate their sense of how they recognize the world that they communicate to each other that they know who they are. They know who each other is, and they know who they as a whole are.

Now fundamentally, our world offers us openings for various kinds of behavior. It is as presentations of horizons of possible action that we experience the things of our world. Our world shows itself to us as the arena for the conduct of our life, and as we saw with Antigone's experience of the corpse, the experience of imperatives to act in this way or that is the immediate experience of things. Our actions thus communicate how we experience the imperatives in things, that is, our actions communicate the sense we immediately have of how things are "to be done." It is thus in our performance of actions that we perform because we simply experience them as "to be done" that we fundamentally establish for ourselves and for each other our identity. Now actions that are performed because they are immediately experienced as "to be done" are rituals, and it is thus in our ritual actions that we establish for ourselves as members of a community a shared sense of who we are.[28]

At the most general level, then, our actions, *qua* culturally embedded practices, are fundamentally ritualized actions or practices that communicate our sense of self-identity. Now there is a special set of ritual practices usually singled out by ethical communities themselves as religious. What is distinctive of these practices is that these are rituals recognized as rituals; these are practices in which we explicitly announce that our identity is based on a shared sense of what is "to be done."[29] This, it seems to me, is how Hegel fundamentally understands religion. Religious actions are the point at which a community enacts its self-consciousness by recognizing a shared set of things "to be done," but the recognition of these values is an immediate recognition, so it is a recognition of a shared identity that does not recognize about itself that in enacting its rituals it is enacting its own communal self-consciousness. Religion is inherently "idolatrous" or committed to *Vorstellungen*—images—in that it is the commitment to the repetition of the practice *qua* un-understood and as a gesture of membership or "belief." In Hegel's words, religion is self-consciousness in the form of consciousness.[30]

So what is the reason that operates behind the back of the members of the ethical substance? It is their own activity of self-recognition as a "we." There is a reason behind their activities: they are effecting a collective self-recognition, and it is a determinate self-recognition, that is, they recognize themselves as this particular community that carries out its relation-to-being in this way and not in that way.[31] This rationality is expressed in all their actions, and it is the reason that these actions need to be performed, yet it is a rationality hidden from the view of the agents themselves. The agents thus experience actions as needing to be done without being able to give an account of that very necessity in precisely the same way that every reflective ego must posit itself in contradistinction to an object and it must do this immediately. This is an ontological and not a moral "must," which means this distinction is the logical precondition (this positing of difference is a presupposition) for any action by this reflective ego, so even if this ego (following, for example, the path I have laid out in this chapter) should come to understand why it posits an object in opposition to itself, this will be subsequent to the positing itself. It is, in other words, only within the context of the immediate participation in the ritual rationality that development is possible. Adequate self-recognition, in other words, must begin in this inadequate self-recognition, that is, in this ritual self-recognition that does not recognize itself as an act of self-recognition. We necessarily begin, therefore, as idolatrous, as committed to a set of *Vorstellungen* that are the images within which the rationality of our existence is enacted, just as we always have a first language that is the set of ritually defined vocalic and gestural behaviors that we and our culture accept as the embodiment of communicable meaning.

What this tells us is that a culture's rituals—both those recognized explicitly as religious and those that simply constitute the day-to-day secular life—are not contingent within a culture but are, rather, the very soil within which that culture's identity can grow, indeed, within which that culture's identity first becomes possible. And *qua* ritual, these practices, these ways of experiencing the immediate sense of a situation, must be, for the members of the culture, practices whose imperative nature is lived and not reflectively posited.[32] The implication of Hegel's argument is thus that a cultural group will necessarily have ritual practices and will necessarily not recognize that they are reflections of cultural identity but will take them instead as demands fixed within the very nature of things. This is, then, a transcendental argument about the necessary conditions for the possibility of culture, and to say that a society must rely on such unreflective practices is not to say "it should not and must not question them," but that "it cannot come into existence without such a basing of itself on an unthematized system of ritual recognition." The ritual life of a culture, then, is something the members immediately participate in; it is their living substance, their immediate embodiment, and not something they experience as an alien set of rules or practices they reflectively endorse.

To be a human being, then, that is, to be a self-conscious member of a community of recognition, requires first and foremost to be integrated into a determinate ritual life. What we as philosophical anthropologists uncover as the decisions, values, and practices by which the community establishes for itself a communal self-identity constitute, therefore, that necessary dimension of human life that we, as members of the ritual community, experience as the significance that is immediately presented to us through our senses. It is the dialectic of this immediate certainty which is always our immediate reality but which is equally always inadequate as a final stance on the nature of truth, which Hegel studies in chapter 1 of the *Phenomenology of Spirit*, "Sense-Certainty."

Sense-certainty (*die sinnliche Gewißheit*) is the name Hegel assigns to the most immediate form of consciousness, that is, the most immediate form of the presentation to a subject of an object. Sense-certainty is the immediate noticing of an other. Ultimately the point of Hegel's phenomenological analysis of sense-certainty is that this experience of "other" is not the truth but is really a kind of idolatry. The object of immediate experience is really an integrated moment in an intelligible totality, and it fundamentally functions as a sign that points to this total context, but sense-certainty treats it as an uncontextualized, immediately meaningful unit with the precise sense of "alien thing," which is really the very notion of *Vorstellung*: something posited as alien and immediately meaningful in independence of the context of subjectivity. Sense-certainty itself, on the other hand, precisely takes the immediate experience of its other to be the truth: "this that I sense right now" comprises experience, according to sense-certainty. Hegel's dialectical phenomenology of sense-certainty proceeds by demonstrating that the here and now of immediate presence exist for us only as contextualized by the there and then, the mediating absences that stand out of sight to let the immediate show itself.

Sense-certainty, says Hegel, equally insists that the truth of experience is "now" when "now it is day" is the truth of its experience and (twelve hours later) when "now it is night" is the truth. At night, a situation that in no way differs in terms of its experiential structures replaces the first situation, for sense-certainty still says the truth is "now," that is, it claims the identical truth for both experiences, and the absolute transformation of all the determinate features of the experience is not recognized in sense-certainty's monotonic intonation of "this, now."[33] Hegel's images are of our most immediate sensible opposition (daylight and darkness of night). We *see* this difference, but this very distinction operative at the level of *sight*—indeed, this opposition is the necessary condition for vision—cannot be accounted for by the very vision it enables. Sense-certainty's efforts to account for its experience are an attempt to say the unique, particular moment of immediacy, but it says instead only the most universal and undifferentiated truth about experience: that it always takes the form of a temporal presentation to a subject—"now." And as the universal form of all experience, it cannot mark out distinctions between experiences, that is, the saying of "now" by itself no more specifies this experience than that.[34]

The point is that what makes our experience determinate and meaningful is the mediation within experience, whereas the way we immediately experience is to find significance appearing seemingly without mediation. In sense-certainty's "now," however, we see how limited would be the recognizable determinacies of experience if it really were the case that the meaningfulness within experience were merely immediate. Our ability to recognize complex determinacies shows that our organization of our experience is actually operating at a level of logical sophistication considerably higher than the level that is explicitly—reflectively—recognized by the sense-certain ego; to say "day" or "night" requires understanding, requires the ability to synthesize and judge a manifold of experience. What is "just present" really points outside itself to what it is not—to its context of mediation, to what is absent—to support its meaning, and for us to recognize the present is for us to equally take up an interpretive stance on the absent, which conceals itself in order to make the present obvious and available.

This concealed mediation takes many forms, but the most significant dimension of this mediation for our purposes is that which we have just been studying: the categories of recognition that are ritually announced and endorsed by a community that, through adopting these ways of being sense-certain, establishes for itself a shared identity. The immediate form our experience takes, then, is the presentation of itself as being immediately and unproblematically in relation to determinate truth, but the dialectic of sense-certainty shows this to be an intrinsically contradictory stance. It is religion, in fact, that provides for us the mediation that structures into things their immediately recognizable identities, but like sense-certainty itself, religion gives an inadequate account of itself, and fails to recognize that it is really the forum for a community's performance of itself as a "we." For Hegel, then, the very immediacy of our vision is constructed through traditional social practices that indoctrinate us into a particular vision, a particular set of images, a particular set of visual expectations: our sensing is inherently religious, that is, it is through ritualized practices that we develop intelligent vision, and this means that the meaning we sense is fundamentally to be understood in the context of the intersubjective pursuit of self-consciousness, but the essential form this activity takes is to conceal the very fact that it is such and to offer up an obvious immediacy that hides the truth of the performance (and it is this contradiction of not being self-conscious in its establishment of self-consciousness that necessitates the overcoming of religion in philosophy).

According to the Hegelian argument, then, religion is that which gives us our already established sense of what the truth of being is, such that this is not in question within experience but is, rather, the very foundational context that makes experience possible. Religion, then, initially determines what, for us, is true: it is this determining that makes meaningful experience possible for us, that illuminates for us the determinacies of the world, and it does this by giving us a system of images. Truth is thus more fundamentally to be identified with the system that provides the illumination of our immediately sensible meaningfulness than with the activities of those determinacies themselves. This is what is announced in what Hegel's *Phenomenology* posits as the most immediate form of religion, *das Lichtwesen*, the religion that says, "God is light."

The most immediate form of religion is precisely the religion that idolizes visual imagery as the ultimate truth. Hegel begins his description by noting the privileging of the illuminating over the illuminated, which is equally the privileging of rituality as such over against the human members whose self-conscious existence is the living substance—the actuality—of the ritual: "Spirit as the essence that is *self-conscious*—or the self-conscious Being that is all truth and knows all reality as its own self—is, to begin with, only its *concept* in contrast to the actuality which it gives itself in the movement of its consciousness."[35] This privileging of the illuminating over the illuminated, the shaping over the shaped, is essentially equivalent to the privileging of the indeterminate over the determinate that characterizes "Sense-Certainty": "In the immediate, first diremption of self-knowing absolute Spirit its 'shape' has the determination which belongs to *immediate consciousness* or to *sense*-certainty. Spirit beholds itself in the form of *being*, though not of the non-spiritual being that is filled with the contingent determinations of sensation, the being that belongs to sense-certainty; on the contrary, it is being that is filled with Spirit. . . . This being which is filled with the concept of Spirit is, then, the "*shape*" of the *simple* relation of Spirit to itself, or the "shape" of "shapelessness." In virtue of this determination, this "shape" is the pure, all-embracing and all-pervading *essential light* of sunrise, which preserves itself in its formless substantiality. Its otherness is the equally simple negative, *darkness*. The movements of its own externalization, its creations in the unresisting element of its otherness, are torrents of light."[36] The truth, then, is posited as the universal form as opposed to the determinate multiplicity it informs.

To simply identify the truth with the illuminating, however, is no better than sense-certainty's identification of the truth with "now." Both stances are right, to be sure, but both equally find themselves in the position of articulating only a formal truth—one that is merely self-same in every situation. In each case, the attempt to say the truth is inarticulate, and, in the case of "God is light" as in the case of "now," the attempt to name the truth of our experience precisely empties our experience of meaning, since the very determinateness—the very substance—of our experience is lost, for it becomes only so many indifferent "examples" of the truth: "The content developed by this pure *being,* or the activity of its perceiving, is, therefore, an essenceless by-play in the substance which merely *ascends,* without *descending* into its depths to become a subject and through the self to consolidate its distinct moments. The determinations of this substance are only attributes which do not attain to self-subsistence, but remain merely names of the many-named One."[37]

Spirit must come to recognize that it is literally the self-consciousness *of* the individual agents who enact it, and religion must come to acknowledge this at the level of the image: the image of the divine must acknowledge the essentiality to the divine of the determinations or articulations, which is to say the image must be of the divine as self-explicating such that the One illuminates the many and requires in turn that it be illuminated (to itself) by them, that is, that it become conscious of itself in and through them: "This reeling, unconstrained Life must determine itself as being-for-self and endow its vanishing "shapes" with an enduring subsistence.... It is thus in truth the *Self;* and Spirit therefore passes on to know itself in the form of self. Pure Light disperses its unitary nature into an infinity of forms, and offers up itself as a sacrifice to being-for-self, so that from its substance the individual may take an enduring existence for itself."[38] It is Christianity, or rather, "the revealed religion," that corrects this by having a god that descends into that which it illuminates and depends on this for its own resurrection.[39]

Revealed religion still insists on the truth of the divine illumination, but like Hegel's own argument, it announces the divinity as the determining power that sacrifices itself to that which it makes possible. Further, it recognizes that that which it makes possible is not a merely superfluous reflection of its own self-sufficient truth, but is, rather, what the divine itself needs for its own completion. Revealed religion is the religion that announces that religion founds sense-certainty: the definitive image of Christ—the divine itself—self-sacrificed and resurrected (in the hearts of the participants in the Christian church) is the image of determining reflection and of determining reflection understood as the logic of the dynamism of the (self-)experiential life of a religious community. It is the image that recognizes the need of the divine—the determining power—to be embodied in that which it determines, to be embodied in the division into immediately experiencing subject and immediately meaningful object, to be embodied in its expressive reflection: the image is the image of the *logos* made flesh, and of the divinity whose embodiment is the community of believers. Just like individual human subjects, the divine light needs to be recognized, and it needs to be recognized in that which it illuminates, as that which it illuminates, and by that which it illuminates. Unlike the light religion, the revealed religion knows the necessity of self-diremption; it knows that the alienation of subject and object is essential, for the divine needs to be known—needs to know itself—and this requires that it first divide itself from itself in order to be able to return to itself in recognition. Human existence must be the comprehension of itself as precisely the divine comprehension of itself; divinity must be the comprehension of itself as precisely the human comprehension of itself. This is absolute knowing, and this is the truth of spirit's self-comprehension.

The revealed or absolute religion is the religion that ritually endorses the necessity for religion. The absolute religion is the commitment to the essentiality of the image that founds a community, that is, it is the ritual endorsement of the image of images as needing to be realized in and as rational interpretation by a human community in pursuit of self-understanding. It is thus the founding commitment to the necessity for an immediate experience of alienation that presents itself as an encounter with an immediate meaningfulness but which is really a sign—a *Vorstellung*—and a sign that points to the need to explicate the images we live by into rational systems of social self-communication. Sense-certainty, the very experience that seems to us immediately to be stepping into the light, is in truth a stepping into the dark, away from the source that illuminates our experience; but this stepping away is necessary for us to be able ultimately to comprehend our truth. It is precisely the goal of knowledge to reconcile these two directions within our experience and to have our immediate experience of the world be the recognition of the truth that animates our experience. It is this fulfilled self-consciousness that is absolute knowing. But this absolute knowing is thus possible only because we have immediate sense experience, and it is only through this route that knowledge can ever complete itself.

We must now complete our story of Hegel's visual images by turning to this absolute knowing, which itself is a vision of a universal humanity. In our study of religion, we have seen that every community, in order to be a community, is unified around a specific vision, a specific set of images. Now we must consider the universality to which each such vision turns. We must turn from human community as imaginative to human community as logical, which will equally mean turning from the specific identity of any community to the universal human identity—on which religion implicitly depends—as rational self-conscious agents.[40] This is the same human identity recognized by enlightenment reflection, but we will now see how Hegel's understanding of the essentiality of the embeddedness of human identity in ritualized cultural practices makes absolute knowing the *Aufhebung* of this enlightenment conception at the same time as it is the *Aufhebung* of religion, precisely by being the synthesis of these two approaches.

IV Speculation, or Absolute Vision

Self-consciousness, according to Hegel, is the human project. Enlightenment reflection tries to gain this too quickly by assuming that its own identity is in clear view, and yet if we rest with the tradition and ritual of "ethical life," our identity is shrouded in darkness, and this clearly cannot be the answer to this human pursuit. Indeed, our very analysis of both enlightenment and religion has been performed from a point of view that can be identified with neither.[41]

Enlightenment reflection wants to see the truth, but it fails to live up to its own ideal because its vision abstracts from its very corporeality. Custom and ritual seek to establish a self-conscious community of mutual recognition but fail to live up to their own ideal because they close their eyes to their own reality. Reflection without custom is empty, and custom without reflection is blind. Each opposes the other, yet for each the other is precisely what it needs. Enlightenment needs to find rationality in its embodiment, and *Sittlichkeit* needs to recognize that it is the single rational ego who must ultimately carry out the task of establishing real human recognition through understanding.[42] What both thus point to is the necessity for a vision that can only be enacted through the rationality of the single ego but sees its own activity as contextualized by the very reality that it "is not": the bodily, cultural, historical context that is the substance of its worldly involvement. In other words, there must be a vision that is, and recognizes itself to be, the vision of the bodily reality itself; that is, it must be the self-consciousness of the cultural community itself. The true vision could only be spirit coming to recognize itself as spirit. Absolute vision must be the point of view of the single ego who recognizes that she sees on behalf of her community: she says "I" always as the voice of "we."[43]

Absolute knowing could be characterized as responsible vision. It requires both a commitment to seeing—to bringing into self-conscious explicitude what confronts one—and a commitment to not abstracting only the obvious and clear features of the situation but instead taking account of the concreteness that normally remains as the implicit mediation in one's perspective. In his *Encyclopedia of the Philosophical Sciences*, Hegel employs two vision-based characterizations of this concrete reason: knowing absolutely he calls "speculation," and spirit's recognition of itself as spirit he portrays as the truth of Aristotle's *noesis tes noeseos.*[44]

"Speculation" is derived from the Latin *speculor*, which means "to spy out," "to examine," or "to explore." It is related to the Latin *specula* (watchtower), *speculum* (mirror), and *species* (a seeing, a sight, a form), and the *spec* root, which all share, indicates a relation to vision.[45] It is cognate with the English "spy," "espionage," and "special." The Greek *noesis* is formed from the verb *noein*, which means "to perceive by the eyes" (as in *Iliad* III.396), and comes to mean "perceive by the mind." It seems to be related to the Greek *nostos*, which means a "return," as typified by Odysseus's return from Troy to his home in Ithaka.[46] In Plato, the proper object for *noein* is form, *eidos*,[47] which, like the Latin *species* that translates it, means "that which is seen," and it is derived from the same *id* root as the "idealism" Hegel uses to name his own and all true philosophy.

How is speculation—absolute vision—different from reflection? The Latin and Greek words give us a clue. Whereas the reflective gaze is fascinated by the immediate show (*Schein*) and (as external reflection) can never get past this appearance (*Erscheinung*) to the real thing because the object it sees only reflects its (reflection's) own presupposition of alienation, speculation spies out what is special to the identity of its other in order to return to itself.

Speculation works with what is not immediately present: it must engage in an act of investigative unmasking to find out what the other keeps hidden. According to Hegel's vision-based vocabulary here, we could say that speculation does not stop at the show the other puts up but explores in the realm of what is not immediately seen. What it sees, however, is that the other is the image of what it (speculation) itself is trying to conceal. The "other," in other words, has as its truth that it is the real substance of the speculating self, and its self-showing as "other" is the crucial concealing mechanism that must be overcome.[48] This is Hegel's version of transcendental philosophy.

Transcendental philosophy is a regressive philosophy seeking the conditions of the possibility of experience by uncovering the unconscious processes of subjective synthesis. Unlike Kant's approach to studying the logic of subjective synthesis in abstraction from all determinate experience, however, Hegel's understanding of the embodiment of reason requires him to approach the structures of subjectivity by way of a comprehension of all experience: philosophical inquiry must not retreat from experience, but must, so to speak, fight its way through experience in its very specificity, and it thus only can see its self when, like Odysseus, it returns after the successful siege. It remains true that the self sought is the self that provides the a priori grounds of experience, but we have no way even to conduct this investigation unless we have already developed a sophisticated relationship to the object so that we can know what we are looking for. (The *Phenomenology of Spirit* is the story of developing this progressively more comprehensive relation to our object in which we gradually come to see just what it is that we are trying to see, that is, the last step is just as much the recognition of what our project is as it is the completion of that project.) The completion of this path of gradually coming to make sense of just what the experience of an object is comes when we recognize the object as precisely that which calls out for us to understand it and to recognize that this is simultaneously its calling to us for our help in bringing it to understand itself: we recognize the object only when we recognize it as calling each of us as an "I" to form with it a "we." As the vision-based terms of Hegel's characterization of absolute knowing suggest, absolute knowing thus means seeing the other as calling for this absolute comprehension. This is what marks out speculative vision from both the clear vision of reflection and the self-blinding of custom and ritual.

Reflection produces its solutions without going by way of an immersion in the other. Like René Descartes's project of solitary meditation, reflection seeks a truth that is universal and necessary without being contaminated by the particularities and contingencies of actuality. For that reason, enlightenment can never show itself to be the truth demanded by its objects, for it has precisely defined itself in exclusion from them.

Religion does not reject the immersion in particularity, and in that respect it can show us the essential dimension of human existence that reflection presupposes and forgets, but it is equally unsatisfactory for it resists admitting that this embodiedness is in the service of self-consciousness. The very premise of customary practices is that they are implicated in a project of mutual recognition, a project of self-consciousness and for that reason these practices whose very logic is to be self-concealing can only complete themselves by undermining themselves, that is, by unconcealing themselves. Ritual life, then, must sublate itself by generating a self-explication in the form of individuals who engage in a self-uncovering discourse in and through which they discover themselves as rational individuals engaged in the universal project of rational self-consciousness within the always necessarily particularized context of natural and cultural embodiment.

Now since the speculative project is to come to recognize oneself qua rational in one's very embodiment, speculation, then, like reflection, still only encounters its own image when it encounters its other, but this mirror, this *speculum speculantis*, is not the static and empty reproduction of an already established identity within an unresisting medium. On the contrary, to understand reality as the mirror of the absolute mind is to see reality as a dialectical process in which a single idea is developing itself through a discourse with itself. The process is then completed when this very project—a project of self-recognition—can turn on itself in its very concreteness and diversity and comprehend this specificity as itself. This speculation sees *sub specie aeternitatis* because it can recognize particularity—specificity—as essential, and it sees this essentiality of particularity when it sees these particularities with respect to "eternity," that is, the universal and necessary—the inescapable—project of any subject who tries to understand, namely, the project of self-understanding. The act of understanding thus ultimately means the act of studying the other as the key to the hidden side of oneself. It is in recognizing the very thing we posit as other as the key to recognizing ourselves that we establish for the first time the possibility of understanding both. Absolute knowing tells us that the truth of this understanding will be that each of us has our specificity precisely as the set of terms in which we are asking to be led to a shared rational self-consciousness, a "we." Therefore the project of understanding must be not the project of reducing all particularity to the same abstract logic but instead the project of leading both ourselves and our others to a shared self-consciousness as rational individuals wherein the cultural specificities of each of us must serve as languages building the route, and wherein we must each become multilingual in order for any of us to be able to succeed in our project of self-understanding.

Hegel says that speculating is reconciling what initially appear as alien realities by way of a dialectical understanding of the human project. This is reflected in his use of speculation and *noesis*, words that suggest a visual paradigm of awareness, but a vision identified with going beyond the immediate in a project of unmasking and return. These images capture nicely the dialectical project of looking behind the back of our everydayness to see the mediating structures that it tries to hide (unmasking) in order to demand of these structures that they fulfill themselves in a self-uncovering that shows itself to be the always already anticipated "homecoming" of the investigative enterprise (return). Reconciling the explicit vision and implicit blindness of enlightenment reflection with the explicit blindness and implicit vision of custom, speculative *noesis* is a vision devoted to eliminating its own blind spots through a threefold commitment to the essentiality of its own singular viewpoint, to the essentiality of the universality of the human project of rational self-consciousness, and to the essentiality of the species, the particularity, of the other.[49]

Conclusion

One might have thought that a philosophy of "absolute knowledge" would have to renounce sensation. On the contrary, we see that absolute knowledge can only be effected through beings who are essentially sensing, that is, essentially constituted by an immediate relation to an apparent other, which is equally to say that we must be embodied. We will always and necessarily be embodied agents, already involved with our others according to a logic that is not immediately apparent, and we will live in a sense-certainty, the implicit intelligence of which conceals its own foundations in the determinate practices that constitute a specific historically embodied community's efforts to say its own identity. This embodiment in determinate cultural ritual means that the truth, for us, will always be expressed in images, in metaphors, but equally our existence as reflective beings means that our task will always be to see how the images a community uses to articulate the truth do offer a route to establishing a universal communication based on the shared human project of rational self-understanding.

Hegel's philosophy of absolute knowledge thus demands of us that we recognize in the practices of those we encounter the expression of truth, but a truth that may well not be understood by the very practitioners. We must approach the cultures of others the way we approach another language, recognizing that, *qua* self-conscious human agents, we share with our others our destiny of self-comprehension as a community, but that this shared sense of self-identity can be performed only through becoming multilingual, so to speak, and we can do this only by letting the language of the other show us its own rationality, while equally demanding that that language have room to accommodate the rational demands of our own reflective experience.[50] Hegel's philosophy is thus neither an unthinking reversion to an unreflective *Sittlichkeit* nor a voyeuristic exotification of an uncomprehended other; rather, it is a conscientious commitment to a single, human, rational discourse of mutually established self-consciousness. Unlike the enlightenment, Hegel demands a political commitment to the rationality of that which appears alien, which means a political vision that begins with the recognition that it is already committed to the essentiality of that which it does not understand, but, unlike traditional custom and religious ritual, this is a commitment to explicit self-consciousness and understanding, and the commitment is thus a demand on the other that that other equally submit itself to rational discourse. Absolute knowing is therefore a political vision that can only endorse a cross-cultural communication that seeks not only to enlighten but to be educated by the other into a new language of self-consciousness within the context of a mutual pursuit of free rationality.[51]

Hegel's position, finally, is consistently and systematically articulated through his use of vision-centered vocabulary. Hegel differentiates three essential stances—reflection, *Sittlichkeit*, and absolute knowing—and these stances are marked through different images, which suggest, respectively, (1) an uncritical trust of the obviousness that attaches to a visual ideal, (2) a recognition of the real determining dimensions of existence as operating out of sight, and (3) a responsible investigative vision that knows that it must see, but that this sight requires it to find what is hidden behind the face the other immediately shows us. Hegel's philosophy is a philosophy of vision, but a vision with its own path of dialectical development.[52]

Notes

1. G. W. F. Hegel, *The Difference Between Fichte's and Schelling's System of Philosophy*, trans. and ed. H. S. Harris and Walter Cerf, (Albany: SUNY Press, 1977), p. 119. See *Science of Logic*, trans. A. V. Miller, (New York: Humanities Press, 1976), pp. 49, 404–405; *Wissenschaft der Logik* (hereafter *WdL*), ed. Eva Moldenhauer and Karl Markus Michel, (Frankfurt: Suhrkamp Verlag, 1986), 1:43, 2:30–32. Periodically, precise line references will be given as a decimal following the page number, with positive numbers referring to lines of text counted from the top of the page and negative numbers referring to lines of text counted from the bottom of the page.

2. "Das reine Selbsterkennen im absoluten Anderssein," in *Phenomenology of Spirit*, trans. A. V. Miller, (Oxford: Oxford University Press, 1977), para. 26; *Phenomenologie des Geistes*, ed. H.-F. Wessels and H. Clairmont, (Hamburg: Felix Meiner Verlag, 1988), p. 19. Hereafter references to the Miller translation will be given as M followed by the paragraph number, and references to the Wessels and Clairmont edition will be given as W/C followed by the page number; hence this reference would be M26, W/C 19. I will consistently alter Miller's translation of *Begriff* from "Notion" to "concept."

3. This and the following quotation are from *Philosophy of Mind*, trans. A. V. Miller, (Oxford: Oxford University Press, 1971), p. 78; *Enzyclopädie der Philosophischen Wissenschaften im Grundrisse* (1830), Dritter Teil, ed. Eva Moldenhauer und Karl Markus Michel, (Frankfurt: Suhrkamp Verlag, 1970), p. 104: "Das eigentlich Materielle der Körperlichkeit dagegen geht uns beim Sehen noch nichts an. Die Gegenstände, die wir sehen, können daher fern von uns sein. Wir verhalten uns dabei zu den Dingen gleichsam nur theoretisch, noch nicht praktisch, denn wir lassen dieselben beim Sehen ruhig als ein Seiendes bestehen und beziehen uns nur auf ihre ideelle Seite. Wegen dieser Unabhängigkeit des Gesichts von der eigentlichen Körperlichkeit kann man dasselbe den edelsten Sinn nennen. Andererseits ist das Gesicht ein sehr unvollkommener Sinn, weil durch denselben der Körper nicht als räumliche Totalität, nicht als *Körper*, sondern immer nur als Fläche, ... an uns kommt."

4. Hegel's account here does not do full justice to his own principles. He knows in general that any coming to unity transforms the identity of its constituent parts, but he does not here treat the various sense modalities as undergoing redefinition from their participation in a unified sensing subject. He needs to see that, as Merleau-Ponty puts it in *Phenomenology of Perception*, trans. Colin Smith, (London: Routledge, 1962), pp. 207–215, we see sounds and hear colors. Likewise, to say we see only the two dimensions, and so forth, is phenomeno-

logically inaccurate, and it is related to an analytic mistake that Hegel criticizes in the Preface to the *Phenomenology*: that anatomy studies a corpse and mistakes its object for the human body. Hegel's account is reasonable for what each sensory modality is singly as a sensitive system, but the senses do not function singly, so he should not talk of actual sight this way, for the senses exist this way only for dismembering reflection. It is also important for Hegel to remember that when he says sight does not affect its object but leaves it at peace, this is a claim about how things work within the parameters established by sight. Metaphysically, sight does alter its object, and this is precisely the point of the Aristotelian epistemology-ontology, which Hegel adopts here, that is, sensation is a simultaneous actualization of seer and seen: we affect the object in that we answer its call to be seen and thereby fulfill it. For an account of vision that Hegel should endorse, see Francisco Varela, Adrian Palacios, and Evan Thompson, "Ways of Coloring: Comparative Color Vision as a Case-Study for Cognitive Science," *Behavioral and Brain Sciences* 15 (1992).

5. *Philosophy of Mind, Zusatz* to sec. 448, p. 197; *Enzyclopädie*, p. 251: ... *Gesicht*, das mit dem Objekte als einem überwiegend *Selbständigen, ideell* und *materiell Bestehenden* sich beschäftigt, zu ihm nur eine *ideelle* Beziehung hat, nur dessen *ideelle* Seite, die *Farbe*, vermittels des *Lichtes* empfindet, die *materielle* Seite aber am Objekt unberührt läß't." Also *Philosophy of Mind*, p. 78: "Light manifests something else and this manifesting constitutes its essential nature"; "colour is what is seen, light is the medium of seeing." *Enzyclopädie* p. 104: "Das Licht manifestiert Anderes, dies Manifestieren macht sein Wesen aus"; "Die Farbe ist das Gesehene, das Licht das Mittel des Sehens."

6. *Faith and Knowledge*, trans. and ed. W. Cerf and H. S. Harris, (Albany: SUNY Press, 1977), p. 57.

7. On this point, and the sense in which even reasoning is rooted in confirmation by others, see my "Hegel's Phenomenology of Reason and Dualism," *Southern Journal of Philosophy* 31 (1993):72–74.

8. This is particularly illustrated through his analysis of the French Revolution, *Phenomenology*, M582–595, W/C 385–394. The revolution is based on the principle of universal rational equality, which means it grants recognition to—accepts as legitimate—individuals *qua* rational, which here means *qua* egos abstracted from all conditioning circumstance, that is, abstracted from all particularity; but only particularity gives distinct identity. Consequently any distinct identity, by being nonuniversal, runs counter to the principle of universal rationality that drives the revolution. The revolution is thus the foe of any distinct individuality, and this abstract goal of universal rational freedom thus reveals its truth in the terror in which all are immediately guilty. See my "Selfhood, Conscience and Dialectic in Hegel's *Phenomenology of Spirit*," *Southern Journal of Philosophy* 29 (1991):538, 542.

9. This is the truth behind "the unhappy consciousness," which Hegel analyzes as the culminating form of self-conscious selfhood. It is the third form of the relationship Hegel lays out in *Phenomenology* M210, W/C 145–146, and that is illustrated in M231, W/C 157.

10. Hegel's study of the logic of reflection is not primarily a study in epistemology, for he is interested in a type of organization of elements that is equally

present in beings other than self-conscious agents. Life, for example, demonstrates the logic of reflection (and, indeed, the more sophisticated logic of "the idea"), as does any relationship of a whole and its parts. Still, it is in cognition that reflection has its paradigmatic realization, and it is as a portrayal of a cognitive stance that I will present reflection. See *Science of Logic*, p. 404, *WdL*, 2:30–31.

11. *Science of Logic* p. 404.15–18, *WdL*, 2:30.12–15: "die Bewegung der Urteilskraft, die über eine gegebene unmittelbare Vorstellung hinausgeht und allgemeine Bestimmungen für dieselbe sucht oder damit vergleicht."

12. *Science of Logic* p. 403.-20–.-19, *WdL*, 2:29.10–12: "Was die äußerliche Reflexion an dem Unmittelbaren bestimmt und setzt, sind insofern demselben äußerliche Bestimmungen."

13. *Science of Logic* (translation modified), pp. 403.-8–404.1, *WdL*, 2:29.-14–.-6: "Aber das Tun der äußeren Reflexion näher betrachtet, so ist sie *zweitens* Setzen des Unmittelbaren, das insofern das Negative oder Bestimmte wird; aber sie ist unmittelbar auch das Aufheben dieses ihres Setzens; denn sie setzt das Unmittelbare *voraus*; sie ist im Negieren das Negieren dieses ihres Negierens. Sie ist aber unmittelbar damit ebenso *Setzen*, Aufheben des ihr negativen Unmittelbaren; und dieses, von dem sie als von einem Fremden anzufangen schien, ist erst in diesem ihrem Anfangen."

14. Compare Merleau-Ponty's discussion of the "tacit *cogito*" in *The Visible and the Invisible*, trans. Alphonso Lingis, (Evanston: Northwestern University Press, 1969), pp. 170–171, 175–176, 179, and in *Phenomenology of Perception*, e.g., p. 402; see also p. 394 for his related discussion of *Fundierung*.

15. Theodor W. Adorno, in "Skoteinos, or How to Read Hegel," in *Hegel: Three Studies*, trans. Shierry Weber Nicholson, (Cambridge: MIT, 1993), pp. 89–148, makes the excellent parallel point that just as much as Hegel's philosophy criticizes the content of rationalism, so is Hegel's style anti-Cartesian. The reflective ideal demands a clear and distinct presentation of a clear and distinct idea (pp. 96–99), but Hegel's text offers instead a demand for an active student who does not "simply look on" (p. 94) but instead becomes immersed in the obscurities of Hegel's text and, adopting a critical stance, works to "illuminate him from behind" (p. 92). See pp. 122–123, 145. For Adorno's own treatment of the images of clarity and enlightenment, see the note to pp. 96–97.

16. Compare Plato, *Republic* Book 7, 518d3–4 on education as "the art of turning around." In general, the account I am here giving of the relation between Hegel's argument and his visual images could equally serve as a commentary on the analogy of the sun in *Republic* 6 and 7.

17. *Phenomenology*, chap. 6, sec. A, pts. a, b, M444–476, W/C 291–316. Strictly speaking, it his only Hegel's allusions to *Antigone* in the *Phenomenology* that we are here considering; his explicit analysis of the tragedy in his *Aesthetics* has slightly different concerns.

I refer to human social life that is "free" to indicate that this is a situation premised on equality of recognition between social members, and not a relationship of master and slave, which Hegel calls not a matter of freedom (*Freiheit*) but a matter of dependence and independence (*Unselbstständigkeit und Selbstständigkeit*). See the titles of *Phenomenology*, chap. 4, sec. A (before M178, W/C

127) and sec. B (before M197, W/C 136). On freedom as equality of recognition, see my "Selfhood, Conscience, and Dialectic" pp. 534–537.

18 I have taken this up directly in "Reading and the Body in Hegel," *Clio* 22 (1993):330–331. Cf. *Phenomenology*, M437, W/C 286–287.

19. *Phenomenology*, M449, 450, W/C 293–294: "Dieser sittlichen Macht und Offenbarkeit tritt aber eine andere Macht, das *göttliche Gesetz*, gegenüber. Denn die sittliche *Staatsmacht* hat als die Bewegung des sich *bewußten Tuns* an dem *einfachen* und *unmittelbaren Wesen* der Sittlichkeit ihren Gegensatz.... Dieses in diesem Elemente der *Unmittelbarkeit* ... die Sittlichkeit ausdrückend ... ist die *Familie*. Sie steht als der *bewußtlose* noch innre Begriff, seiner sich bewußten Wirklichkeit ... gegenüber."

20. *Phenomenology*, M457, W/C 299: "Das Weibliche hat daher als Schwester die höchste *Ahndung* des sittlichen Wesens; zum *Bewußtsein* und der Wirklichkeit desselben kommtes nicht, weil das Gesetz der Familie das *ansich*seiende, *innerliche* Wesen ist, das nich am Tage des Bewußtseins liegt."

21. *Phenomenology*, M460, W/C 301.39–40, M469, W/C 309.22, M477, W/C 316.12–13.

22. Compare Pierre Bourdieu, *Outline of a Theory of Practice*, trans. Richard Nice, (Cambridge: Cambridge University Press, 1977), p. 72, on the need "to pass from the *opus operatum* to the *modus operandi*, ... to the principle of the production of this observed order."

23. This and the preceding passage are from Robert S. Hartman's translation of Hegel's introduction to the *Lectures on the History of Philosophy*, entitled *Reason in History*, (Indianapolis: Bobbs-Merrill, 1953), pp. 13–14. *Vorlesungen über die Philosophie der Geschichte*, ed. Eva Moldenhauer und Karl Markus Michel, (Frankfurt: Suhrkamp, 1986), pp. 23–24: "Anaxagoras zuerst gesagt hat, der *nous*, der Verstand überhaupt, oder die Vernunft, regiere die Welt—nich eine Intelligenz als selbstbewußte Vernunft, nicht ein Geist als solcher; beides müssen wir sehr wohl voneinander unterscheiden. Die Bewegung des Sonnensystems erfolgt nach unveränderlichen Gesetzen, diese Gesetze sind die Vernunft desselben; aber weder die Sonne noch die Planeten, die in diesen Gesetzen um sie kriesen, haben ein Bewußtsein darüber.... Man sieht, das Ungenügende, welches Sokrates an dem Prinzip des Anaxagoras fand, betrifft nicht das Prinzip selbst, sondern den Mangel an Anwendung desselben auf die konkrete Natur, daß diese nicht aus jenem Prinzip verstanden, begriffen ist, daß überhaupt jenes Prinzip abstrakt gehalten blieb, daß die Natur nicht als eine Entwicklung desselben, nicht als eine aus der Vernunft hervorgebrachte Organisation gefaßt ist. Ich mache auf diesen Untershied hier gleich von Anfang an aufmerksam, ob eine Bestimmung, ein Grundsatz, eine Wahrheit nur abstrakt festgehalten oder aber ob zur näheren Determination und zur konkreten Entwicklung fortgegangen wird." These concepts of the "concrete" and "development" are also given special focus in Hegel's Introduction to the *Lectures on the History of Philosophy*, in pt. A, "The Notion of the History of Philosophy," sec. 2, "Explanatory Remarks upon the Definition of the History of Philosophy."

24. Consequently we can see that the very attempt to separate form and content itself is an approach to form that does specify a content. Hegel discusses this in

John Russon

Phenomenology of Spirit, chap. 5, "Reason," in the section of "Observing Reason" entitled "Observation of Self-Consciousness in its Purity and in Its Relation to External Actuality: Logical and Psychological Laws," M299–300, W/C 201–202. See also *Science of Logic,* pp. 43–45 ff., *WdL,* 1:36–38 ff.

25. Indeed, this articulation is what each of Hegel's systematic books does. The *Phenomenology* articulates its own principle only through the exposition of that which this principle explains, the *Logic* develops the idea of logic only as it develops its determinations, the *Philosophy of Nature* shows how the very concept of nature comes to be articulated only through the development of the determinations of nature, and so on.

26. To have the experience of other selves (*as* selves) is to have the experience that I am subject to the judgment of others, just as they, and the rest of the stuff of the world, are subject to my judgment, my consciousness. The presence within my experience of other self-conscious selves means, thus, that my actions in the world are always necessarily public. What I do defines who I am, but it is not simply up to me to decide what I did. My actions and my experience are the very stuff of my existence, and who I really am is whatever the source is that will adequately explain this. We are what our actions show us to be, and one of the most important sides of our action—what makes it what it is, when we are in a social context—is how it has impact on others. But if one's substance, one's "stuff," itself is all "public domain" material, then what it is of which the real "I" is the source has its reality established publicly. What that stuff is is how it functions in the experience of those others who equally have it as their substance. It is all of our substance, and one's real self will be the thing that is the explanatory source of what it turns out to be (or to have been) in this public context. But that means my reality is established socially, and whether my intent or my interpretation—who I appear to be—is who I really am depends on my ability to interpret and intend what actually is. It is when I see things as my fellows must see them that my view of me is right. On these points, see especially *Phenomenology,* chap. 5, pt. C, sec. A, "The Spiritual Animal Kingdom and Deceit, or, *die Sache selbst.*"

27. Compare Bourdieu, *Outline,* p. 22, on the double goal in rule following of both accomplishing the manifest objective of the rule and winning the honor of living up to the rules, and p. 81, on the notion that "interpersonal" relations are never strictly "individual to individual" but involve the mediation of a sense of the objects that is communally established through traditional systems of practice.

28. Compare Bourdieu, *Outline,* on the notion of "habitus," which he defines as "systems of durable, transposable *dispositions,* structured structures predisposed to function as structuring structures, that is, as principles of the generation and structuring of practices and representations which can be objectively 'regulated' and 'regular' without in any way being the product of obedience to rules" (p. 72). See especially p. 80: "One of the fundamental effects of the orchestration of habitus is the production of a commonsense world endowed with the *objectivity* secured by consensus on the meaning (*sens*) of practices and the world, in other words, the harmonization of agents' experiences and continuous reinforcement that each of them receives from the expression, individual or collective (in festivals, for example), improvised or programmed (commonplaces, sayings), of similar or identical experiences." See also Clifford Geertz, *The*

Interpretation of Cultures (New York: Basic Books, 1973), p. 112: "For it is in ritual—that is, consecrated behavior—that this conviction that religious conceptions are veridical and that religious directives are sound is somehow generated. It is in some sort of ceremonial form ... that the moods and motivations which sacred symbols induce in men and the general conceptions of the order of existence which they formulate for men meet and reinforce each other." Hegel's understanding of the origins of ritual in the dialectic of recognition has the advantage of being able to answer the question of motivation for religious participation that Geertz (p. 109) describes as being "of all the problems surrounding attempts to conduct anthropological analysis of religion ... the one that has perhaps been most troublesome and therefore the most often avoided." Like Geertz (pp. 109–110), Hegel locates the source in a cultural demand for faith in its values and images. See my "Heidegger, Hegel and Ethnicity: The Ritual Basis of Self-Identity," *Southern Journal of Philosophy* 33 (1995):509–532.

29. See Geertz, *Interpretation*, p. 113, for a comparable distinction.

30. *Phenomenology*, M677–682, 788, W/C 444–449, 516–517.

31. It is precisely this determinateness that is the core of the self-contradiction of religion. The very thesis of religion, as I have here argued, is that it serves to establish a shared recognition, a communal self-consciousness. Yet precisely what the determinateness of a society's ritual practices creates is a situation in which those who do not practice the same rituals cannot be recognized. Consequently, the very same practices that make a shared self-consciousness possible within a community preclude its possibility outside the community. Religious rituals thus establish boundaries between communities and actually hinder their own constitutive project of establishing a universal self-consciousness. This last can be done only in the absolute knowing that moves beyond the insistence on the immediacy of the ritual practice, the immediacy of the image in which the spiritual self-consciousness is established, and endorses instead the mediation, the universal rationality of self-consciousness, which gives the image its power.

32. Compare Bourdieu, *Outline*, pp. 5–6, on why a ritual practice requires to be not understood (p. 80), on the production of a "commonsense" world, and pp. 166–167, on what "goes without saying."

33. *Phenomenology*, M95, W/C 71.

34. Ibid., M96–100, W/C 71–72.

35. Ibid., M685, W/C 452: "Der Geist, als das *Wesen*, welches *Selbstbewußtsein* ist,—oder das selbstbewußte Wesen, welches alle Wahrheit ist und alle Wirklichkeit als sich selbst weiß, ist gegen die Realität, die er in der Bewegung seines Bewußtseins sich gibt, nur erst *sein Begriff*." Hegel adds: "and this concept is, as contrasted with the daylight of this explicit development, the night of its essence"; "und dieser Begriff ist gegen den Tag dieser Entfaltung die Nacht seines Wesens."

36. Ibid., M686, W/C 542–453: "In der unmittelbaren ersten Entzweiung des sich wissenden absoluten Geistes hat seine Gestalt diejenige Bestimmung, wel-

che dem *unmittelbaren Bewußtsein* oder der *sinnlichen* Gewißheit zukommt. Er schaut sich in der Form des *Seins* an, jedoch nicht des geistlösen mit zufälligen Bestimmungen der Empfindung erfüllten *Seins*, das der sinnlichen Gewißheit angehört, sondern es ist das mit dem Geiste erfllte Sein.... Dies mit dem Begriffe des Geistes erfüllte *Sein* ist also die *Gestalt* der *einfachen* Beziehung des Geistes auf sich selbst, oder die Gestalt der Gestaltlösigkeit. Sie ist vermöge dieser Bestimmung das reine, alles enthaltende und erfüllende *Lichtwesen* des Aufgangs, das sich in seiner formlosen Substantialität erhält. Sein Anderssein ist das ebenso einfache Negative, die *Finsternis*; die Bewegungen seiner eignen Entäußerung, seine Schöpfungen in dem widerstandslosen Elemente seines Andersseins sind Lichtgüsse."

37. Ibid., M687, W/C 453: "Der Inhalt, den dies reine *Sein* entwickelt, oder sein Wahrnehmen ist daher ein wesenloses Beiherspielen an dieser Substanz, die nur *aufgeht*, ohne in sich *niederzugehen*, Subjekt zu werden und durch das Selbst ihre Unterschiede zu befestigen. Ihre Bestimmungen sind nur Attribute, die nicht zur Selbstständigkeit gedeihen, sondern nur Namen des vielnamigen Einen bleiben."

38. Ibid., M688, W/C 453–454: "Dies taumelnde Leben ... muß sich zum *Fürsichsein* bestimmen, und seinen verschwindenden Gestalten Bestehen geben.... Es ist also in Wahrheit das *Selbst*; und der Geist geht darum dazu über, sich in der Form des Selbsts zu wissen. Das reine Licht wirft seine Einfachheit als eine Unendlichkeit von Formen auseinander und gibt sich dem Fürsichsein zum Opfer dar, daß das Einzelne das Bestehen an seiner Substanz sich nehme."

39. Ibid., M748–787, W/C 488–515.

40. Treating religion thus as spirit's "imagination" is Hegel's appropriation of Aristotle's claim that all thought takes place in a *phantasm*; see Aristotle, *De Anima*, III.8.432a8–9.

41. Compare Andrew Buchwalter, "Hegel's Concept of Virtue," *Political Theory* 20 (1992):548–583, who shows, within the context of Hegel's *Philosophy of Right*, that Hegel's speculative return to a Greek notion of virtue cannot be understood as a rejection of the modern notion of the primacy of individual subjectivity but is in fact premised on the respect for individual rational autonomy. Hegel's position is thus the speculative synthesis of the otherwise opposed ideals of Enlightenment and *Sittlichkeit*. See especially pp. 552–553, 562, 576. See also my "Reading and the Body in Hegel," p. 333 n. 14. Adorno makes a comparable point: "But once it is acknowledged that clarity and distinctness are not mere characteristics of what is given, and are not themselves given, one can no longer evaluate the worth of knowledge in terms of how clearly and unequivocally individual items of knowledge present themselves.... Of course one cannot grossly neglect the demand for clarity; philosophy should not succumb to confusion and destroy the very possibility of its existence. What we should take from this is the urgent demand that the expression fit the matter expressed precisely" (p. 100).

42. See Buchwalter, "Hegel's Concept of Virtue," pp. 563–564.

43. *Phenomenology*, M177, W/C 127.

44. Hegel discusses speculation in *Enzyclopädie*, sec. 82. In the *Zusatz* to this section, Hegel discusses the meaning of the word in terms of transcending what is immediately given and in terms of uniting into a concrete totality the determinations that the reflective understanding holds in mutual alienation. Compare his discussion of speculation in *The Difference Between Fichte's and Schelling's System of Philosophy*, pp. 102–103; this passage is discussed by Adorno, "Skoteinos," pp. 90–91. The reference to Aristotle is in *Enzyclopädie*, sec. 577. Here Hegel discusses how the unity of absolute mind is revealed in a duality of appearances.

45. It is derived from the Indo-European root *spek* and is cognate with the Greek *skeptomai* from which we get such words as *skeptic, scope*, and *episcopal*. It is also related to other words for *seer*, as, for example, *haruspex*, which is the name for one who looks at the entrails of animals. See *The American Heritage Dictionary of Indo-European Roots*, ed. Calvert Watkins (Boston: Houghton Mifflin, 1985); *Origins: A Short Etymological Dictionary of Modern English*, ed. Eric Partridge (New York: Greenwich House, 1983); *A Latin Dictionary*, ed. Charlton T. Lewis and Charles Short (Oxford University Press, 1984); *Greek-English Lexicon*, ed. Henry G. Liddell, Robert Scott, and Henry S. Jones (Oxford University Press, 1968).

46. On the connection of *noein* with *nostos* and with the Odyssey in general, see Douglas Frame, *The Myth of Return in Early Greek Epic* (New Haven: Yale University Press, 1978).

47. *Republic*, 6.511b3–c2.

48. See *Science of Logic*, pp. 826–827, esp. p. 826.-3 to .-4, *WdL*, 2:551–553.

49. Hegel's project thus dovetails with Geertz's "semiotic" approach to culture according to which "the aim of anthropology is the enlargement of human discourse" (p. 14).

50. See Geertz, *Interpretation*, p. 13: "We [anthropologists] are not ... seeking either to become natives ... or to mimic them.... We are seeking, in the widened sense of the word in which it encompasses very much more than talk, to converse with them, a matter a great deal more difficult, and not only with strangers, than is commonly recognized." In this project we cannot simply trust our own sense of what another's images "obviously" mean, and neither can we immediately trust the account given by the reflective ego of the other: that account is not the truth of these images but is itself part of the system of images—a piece of evidence but not the solution. Compare Bourdieu, *Outline*, pp. 18–19, on why the vision of a native of some culture on that culture is not necessarily adequate; in particular, such an "informant's" discourse "tends to draw attention to the most remarkable 'moves' ... rather than to the principle from which these moves and all equally possible moves can be generated and which, belonging to the universe of the undisputed, most often remain in the implicit state."

51. Compare Adorno, "Skoteinos," p. 94: "Hegel's logic is not only his metaphysics; it is also his politics."

52. Compare Geertz's discussion of the difference between the religious, the scientific, the commonsense, and the aesthetic perspectives in terms of "seeing," in *Interpretation*, pp. 110–112.

7

Sighting the Spirit: The Rhetorical Visions of *Geist* in Hegel's *Encyclopedia*

John H. Smith

Although Hegel's philosophy develops a clear priority of the conceptual over the visual (e.g., in his emphasis on *Begreifen* over the contemporary notions of *intellektuales Anschauen*), the problem of how to visualize the Spirit persists in crucial and ironic ways even in his later, more abstract philosophical systems. This problem links and complicates matters of form and content, since the formal question of how Hegel can possibly enable an audience to "see" the (logic of the) Spirit can never be dismissed as unphilosophical once the fundamental principle of the reality of the Spirit has been formulated. That is, given the basic tenet of Hegel's philosophy—that the Spirit exists in the world—we (in the world) must be capable of "seeing" it and Hegel must be able to give us (his readers) images of it. At the same time, we and he must be very careful not to reduce Spirit to the visible, lest the conceptual lose its priority. Thus we encounter at the core of Hegel's thought a series of basic tensions between images of seeing and concepts of invisible thought. Hegel must resolve these tensions dialectically, maintaining and cancelling the opposition between the seen and the unseen. Hegel's powerful and effective arguments accomplish his dialectical task by using the rhetorical strategy of simultaneously depicting and then negating the visual in order to render the "Spiritual" indirectly visible through the negation. Specifically, in his discussion of visions aroused by animal magnetism, Hegel argues for, and rhetorically performs, a different kind of visualization, which he calls "speculative," by ironically presenting accounts of quasi-miraculous sightings. He can thereby not only have his Spirit and see it too, but also move his readers to engage in a new mode of speculation.

Hegel opens what must be considered the culmination of his philosophical carreer, the third part of the *Enzyklopädie der philosophischen Wissenschaften im Grundrisse* (1830), *Die Philosophie des Geistes*, with a blanket statement of the importance and difficulty involved in understanding his central concept, Spirit: "Die Erkenntnis des Geistes ist die konkreteste, darum höchste und schwerste" ("The knowledge of Mind is the highest and hardest, just because it is the most 'concrete' of sciences"; sec. 377).[1] By the difficulty of the "concrete" he means that Spirit, properly comprehended, needs to be recognized as the making real and identical of opposites. Two brief sections later, he raises an essential characteristic of our experience of Spirit—"das Selbstgefühl von der *lebendigen* Einheit des Geistes" ("our own sense of the mind's *living* unity")—and points to a broad category of phenomena that will show the reader how to grasp, or literally see, the nature of that "unity":

In modern times especially the phenomena of *animal magnetism* have given, even in experience, a lively and visible confirmation of the underlying unity of soul, and of the power of its "ideality." Before these facts, the rigid distinctions of practical common sense are struck with confusion; and the necessity of a "speculative" examination with a view to the removal of difficulties is more directly forced upon the student.

[Insbesondere haben die Erscheinungen des *animalischen Magnetismus* in neueren Zeiten auch in der Erfahrung die *substantielle Einheit* der Seele und die Macht ihrer Idealität zur Anschauung gebracht, wodurch alle die festen Verstandesunterschiede in Verwirrung gesetzt [werden] und eine spekulative Betrachtung für die Auflösung der Widersprüche unmittelbar als notwendig gezeigt werden.] (sec. 379)[2]

We are thus truly at the heart of Hegelian dialectical idealism since the task he sets for his philosophy is to comprehend Spirit as a unity of contradictions. And what I wish to pursue in this chapter is some of the rhetorical means Hegel would use for achieving such a comprehension. My fundamental concern is Hegel's argument that phenomena (appearances, *Erscheinungen*) of a particular sort can make a visualization of the ideal possible (*zur Anschauung bringen*), a visualization that in turn creates a confusion of the viewer's categories of understanding so that a different kind of viewing (*spekulative Betrachtung*) becomes necessary. We shall pursue the techniques whereby the reader is brought to experience a "shift of vision," ironically on the basis of a discussion of amazing and dazzling visions.[3] He gives us the strands to follow. The sections on the "feeling soul" (*die fühlende Seele* and *Selbstgefühl*), with their depictions of peculiar phenomena of a disruptive, disrupted, and disrupting vision, attain a special place in Hegel's system, not just because of their content but because of their (rhetorical) *effect* on the reader's structures of thought.

Before turning to the actual analysis, however, we should be clear on Hegel's unbridled emphasis on the impact of the range of phenomena subsumed under "animal magnetism."[4] In the Addition to section 379, we hear of the two major forces that have overcome the limited conceptualizations of Spirit: the tremendous transformations (*ungeheure Umgestaltungen*) in contemporary philosophy and the fact that in the empirical sciences narrow conceptions of Spirit "have been repressed (or pushed aside) by the phenomena of animal magnetism that have left finite thought dazed" ("durch die das endliche Denken vor den Kopf stoßenden Erscheinungen des animalischen Magnetismus verdrängt worden").[5] And a bit further on, he refers to the effect (*Wirkung*) of animal magnetism, which has contributed to the repressing or "ousting" (*verdrängen*) of "the untrue, finite interpretation of mind from the standpoint of the merely abstractive intellect" ("die unwahre, endliche, bloß verständige Auffassung des Geistes"). This effect is produced because in the phenomena linked to animal magnetism, something appears or comes into view (*zum Vorschein kommt*) that the understanding cannot grasp or even believe, even though it arises "in the realm of the senses" (*innerhalb des sinnlichen Daseins*). The additions nuance very carefully the significance of such phenomena in a passage I shall quote at length because it provides the major elements for my analysis:

Now although it would be very foolish to see in the phenomena of animal magnetism an elevation of mind above even Reason with its ability to comprehend, and to expect from this state a higher knowledge of the eternal than that imparted by philosophy, and although the fact is that the magnetic state must be declared pathological and a degradation of mind below the level even of ordinary consciousness in so far as in that state mind surrenders its thinking as an activity creative of specific distinctions, as an activity contradistinguished from Nature: yet, on the other hand, in the visible liberation of mind in those magnetic phenomena from the limitations of space and time and from all finite association, there is something akin to philosophy, something which, as brute fact, defies the scepticism of the abstractive intellect and so necessitates the advance from ordinary psychology to the comphrehension afforded by speculative philosophy for which alone animal magnetism is not an incomprehensible miracle.

[Obgleich es nun sehr töricht wäre, in den Erscheinungen des tierischen Magnetismus eine Erhebung des Geistes sogar über seine begreifende Vernunft zu sehen und von diesem Zustande über das Ewige höhere Aufschlüsse als die von der Philosophie erteilten zu erwarten—obgleich der magnetische Zustand vielmehr für eine Krankheit und für ein Herabsinken des Geistes selbst unter das gewöhnliche Bewußtsein insofern erklärt werden muß, als der Geist in jenem Zustand sein in bestimmten Unterscheidungen sich bewegendes, der Natur sich gegenüberstellendes Denken aufgibt—, so ist doch andererseits das in den Erscheinungen jenes Magnetismus sichtbare Sichlosmachen des Geistes von den Schranken des Raums und der Zeit und von allen endlichen Zusammenhängen etwas, was mit der Philosophie eine Verwandtschaft hat und das, da es mit aller Brutalität einer ausgemachten Tatsache dem Skeptizismus des Verstandes Trotz bietet, das Fortschreiten von der gewöhnlichen Psychologie zum begreifenden Erkennen der spekulativen Philosophie notwendig macht, für welche allein der tierische Magnetismus kein unbegreifliches Wunder ist.]

Hegel clearly wants to put such phenomena in their place. They should not be considered as rising above the realm of philosophy, as if they were unlocking a door to the eternal. Indeed, they are in fact forms of pathology, since they represent the Spirit in a state perilously undifferentiated from nature. And yet, even as pathology, such phenomena do have their place within philosophy. And at that place, they have a unique function of making the Spirit's essential independence from space and time *visible* ("das ... sichtbare Sichlosmachen des Geistes"). Such a sighting of the Spirit has, for the understanding and for the reader at that stage, the status of a miracle or the marvelous (*Wunder, wunderbar*); that is, it leads the viewer to marvel and thus to see differently, namely, "speculatively."[6] Despite Hegel's denial of the significance of these visions, then, and his attempt to assign them to a limited place, their effect on the reader is essential to the development of true speculative philosophy.[7]

It may be helpful to locate briefly the place of such visualizations of Spirit in the systematic unfolding of the system. The *Encyclopedia*, like so many other of Hegel's later works, reveals the near-mechanical unfolding in tripartite structures.[8] The largest three parts deal with the subjective Spirit (modes of conscious being in the broadest sense), the objective Spirit (modes of public being), and the absolute Spirit (self-conscious representations in art, religion, and philosophy). The first of these parts is the only one that concerns us here, and it treats subjective Spirit in three forms: as "soul" (or psyche, *Seele*), consciousness (*Bewußtsein*), and *Geist* proper. The first of these, "Anthropologie. Die Seele," is concerned with the mind as it relates intimately to its environment, including some of Hegel's most notorious passages on the different races' ties to geographical formations and fascinating passages on the "preconscious" states of mind like childhood, dreams, hypnosis, and habit, in which we are immersed in ourselves and (our) nature. The section that interests us here, on the "feeling soul" or consciousness merely as "sentient," makes up the large middle section of this part. The entire treatment of psyche is, because of the inclusion of the lengthy Additions, by far the longest of the book (over five times longer than the section on "The Phenomenology of Spirit. Consciousness" ["Die Phänomenologie des Geistes. Das Bewußtsein"] and nearly three times longer than the entire part on objective Spirit).[9] As such, it clearly supersedes the structural and conceptual role it should play in Hegel's system (since he ought to have been least interested in this "lower" form of Spirit). While the amount of attention brought to bear on the soul could in part be explained by the fact that Hegel had lectured in the past on the philosophy of right and aesthetics and did not feel the need to cover that ground again, the fact is, as we shall see, that the discussion of the soul also has a crucial argumentative and rhetorical function to play. I use the term *rhetorical* in the sense of Aristotle: "The faculty of *observing* in any given case the available means of persuasion" (*Rhetoric*, Book I, Chapter 2), since Hegel's discussion of the soul does persuade by making a different kind of observation possible. The exceedingly long Additions to this section on the soul, even if they were not composed in this form by Hegel, nonetheless represent the importance he did give to such phenomena as visions and animal magnetism and accomplish with their detail an effect on the reader that Hegel referred to abstractly at the opening of the volume as a turn to a "speculative point of view."

Turning more specifically to the sections on the "feeling soul," we see first that they are contained within a structure of ironically arranged binarisms, especially those of darkness and light, sleep and wakefulness. The phenomena that lead the reader to the necessity of a more enlightened speculative philosophy are paradoxically not associated with light. On the contrary, we find ourselves dealing with the stage of the Spirit's darkness ("die Stufe seiner Dunkelheit," sec. 404), where sleep reigns. The soul in general, as Hegel said earlier, is the Spirit in a state of sleep ("der Schlaf des Geistes," sec. 389).[10] The elements of the visions will arise out of the deepest recesses of the self, which is not yet fully conscious (also of itself) but remains a dark, indeterminate shaft or pit ("ein bestimmungsloser Schacht," sec. 403).[11] Only later will there be an awakening of the soul, which then takes the form of a differentiated ego ("das höhere Erwachen der Seele zum *Ich*," sec. 412); and this ego appears as light ("*das Licht*, das sich und noch anderes manifestiert," sec. 413). Thus, what we have here is not just a metaphorics of light and darkness but a crucial ironic inversion, since it is precisely in the dark sleep of the Spirit, in the "feeling soul" experiencing magnetic somnambulism and related states ("*magnetischer Somnambulismus* und mit ihm verwandte Zustände," sec. 406), that the most powerful, indeed miraculous visions will appear.

That the sighting of the Spirit is connected to a rhetorical problem of persuading the reader (as viewer) to see things differently is clear from the early sections of *die fühlende Seele*. Hegel admits that he will be presenting some peculiar things without being able to provide the appropriate "verification" that they correspond to real experiences (sec. 406).[12] And yet, he goes on in his own defense, precisely those who would find the "facts" (*das Faktische*) in need of proof are in the position of further denying all the incontrovertible witnesses. Those who are in doubt, he claims, are fixed in their categories of understanding; "the *a priori* conceptions of these inquirers are so rooted that no testimony can avail against them, and they have even denied what they have seen with their own eyes" ("in ihrem apriori-sichen Verstande so fest sind, daß nicht nur gegen denselben alle Beglaubigung nichts vermag, sondern daß sie auch schon das geleugnet haben, was sie mit Augen gesehen"). The reason for their denial is that in this particular area, even what one sees with one's own eyes has no weight against the categories of understanding since one must have already abandoned them in order to believe (grasp, see) what is there before one's eyes. He writes: "In order to believe in this department even what one's own eyes have seen and still more to understand it, the first requisite is not to be in bondage to the hard and fast categories of the practical intellect" ("Um auf diesem Felde selbst das, was man mit seinen Augen sieht, zu glauben, und noch mehr, um es zu begreifen, dazu ist die Grundbedingung, nicht in den Verstandeskategorien befangen zu sein"). In other words, Hegel is arguing in a fundamentally circular fashion (*petitio principii*).[13] The whole point of including these visions is that they make something visible that has contributed to the undermining of (philosophies of) the understanding. And yet for someone still operating according to those categories of the understanding, these visions are literally invisible. Thus, one needs to see these phenomena to have one's mind changed but needs to have already adopted a new perspective in order to see the phenomena. I do not wish to cast this circular reasoning as vicious but, rather, as a necessary turn of Hegel's argumentation.

Hegel finds himself here in the position of the scientist according to Kuhn, stationed in a new paradigm (recall Hegel's reference to *Umgestaltungen* in *Wissenschaft*), able to see things differently, and talking to those "outside."[14] Hegel knows that once his readers see what he sees—the reality of the ideal, the existence of the Spirit—they will never be able to go back to doubting it; they will have made the "paradigm shift." And yet he must somehow persuade them to move into his paradigm so that they will be able to see what he sees, as he sees it, in the first place.[15] Kuhn describes this by using the "useful elementary prototype" of the "switch of gestalt," with a minor difference: "the marks on paper that were first seen as a bird are now seen as an antelope, or vice versa. That parallel can be misleading. Scientists do not see something as something else; instead, they simply see it" (p. 85). And Kuhn points out how this shift occurs through rhetorical persuasion:

Like the choice between competing political institutions, that between competing paradigms proves to be a choice between incompatible modes of community life. Because it has that character, the choice is not and cannot be determined merely by the evaluative procedures characteristic of normal science, for these depend in part upon a particular paradigm, and that paradigm is at issue.... [Thus, the argument for a paradigm] cannot be made logically or even probabalistically compelling for those who refuse to step into the circle.... To discover how scientific revolutions are effected, we shall therefore have to examine not only the impact of nature and of logic, but also the techniques of persuasive argumentation effective within the quite special groups that constitute the community of scientists. (p. 94)

For Hegel, it means presenting the visions in such a form that the reader is "moved" simultaneously to "see" them and to drop traditional categories. Now we can understand why these Additions are the longest in the entire *Encyclopedia*. They (regardless of authorship) function in fact for the reader as the major rhetorical turning point, allowing the reader thenceforth to visualize the Spirit. They are "about" observing the Spirit, and they allow the reader to learn to observe it. To the extent that they can accomplish that rhetorical feat, they are essential and successful.

Let us now consider Hegel's visions, first within the context of his wider argument on the soul. His overall discussion of the "anthropological" consideration of the soul has not received the attention it deserves. Hegel is not concerned with the psyche as it is in direct contact with nature—the senses as the boundary between inside and outside. That was the topic of the "natural soul" in the previous section. Nor is he concerned with the mind as it "stands against" its objects (*Gegenstand*) in the world. That is the topic of the next section on consciousness. Rather, he is presuming a state of individuation without (self)reflexive subjectivity. He writes: "Though the sensitive individuality is undoubtedly a monadic individual, it is, because immediate, not yet as *its self*, not a true subject reflected into itself, and is there-fore passive" ("Die fühlende Individualität zunächst ist zwar ein monadisches Individuum, aber als *unmittelbar* noch nicht als *es selbst*, nicht in sich reflektiertes Subjekt und darum *passiv*," sec. 405). The general state of consciousness that he is describing here can perhaps best be approached by thinking of parallels to the more accessible conception of modern object-relations psy-chology.[16] Hegel presents us with a brute subject in the process of establishing an "inner world" of internalized objects at the order of fantasy. This world of the proto-subject consists of the totality of internalized perceptions (grouped, we could say, around key "partial objects"). They are the memory traces, complexes of cathected mnemic elements, from all experiences, stored yet not fully appropriated by consciousness and therefore not separated out and organized according to categories of the understanding, or even the primal distinction between self and other. ("All the general determinations of the soul individu-alized in me and experienced by me constitute my actuality. . . . I *am* this whole circle of determinations" ["Alle die in mir indi-vidualisierten und von mir durchlebten allgemeinen Seelenbes-timmungen machen meine Wirklichkeit aus. . . . Ich *bin* dieser ganze Kreis von Bestimmungen"]; Addition, sec. 406, English

p. 110; German p. 144.) These internal objects remain throughout the life of the mind the core of individuality, even as they are
in priniciple unknowable and unconscious:

> Thus a person can never know how much of things he once learned he
> really has in him, should he have once forgotten them: they belong not
> to his actuality or subjectivity as such, but only to his implicit self. And
> under all the superstructure of specialized and instrumental conscious-
> ness that may subsequently be added to it, the individuality always
> remains this single-souled inner life.

> [So kann der Mensch nie wissen, wie viele Kenntnisse er in der Tat *in
> sich hat,* sollte er sie gleich vergessen haben;—sie gehören nicht seiner
> Wirklichkeit, nicht seiner Subjektivität als solcher, sondern nur seinem
> an sich seienden Sein an. Diese *einfache Innerlichkeit* ist und bleibt die
> Individualität in aller Bestimmtheit und Vermittlung des Bewußtseins,
> welche später in sie gesetzt wird.] (sec. 403)

Only by putting these internal objects into some reflexive order
can consciousness emerge; but these unmediated experiences—
raw and resistant elements of organizing consciousness—reveal
the possibility of a primal unity, a state of undifferentiation, since
they are not separated out as "objects in the world" or as "*my*
objects as opposed to anyone else's." They are me, and I am
them. Like Kleinian partial objects, they are not localizable in
space, not isolatable bodily phenomena. Their reality and internal status are unseparated for the "feeling psyche." And as such,
they are (an example of) the existence of the speculative unity
of the objective and subjective; in Hegel's words:

> Just as the number and variety of mental representations is no argu-
> ment for an extended and real multeity in the ego; so the "real" out-
> ness of parts in the body has no truth for the sentient soul. As sentient,
> the soul is characterized as immediate, and so as natural and corporeal:
> but the outness of parts and sensible multiplicity of this corporeal
> counts for the soul (as it counts for the intelligible unity) not as any-
> thing real, and therefore not as a barrier: the soul is this intelligible
> unity *in existence*—the existent speculative principle.

> [Sowenig die *Mannigfaltigkeit* der vielen *Vorstellungen* ein Außereinander
> und reale Vielheit in dem *Ich* begründet, so wenig hat das reale
> Auseinander der Leiblichkeit eine Wahrheit für die fühlende Seele.
> Empfindend ist sie *unmittelbar* bestimmt, also natürlich und leiblich,

aber das Außereinander und die sinnliche Mannigfaltigkeit dieses Leib-lichen gilt der Seele ebensowenig als dem Begriffe als etwas Reales und darum nicht für eine Schranke; die Seele ist der *existierende* Begriff, die Existenz des Spekulativen.] (sec. 403)

That unity of the feeling soul is thus a preview of the speculative unity Hegel is interested in and stands, like the latter, in opposi-tion to the understanding. For this reason, the "sighting" and seeing of the former can allow us, according to Hegel, to see beyond the fixed notions of the understanding, even if the visions of a feeling soul are, for consciousness, "pathological." The feeling psyche offers a "royal road" to an understanding of *Geist*.[17]

Since I cannot possibly unfold all the incredible examples and formulations Hegel has for this primal vision of the soul, I will isolate a few to focus on the way they function in Hegel's argu-ment to lead us to a different kind of speculation. Consider the phenomena associated with clairvoyance (*Hellsehen*). The status of such visions is uniquely disruptive of our traditional mode of thought, and hence we are led to adopt Hegel's. He writes:

But such clairvoyance—just because its dim and turbid vision does not present the facts in a rational interconnection—is for that very reason at the mercy of every private contingency of feeling and fancy etc.—not to mention that foreign *suggestions* (see later) intrude into its vision. It is thus impossible to make out whether what the clairvoyants really see preponderates over what they deceive themselves in.—But it is absurd to treat this visionary state as a sublime mental phase and as a truer state, capable of conveying general truths.

[Dies Anschauen ist insofern ein *Hellsehen,* als es Wissen in der unge-trennten Substantialität des Genius ist und sich im *Wesen* des Zusam-menhangs befindet, daher nicht an die Reihen der vermittelnden, einander äußerlichen Bedingungen gebunden ist, welche das beson-nene Bewußtsein zu durchlaufen hat und in Ansehung deren es nach seiner eigenen äußerlichen Einzelheit beschränkt ist. Dies Hellsehen ist aber, weil in seiner Trübheit der Inhalt nicht als verständiger Zusam-menhang ausgelegt ist, aller eigenen *Zufälligkeit* des Fühlens, Einbildens usf. *preisgegeben,* außerdem daß in sein Schauen *fremde* Vorstellungen (s. nachher) eintreten. Es ist darum nicht auszumachen, ob dessen, was die Hellsehenden richtig schauen, mehr ist, oder dessen, in dem sie sich täuschen.—Abgeschmackt aber ist es, das Schauen dieses Zustandes für eine Erhebung des Geistes und für einen wahrhafteren, in sich *allgemeiner* Erkenntnisse fähigen Zustand zu halten.] (sec. 406, English p. 103 f.; German p. 135 f.)

If the clairvoyance of the feeling psyche does not operate according to the categories, differentiations, and relationships of the understanding, then we confont a peculiar problem: a radical arbitrariness and undecidability in evaluating the visions. Implicitly we are therefore thrust onto Hegel's authority, which is grounded not on logical categories but on such ones as "taste" and effectiveness. (In fact, the footnote by Hegel to the passage just quoted challenges the common use of Plato as *Autorität* for a, in Hegel's view false, overestimation of the meaning of visions.) Thus, what is at stake here is a discussion of visions that need to be "seen" in their "proper" light, whereby the very presentation of the visions is crucial for organizing the reader's gaze and focus.

This mixture of levels of argumentation—visions as the content and the organization of the reader's vision—occurs numerous times explicitly in Hegel's use of visual images. Consider the passage in the Addition to section 406 on the ability to "see" objects that are not there before the eyes. He rules out merely physically caused illusions (e.g., hallucinations due to fevers) since he is concerned with the ability to see something real, even if it is out of the field of vision. The following is the transition from the first (uninteresting) to the second kind:

> But what we have mainly to keep in view in our anthropological exposition is the second kind of visions, those which relate to actually existent objects. In order to understand the miraculous aspect of this class of phenomena it is important to bear in mind the following points of view relative to the soul.

> [In unserer anthropologischen Betrachtung haben wir aber vorzugsweise die zweite Art der Visionen, diejenigen, welche sich auf *wirklich* vorhandene Gegenstände beziehen, ins Auge zu fassen. Um das Wunderbare der hierher gehörigen Erscheinungen zu begreifen, kommt es darauf an, in betreff der Seele folgende Gesichtspunkte festzuhalten.] (Addition, English, p. 109; German, p. 143)

What interests me here is not just his fascination with such phenomena but the way his rhetoric is engaged in the exact same activity. He, like the visionary, calls on the reader to conceptualize (*begreifen*) this phenomenon by contemplating it visually (*ins Auge fassen*). The reader can appreciate the marvel and wonder of the phenomenon only by following Hegel's own "point of view" (*Gesichtspunkt*) on the matter.

Likewise, Hegel deals with different forms of "intuition" (*schauendes Wissen*), pointing to both the problems associated with it and its necessity for a philosophical understanding if it is understood philosophically. Intuition involves recalling something long since forgotten, or seeing beyond the framework of space and time, or experiencing a heightened sensitivity toward one's own bodily states. Throughout these discussions, Hegel stresses time and again the possibilities for "endless deceptions" (*unendliche Täuschungen*, p. 148) and the need for the greatest skepticism in regard to such claimed experiences. At the same time, he stresses their undeniability. It is this opposition inherent in the persuasive status of these phenomena (not the phenomena themselves) that plays the crucial role in his argument. Thus he writes:

However, in these as in similar phenomena, philosophy obviously cannot set out to explain all the particular details which often are not properly authenticated but, on the contrary, extremely doubtful; rather must we restrict ourselves in a philosophical treatment, as we have done above, to bringing into prominence the main points of view of the phenomena in question which are to be borne in mind.

[Es versteht sich indes bei dieser wie bei ähnlichen Erscheinungen von selber, daß die Philosophie nicht darauf ausgehen kann, alle einzelnen, häufig nicht gehörig beglaubigten, im Gegenteil äußerst zweifelhaften Umstände erklären zu wollen; wir müssen uns vielmehr in der philosophischen Betrachtung, wie wir im Obigen getan haben, auf die Hervorhebung der bei den fraglichen Erscheinungen festzuhaltenden Hauptgesichtspunkte beschränken.] (Addition, English, p. 113 f.; German, p. 148 f.)

His concern, in other words, with these visions is neither their truth nor untruth, their inexplicability nor ultimate explanation. He does not care if we believe any given example. Rather, the force of these examples, their simultaneous credibility and incredibility, facticity and marvelousness, serves to keep our sights on a philosophical consideration or mode of observation and the emphasis of a particular point of view. The "second sight" or double vision of present and future, which he says is common among the (somewhat primitive) Scots, is thus a perfect figure for Hegel's own practice: He wants us to see his point and to see beyond it, accept a visionary possibility, even necessity, even as we reject it as inadequate to our speculation.[18]

The phenomenon of "animal magnetism," which Hegel considered fundamental to the move toward speculative philosophy, is subsumed under the general category of *schauendes Wissen*. The differentiating characteristic of magnetism is the possibility of calling it forth intentionally, as it were with foresight (*absichtlich*) (p. 150). Since we know that the problem confronting Hegel is that he must use these examples to convince the reader of the necessity of a "speculative" comprehension of the Spirit's reality at the same time as he recognizes that they would be incomprehensible examples for anyone who does not already view them speculatively, we should consider his rhetorical organization of the discussion to see how he would accomplish both tasks. I would isolate three techniques that convince the reader of the "comfortability" of occupying a position of belief. The first is the extensive use of detail. Hegel's descriptions of the different possibilities for bringing on a "magnetic" or hypnotized state, like touching or stroking the subject, take the reader through the motions in what for the *Encyclopedia* amounts to extraordinary realistic detail.[19] One might almost be tempted to say that he is putting the reader into the state of accepting his way of seeing by putting us into his head as he describes the movements of the *Magnatiseur* (esp. p. 153 f.).

A second technique is the appeal to authority. A brief review of the *Encyclopedia* reveals that nowhere else does Hegel (and his editor) rely so heavily on providing references for his views. In this section, he grants such scientists a considerable, indeed superlative ethos to lend them greater credibility, as they are "Männer edelster Gesinnung und größter Bildung" (p. 154).[20] Ironically, he even attributes—in this case only—a greater reliability on the part of the French, despite their "naive" metaphysics otherwise.[21] The clear implication is thus not that these examples are in themselves so persuasive but that the reader who does not allow himself or herself to be persuaded, to see them as Hegel would, is going against a certain authority. Given the circle within which Hegel is operating—you've gotta see it to believe it, but you've gotta believe in order to see it—he must use the appeal to *auctoritas* as one of the different techniques to help us make the leap to seeing and believing, simultaneously, as he does.[22]

Finally, by the end of the section, Hegel has accomplished an inversion of perspective, such that what began as the miraculous for the man of understanding becomes the self-evident to the objective and scientific observer. In speaking of the uses of magnetism for curing illness, he says:

Undoubtedly many cases of ancient times which were considered miraculous must be regarded as nothing else but the results of animal magnetism. But there is no need to appeal to marvellous tales wrapped in the obscurity of the distant past; for in modern times men of unimpeachable integrity have performed so many cures by magnetic treatment that anyone forming an unbiassed judgment can no longer doubt the curative power of animal magnetism.

[Ohne Zweifel müssen viele in älterer Zeit geschehene Heilungen, die man als Wunder betrachtete, für nichts anderes angesehen werden als für Wirkungen des animalischen Magnetismus. Wir haben aber nicht nötig, uns auf solche in das Dunkel ferner Vergangenheit eingehüllte Wundergeschichten zu berufen, denn in neuerer Zeit sind von den glaubwürdigsten Männern durch die magnetische Behandlung so zahlreiche Heilungen vollbracht worden daß, wer unbefangen darüber urteilt, an der Tatsache der Heilkraft des animalischen Magnetismus nicht mehr zweifeln kann.] (Addition, English, p. 121; German, p. 159)

In other words, whereas Hegel at the beginning of the section had presented the acceptance of the "miraculous" nature of such "magnetic" phenomena as possible only if one adopted a "speculative" viewpoint, here such acceptance is presented as a matter of fact, beyond doubt for any reasonable person with the minimal condition of being without prejudice (*unbefangen*; this opposed to the person "caught" [*befangen*] in the categories of the understanding as we saw above, sec. 403). This means that implicitly we have entered a sphere in which the fantastic has been normalized and speculative has become *the* mode of vision. We are on our way out of darkness into the light of a higher consciousness. In accepting Hegel's account of *Hellsehen*, we ourselves become *Hellseher* of the Spirit.

I conclude this analysis by returning to a passage from the first paragraph on the feeling soul, which states in abstract terms an essential relationship between the ideal and the real according to Hegel. The passage justifies on many levels the centrality of a rhetorical reading of the soul:

> Nowhere so much as in the case of the soul (and still more of the mind) if we are to understand it, must that feature of "ideality" be kept in view, which represents it as the *negation* of the real, but a negation, where the real is put past, virtually retained, although it does not *exist.*
>
> [Nirgend so sehr als bei der Seele und noch mehr beim Geiste ist es die Bestimmung der *Idealität,* die für das Verständnis am wesentlichsten festzuhalten ist, daß die Idealität *Negation* des Reellen, dieses aber zugleich *aufbewahrt,* virtualiter erhalten ist, ob es gleich nicht existiert.] (sec. 403)

On one level, Hegel is saying with this peculiar comparative ("nirgend so sehr ... und noch mehr ...") that he does want to grant the analysis of the soul a special status in terms of idealist thought because the soul is both the negation of assumed realities and itself an all-too-real version of Spirit. On another level, the soul plays a special role in developing our understanding (*das Verständnis*). That is, Hegel is early on warning us that the analysis of the soul is essential as much for its content as for its function in engendering our comprehension. Because the soul is a prime example of "ideality," its analysis will allow us to experience in ourselves the unique form of speculative understanding Hegel is after. (Note how the English translation provides an additional sight metaphor, "kept in view," itself only present, one could say, *virtualiter* in the German.) And finally, concretely, that understanding will consist of a rhetorical determination that makes possible simultaneous negation and conservation. The visionary phenomena of the soul may seem like bizarre aberrations, but their presentation to the reader opens up the essential experience of doubleness that is absolute philosophy for Hegel; it offers the key shock (negation) to the understanding that makes speculative understanding possible. "See the reality of these visions," Hegel seems to be saying, "so that in seeing it you will accept the negation of reality they entail, and thereby change your notion of reality. And if you do that, you will have experienced the doubleness which is ideality." The visions of the soul and their rhetorical presentation are thus paradigmatic for the way the gestalt shift to speculative philosophy is to be attained.

Let me illustrate my argument about the rhetorical function of Hegel's treatment of phenomena like animal magnetism by briefly relating it to somewhat better-known passages from the *Phenomenology* on the pseudoscience of phrenology.[23] Here, too, my point is to use apparently tangential arguments in Hegel to locate the way the text brings about dialectical shifts of vision in the eyes of the reader. Donald Verene has pointed out in his superb reading of the rhetorical figures in the *Phenomenology* that the chapter on phrenology gains in significance if it is neither dismissed nor reduced to a "historical" interest of Hegel but, rather, seen as "an ironically stated version of the philosopher's position."[24] In this case, Verene sees this section of the *Phenomenology* as highlighting and grappling with the fundamental issue for Hegel: the relationship between pictorial and conceptual thought (*vorstellen* and *begreifen*). The chapter on phrenology is Hegel's opportunity to show graphically the "unphilosophical" nature of thought that would reduce concepts to images, the absolute to the concrete. Hegel concludes the chapter with the infamous line that for phrenology to take the truth of Spirit's reality and turn it into the belief that it is thus visible in the shape of a person's skull is like taking the duality of the male sexual organ's functions and reducing it to its "pissing" (*Pissen*).

Verene raises a perfectly legitimate question in response to Hegel's reading: "Why does Hegel use such strong language here?" (p. 87). After his excellent analysis, Verene offers the answer that Hegel needs to "make clear" the difference between his own version of phenomenology and other (inadequate, overly concrete) sciences of the mind: "Hegel must make clear the difference between the science of the experience of consciousness and the science of psychology in any of its forms. If this is not done, phenomenology will be seen as a kind of psychological science or as a type of thinking that works with psychology in some fashion." (p. 91). Although I fully agree that much of Hegel's polemic is aimed at such a process of differentiating his own philosophical position from somewhat related forms of science, I would like to point to a different rhetorical use of such graphic, that is, visually powerful critiques of vision.[25] What we have in both this section of the *Phenomenology* and in the key passages of the *Encyclopedia* is the use of techniques of visualization to draw the reader, as Kuhn argues, "into his circle." Hegel would have us look at powerfully presented examples of absurd and marvelous phenomena (phrenology and magnetism, respectively). If we can see their absurdity and miraculousness (and Hegel or his editors will write as graphically as possible so that we can), then he already has us where he wants us: in a position of the speculative Spirit. It is therefore not just a question of using visual images to "make clear" a distinction between two modes of thought, because those very images need to be seen from the right perspective in order for that distinction to have meaning. The images need to be presented in such a way that the reader will be led to want to see them as Hegel does, and thereby to adopt the distinction he is aiming for. And once the reader has "stepped into the circle" of the Spirit and sees "speculatively," the visual ladder used to get there can be *aufgehoben* (which is not the same as tossing it aside).

By placing Hegel's discussion of visions in this rhetorical context, we avoid a number of pitfalls. I hope not to be "tasteless" in Hegel's sense, because I do not intend to inflate the mode of the soul's seeing with that of the Spirit. On the contrary, I would maintain the difference at the level of Hegel's argumentation (he needs both for different reasons). Moreover, I also hope to avoid an idealized conception of speculative thought that would be independent of modes of seeing and arguing that are more "concrete." And finally, I would also strive to emphasize the strength of Hegel's argumentation not on the basis of the "truth" of the speculative but in terms of how he moves us into a "paradigm" shift. He is right that one can appreciate his vision only if one is already beyond the dichotomies of the understanding, and he is using rhetorical techniques to bring about a literal shift in gestalt in our minds. He cannot be "deconstructed" by pointing this out, since by definition the two paradigms are mutually exclusive. In other words, the circular reasoning we saw earlier (seeing the visions helps us see speculatively, but we need to adopt a speculative perspective to see the visions) does not undermine Hegel's argument but, rather, indicates the place where his argument depends on other, rhetorical devices to shift the reader's vision.[26]

In conclusion, what we have here is a radical, rhetorical inversion and ironization of the proverb "out of sight, out of mind" (*aus den Augen, aus dem Sinn*). For Hegel, the necessary inversion would mean that to be in the realm of the mind as Spirit, we need to be able to "see" its reality. But this implies a proper mode of vision, namely, speculative. And ironically, the only way to come to see speculatively is to learn to see what is not there, to accept the possibility of visions. Those visions, however, are not yet, for Hegel, philosophy in its full form. They are products of the "feeling psyche" and hence pathology. His speculative philosophy of Spirit thus cannot be reduced to a spooky sighting of spirits (*Geisterseherei*). And yet these visions have an indispensable rhetorical function if they teach us a double vision, one that allows us to see (*einsehen*, accept) visions as graphically and persuasively real, even as we reject their ultimate legitimacy.[27] We must be made to see in order to get into the proper state of mind from which, ironically, we can then claim to be truly, speculatively, seeing for the first time.

Notes

1. Citations all from Hegel, *Enzyklopädie der philosophischen Wissenschaften im Grundrisse* (1830), *Dritter Teil: Die Philosophie des Geistes*. Mit den mündlichen Zusätzen (Frankfurt: Suhrkamp, 1981). All translations, with minor variations, are from *Hegel's Philosophy of Mind. Part Three of the Encyclopedia of the Philosophical*

Sciences (1830), trans. William Wallace; together with the *Zusätze* in Boumann's Text (1845), trans. A. V. Miller (Oxford: Clarendon Press, 1971). I have quoted in both English and German since the metaphors of vision are clearer at times in the one language, at times in the other. In the case of longer sections or Additions, I have also provided the page numbers of the English and German to make location of the passages easier.

The *Zusätze* are largely reconstructions by the editor, Ludwig Boumann, taken from Hegel's notes, marginalia, students' notebooks, and other lectures. Their precise philological status is thus questionable, and they certainly betray a stylistic reworking by the editor. Thus, all references to "Hegel" as the author of the Additions should in fact be in quotation marks. A significant problem arises for my rhetorical analyses based on these later Additions. My justification must in part disregard the notion of authorial unity and focus on the impact of the Additions on the reception of the *Philosophy of Spirit*. Consider Boumann's statement that he was guided by the intention "daß ihm die unerläßliche Pflicht oblag, den vergleichungsweise rohen Stoff gedachter Vorlesungen in diejenige *künstlerische Form* zu bringen, die auch von einem wissenschaftlichen Werke mit Recht gefordert wird. Ohne eine solche *Umgestaltung* würde in dem vorliegenden Falle eine widerwärtige Disharmonie zwischen dem zu erläuternden Buche und den zu demselben gemachten Zusätzen entstanden sein" (p. 429 f., my emphasis). And Findlay's comment: "There can, however, be no doubt that the material assembled in the *Zusätze* to the *Philosophy of Mind* is of absolutely prime importance for the understanding of Hegel's thought, and that it shows that thought venturing into regions not at all charted in his other writings. To read the paragraphs of the *Philosophy of Mind* together with the *Zusätze* is to see many of Hegel's opinions in a surprisingly fresh, 'modern' light" (v). Both of these comments point to the fact that the Additions, regardless of questions of "authenticity" and philological accuracy, have had, and continue to have, an impact on the way Hegel is received. And this is precisely the point I wish to make. Hegel's own text, we shall see, explicitly states the need for the reader to have a "shift of vision," and the Additions have helped make that possible. I would even argue that it is only thanks to the Additions that we could now, so to speak from our position in a Hegelian paradigm, consider reading Hegel without them. Had we not had the Additions from the start, however, the leap into the Hegelian paradigm would have been that much more difficult. Furthermore, as I will try to indicate at times, many of the key formulations did indeed stem from Hegel's pen and can be found, for example, in the "Fragment zur Philosophie des subjektiven Geistes," reprinted in the critical edition, *Schriften und Entwürfe I (1817–1825)*, ed. Friedrich Hogemann and Christoph Jamme (Hamburg: Felix Meiner Verlag, 1990), vol. 15; as well as the Theoriewerkausgabe (Suhrkamp), vol. 11. Thus, although the actual organization of material by Boumann may not have been the same as Hegel's (see Petry's notes, p. 557), the preoccupation with and argumentative significance of the topic, as well as the focus on visions and visualizations, are all Hegelian to the core. Finally, the fact that the Additions were largely put together by the notes of Hegel's students (notes that he also used when he repeated the lectures) indicates that we have here precisely the closest re-creation of the devices that were so effective in the persuasion of potential young Hegelians.

2. See the "Fragment" (probably written 1822/23), in which Hegel refers to two conditions that have led to a new *Betrachtungsweise* of Spirit: "die völlige Veränderung des Begriffs der Philosophie" and "Der andere Umstand kommt von der empirischen Seite selbst, und ist der *animalische Magnetismus*, welcher

in der Welt des Geistes ein Gebiet von *Wundern* entdeckt, und uns damit bekannt gemacht hat. Für die Auffassung der verschiedenen Zustände und sonstiger natürlicher Bestimmungen des Geistes, welche den Zusammenhang der Natur und des Geistes enthalten, wie für die Auffassung seines Bewußtseyns und seiner geistigen Tätigkeit, reicht, wenn man bey den Erscheinungen stehen bleibt, nothdürftig die *gewöhnliche endliche Betrachtungsweise* hin, und der *verständige* Zusammenhang von *Ursache* und *Wirkung*, den man den *natürlichen Gang* der *Dinge* nennt, findet in diesem äusserlichen Gebiete sein Auskommen. Aber in den Erfahrungen des thierischen Magnetismus ist es die *Region der äusserlichen Erscheinungen* selbst, in welcher der verständige Zusammenhang von Ursachen und Wirkungen, mit seinen Bedingungen von den räumlichen und zeitlichen Bestimmungen seinen Sinn verliert, und innerhalb des sinnlichen Daseyns selbst und seiner Bedingtheit die höhere Natur des Geistes sich geltend macht und zum Vorschein kommt" (pp. 213–215). This description captures nicely one of the points I wish to make below: Hegel will use the graphically and visually persuasive force of phenomena associated with animal magnetism to help bring about a shift from "normal" to "revolutionary" philosophical *Wissenschaft*.

In this fragment we also see at least one clear source of Hegel's ideas, since the next paragraph introduces the psychological study by Eschenmeyer, who also edited the *Archiv für den thierischen Magnetismus* (Leipzig).

3. Findlay's foreword to the translation of the *Encyclopedia* (p. xi). I find this notion of vision more interesting than the one just prior to it that sees the "Absolute Idea defined by Hegel as the eternal *vision* of itself."

4. One way of measuring Hegel's interest in this field is to consider the number of books in his library at the time of his death that dealt specifically with animal magnetism. See the list compiled by Wolfgang Neuser, published in Michael John Petry, ed., *Hegel und die Naturwissenschaften* (Stuttgart-Bad Cannstatt: Frommann-Holzboog, 1987), pp. 479–499 (esp. the high percentage of books that deal with animal magnetism among those relevant for the anthropology).

I cannot deal here with the general historical significance of animal magnetism for the late eighteenth and early nineteenth centuries. One colleague of mine has called it the "chaos theory" or "relativity theory" of the age given the impact it had on so many areas of thought. For a fascinating overview of the kinds of views dominating the early nineteenth century, consider the *Report of the Experiments on Animal Magnetism* presented to the Committee of the Medical Section of the French Royal Academy of Sciences in June 1831, published in an English translation with an extensive introduction by J. C. Colquhoun (Edinburgh: Robert Cadell, 1833; reprinted New York: Arno Press, 1975). This report stands in stark contrast to findings of the earlier commission (1784) that denied the existence of animal magnetism. The parallels to Hegel's discussion are at times astonishing and reveal the common store of knowledge of these phenomena. For a more recent treatment, see Ernst Benz, "Franz Anton Mesmer und die philosophischen Grundlagen des 'animalischen Magnetismus'" (*Akademie der Wissenschaften und Literatur. Abhandlungen der geistes- und sozialwissenschaftlichen Klasse,* Jahrgang 1977, Nr. 4). While the former work indicates that in Germany in general "the treatment [of animal magnetism] is almost universally employed and recommended by the most intelligent physicians; much attention is bestowed upon the magnetic phenomena, and great ingenuity is displayed in the formation of theories to account for the results" (p. 78), the latter points specifically to the importance of Berlin: "Nach der Jahrhundertwende regte sich vor allem in Berlin bei jüngeren Ärzten ein praktisches und theoretisches Interesse an dem tierischen Magnetismus'' (p. 6). See in the same series by the Akademie der Wissenschaften und Literatur: Walter Artelt, "Der Mesmerismus in Berlin" (1965, Nr. 6).

5. These formulations were present in Hegel's own manuscripts for his planned publication of a philosophy of spirit from 1822/23. It is interesting that animal magnetism is related to a series of (false) dichotomies (freedom versus determinism, body versus soul) that point to the "Bedürfnis, hier *zu begreifen*" (sec. 379). This notion of some state of knowledge generating a "need" of/for philosophy has accompanied Hegel's thoughts since his youth. See Kunio Kozu, *Das Bedürfnis der Philosophie. Ein Überblick über die Entwicklung des Begriffkomplexes 'Bedürfnis,' 'Trieb,' 'Streben,' und 'Begierde' bei Hegel* (Hegel-Studien, Beiheft 30; Bonn: Bouvier Verlag, 1988).

6. John Sallis, "Imagination and Presentation in Hegel's Philosophy of Spirit," in Peter G. Stillman, ed., *Hegel's Philosophy of Spirit* (Albany: State University of New York Press, 1987), points to the passage in the Addition to sec. 449 where Hegel reminds us of Aristotle's statement that all knowledge (*Erkenntnis*) has its beginning in wonder (*Verwunderung*). See that book for other recent essays in English on the *Encyclopedia*.

7. Even if one does not consider the Additions, Hegel's own published words indicate a unique significance that he attributed to these phenomena. Consider the fact that sec. 406, which deals with animal magnetism and related states of mind, is the longest single paragraph (over four pages compared to most which are a page or so long) besides the two near the end on art and philosophy (secs. 563 and 573, respectively). The same is true for the 1830 *Encyclopedia*.

8. See Allen W. Wood, *Hegel's Ethical Thought* (Cambridge: Cambridge University Press, 1990), for a critique of the reduction of these structures to the pseudo-Hegelian mold of "thesis-antithesis-synthesis" (pp. 1–4).

9. The "Verein des Verewigten" indicated that Boumann need not include Additions for the sections on "objective Spirit" because the *Philosophy of Right* included much of that material. The same was true for the sections on absolute Spirit, since the lectures on aesthetics, religion, and philosophy of history had already been published. See the editorial comments in the German edition, p. 429.

10. See also the discussion of sleeping and waking, sec. 398.

11. See also the discussion of the ego as a *Schacht* in sec. 462 and, of course, Derrida's treatment of that later reference (no mention of the earlier one) in "Le puits et la pyramide," "The Pit and the Pyramid: Introduction to Hegel's Semiology," in *Margins of Philosophy*, trans. Alan Bass (Chicago: University of Chicago Press, 1982).

12. "In this summary encyclopaedic account it is impossible to supply a demonstration of what the paragraph states as the nature of the remarkable condition produced chiefly by animal magnetism—to show, in other words, that it is in harmony with the facts." ("In dieser enzyklopädischen Darstellung kann nicht geleistet werden, was für den Erweis der gegebenen Bestimmung des merkwürdigen, durch den animalischen Magnetismus vornehmlich hervorge-

rufenen Zustands zu leisten wäre, daß nämlich die Erfahrungen entsprechend seien," sec. 406). The indirect discourse (*seien*) indicates a fictional dialogue with some doubting reader.

13. That Hegel was aware of and indeed mastered such modes of argumentation, see my study, *The Spirit and Its Letter: Traces of Rhetoric in Hegel's Philosophy of Bildung* (Ithaca: Cornell University Press, 1988), esp. chap. 3 on the Jena writings in which Hegel was engaged in preparing for the "paradigm shift," or in his words, "clearing the ground" for Absolute Idealism.

14. Thomas S. Kuhn, *The Structure of Scientific Revolutions.* (Chicago: University of Chicago Press, 1970).

15. Michael J. Petry, in his long review essay, "Hegel's Philosophy of Nature: Recent Developments," *Hegel-Studien* 23 (1988), points to Hegel's use of rhetoric in his lectures in a somewhat more disparaging tone, referring to the "frequently specious arguments by means of which Hegel attempted to persuade his students of the plausibility of his progressions" (p. 322). My concern here is not to reduce such argumentation to "mere" rhetoric but to see it as an indispensable part of argumentation.

16. The point of this parallel is to lend credence to Hegel's often abstract conceptualizations. For a brief summary of object relations theory, with references to Freud's theory of the drive, Melanie Klein, Ronald Fairbain, and Donald Winnicott, see Elizabeth Wright, ed., *Feminism and Psychoanalysis: A Critical Dictionary* (Oxford: Blackwell, 1992). See Eckhard Hammel, "Hegel und die Dingproduktion: Ein Einblick in Lacans Hegel-Rezeption," *Hegel-Studien* 23 (1988):227–244. He comes closest of anyone I know to pointing to these sections in the *Encyclopedia* as related to certain theories of subject formation in psychoanalysis (esp. pp. 227–233).

17. The parallels between Hegel's analysis and Freud's, esp. in chap. 7 of the *Interpretation of Dreams*, would deserve fuller analysis. It is also not by chance that we find shared interests. Hegel here is interested in dreams and infantile life, and Freud was interested in such phenomena as "magical thinking" and telepathy. Similarly, both considered "pathology" as a form of "regression" or fixation on earlier stages. This connection would lead to a different one from that proposed by Ricoeur.

18. Again, on the historical background to this phenomenon in the literature of Hegel's day, see Petry's translation and notes (pp. 538–543).

19. Here the parallels to such contemporary treatises as the "Report" to the French Academy of Sciences and the Introduction to the English translation are remarkable.

20. Also his characterization of Pierre Gabriel von Ghert (one of Hegel's friends), as a "reliable man rich in ideas and well read in recent philosophy" ("ein[] zuverlässige[r] und zugleich gedankenreiche[r], in der neuesten Philosophie gebildete[r] Mann"; English, p. 118; German, p. 154). Aristotle, of course, sees *ethos*, the appeal to the character of the speaker, as one of the main means of achieving persuasion.

21. "When the Germans ridicule, as they often do, the faulty theories of the French, it can be asserted, at least as regards animal magnetism, that the naive metaphysics employed by the French is more satisfactory than the often fanciful explanations and the lame as well as erroneous theorizing of German savants." ("Wenn die Deutschen sich häufig über die mangelhaften Theorien der Franzosen lustig machen, so kann man wenigstens in bezug auf den animalischen Magnetismus behaupten, daß die bei Betrachtung desselben von den Franzosen gebrauchte naive Mataphysik etwas viel Erfreulicheres ist als das nicht seltene Geträume und das ebeso schiefe wie lahme Theoretisieren deutscher Gelehrter"; English, p. 117 f.; German, p. 154).

22. On *auctoritas*, see, for example, Heinrich Lausberg, *Handbuch der literarischen Rhetorik* (Munich: Max Hueber, 1960), sec. 426 ff.

23. In the *Encyclopedia* both phrenology and physiognomy are dealt with (briefly and dismissively) just a few paragraphs later, at the end of the section on Anthropology ("Die wirkliche Seele," sec. 411). This shift in location (recall that in the *Phenomenology* they are dealt with near the end of the chapter on Reason) indicates that there is a close connection in Hegel's mind between the visionary realities of the soul and the belief in the skeletal thingness of Spirit. On the connection between Lavater and animal magnetism, see the Report to the French Royal Academy, p. 71 f.

See Eric von der Luft, "The Birth of Spirit for Hegel out of the Travesty of Medicine" and the comment on this paper by Quentin Lauer, in Stillman, *Hegel's Philosophy of Spirit*. Von der Luft focuses largely on the transition to *Geist* in the *Phenomenology* via the critique of phrenology and other pseudosciences, and links this to the end of the book of the *Encyclopedia* on Nature and the transition to the *Philosophy of Spirit*. No mention is made, however, of Hegel's use of animal magnetism as a visualization of Spirit.

24. Donald Phillip Verene, *Hegel's Recollection: A Study of Images in the Phenomenology of Spirit* (Albany: State University of New York Press, 1985), p. 81.

25. I argued this in *The Spirit and Its Letter*, pp. 234–236.

26. This stance in regard to Hegel is not unlike that of William Desmond. See his most recent study, *Beyond Hegel and Dialectic: Speculation, Cult, and Comedy* (Albany: State University of New York Press, 1992). Desmond formulates a fundamental paradox in Hegel's thought that he strives to maintain, occasionally even against Hegel: "Hegel wants to think the dialectical togetherness of philosophical reason and its recalcitrant others. The paradox consists in the tense coexistence of systematic philosophical completeness and philosophical openness to what is other to philosophy" (p. 4). This kind of thinking is, according to Desmond, "speculative" in the widest sense (e.g., p. 9). My reading contributes to such a perspective on Hegel by highlighting the double vision inherent in the speculative.

27. Petry points out the remarkable (and perhaps not simply coincidental) similarity between the formulation of the overall purpose of the periodical, *Archiv für den thierischen Magnetismus* (announced in 1817), and the opening theme of Hegel's inaugural lecture delivered at Berlin on October 22, 1818. I hope to have accounted for the argumentative significance of this similarity.

8

Perspectives and Horizons: Husserl on Seeing the Truth

Mary C. Rawlinson

Even the mind's eye has its blind spot.
—Maurice Merleau-Ponty, *The Visible and the Invisible*

Famously, Husserl's philosophy invokes a "return to the things themselves," presents itself as a "presuppositionless science," and promises access to the "absolute." Against Kant, Husserl argues that the objects of experience, conditioned by subjective constitution, are in fact the "things themselves." And Husserl does not doubt the capacity of language—of his own language—to articulate this reality so that "nothing is left over." Through a system of metaphors and (dis)analogies, Husserl institutes a parallel between the experience of sensuous seeing and the non-sensuous vision of the phenomenologist. In this paradoxical parallel—at once constituted in language and making a place for that very language, even authorizing it—Husserl unfolds, as if explicating the perspectives and horizons of a perceptual thing, the program of phenomenology.

Phenomenology establishes its legitimacy by exposing the false pretensions of any philosophy that constitutes itself as an objective science. The issue is not one of technique or method but vision. Such a pseudophilosophy "remains blind to the full concrete being and life that constitutes [its objects] transcendentally" (*Crisis*, p. 176).[1] This philosophical blindness reflects the natural blindness of the man in the world who is so dazzled by things that his vision terminates in them.[2] Considering these objects in relation to interest and need, he is "born blind" to their genesis in acts of synthesis. Seeing only them, he does not really see, for he is blind to the very processes from which these things result.

Through phenomenological analysis, however, objects "pass into the brightly lit circle of perfect presentation" (*Ideas*, sec. 69). Explicitly likened to the explication of perceptual perspectives, this analysis or "unfolding" reveals the subjective acts of constitution in which objective sense is determined. His eyes opened by phenomenology, the "man in the street" is transformed and elevated to a perspective "above the world," where he discovers the absolutely foundational activity of the transcendental ego illuminating every level of sense or being. Thus, Husserl argues, a "presuppositionless" philosophy is possible, one that reveals what is hidden in ordinary experience by exposing in what appears merely "given" the generative acts that condition it.

This philosophical confidence secures itself in a chiasm of vision and voice. Elaborating itself through the metaphorical appropriation of visual perception, phenomenological analysis produces at once a nonsensuous seeing and a "univocal language" of the general. The phenomenologist describes visual perception only in order to recapitulate certain of its features in a strictly nonperceptual register, and the descriptions of perception themselves already reflect this theoretical itinerary.

It is as if Husserl writes with two hands. On the one hand, the being before consciousness of the visual thing provides the positive model for "immanent perception" and for the presentation of essences in "eidetic seeing." On the other, visual perception supplies an alien alterity against which the phenomenologist's "volitionally directed glance" unfolds. Elaborating this system of (dis)analogies, Husserl speaks repeatedly of paradoxes, enigmas, and "tempting parallels." (See, e.g., *ITC*, sec. 9, n. 7; also, sec. 44 on the "ambiguity" of the term "inner perception," which Husserl employs regularly. See also *CM*, Fifth Meditation, where the main theme is the "enigma" or "riddle" involved in seeing another human body.) Though one speaks "rightly" of transcendental self-*perception* or eidetic *seeing* or the shifting *glance* of the phenomenologically reduced ego or the *horizons* of time-consciousness, nevertheless, in doing so, one does not speak "strictly." (See, e.g., *CM*, p. 46.) And the invocation of the metaphor or parallel brings with it an insistence on the absolute difference of phenomenological seeing and sensuous seeing: "This having in one's glance, in one's mental eye, which belongs to the *essence* of the *cogito* ... should not be confused with perceiving (in however wide a sense this term be used), or with any other types of act related to perceptions" (*Ideas*, sec. 37; see also sec. 35). The analogy between phenomenological analysis and transcendental reflection, on the one hand, and visual perception, on the other, is both necessary and dangerous.

Through this system of metaphors, Husserl arrogates to the apprehension of essences and to the self-apprehension of the transcendental ego the qualities of vision: most important, its credibility and immediacy—the being before the object of the perceiver—but also its *horizonality*, directionality, and action at a distance. Yet this strategy of metaphor and analogy succeeds only through its own self-denial: by asserting and reasserting that the horizonality of time-consciousness is not that of visual perception, that the "volitionally directed *glance*" of the phenomenologist is not the vision of the man of the world looking at things, that eidetic *seeing* is "not a sensuous seeing," that the multiple presentations in which we *see* the unity of the essence are not like the multiple perspectives in which the unity of the thing is apprehended, and so on. Employing this strategy of identification and differentiation, Husserl endeavors to transfer to philosophical analysis the irresistible credibility of sensuous immediacy and, at the same time, to protect phenomenological seeing from the incompleteness and revisibility that characterize the evidence of visual perception.

This strategy requires its own blindness. While Husserl, like Hegel, insists on perception, and specifically visual perception, as a methodological starting point—both in the sense that the analysis of visual perception provides a model for all phenomenological analysis and insofar as the language articulating eidetic and transcendental apprehension is borrowed from the experience of seeing—phenomenology cannot accept this perception in its "natural" state. It must be treated by the "reductions," subjected to the "modifications of the pure imagination," and disconnected from the life-world, so as to be detached from actuality and rendered "only an example." (See, e.g., *EJ*, sec. 87a.) In the method of eidetic variation the philosopher assumes this blindness to contingency in order to "see through" the actual examples to the essential form of which they are only instances. Blinded to the specificity and interests of actual perception, the phenomenologist's gaze nonetheless dissects and remembers perception, so as to exhibit its truth in an order that is, strictly speaking, nonperceptual.[3] The mobile eye is made to say "I," but in the voice of the general, where its specificity is always reduced and it is no more than an instance.

Via the multiple gestures of this metaphorical appropriation of sensuous seeing, Husserl revisions the spectacle of the other's body in motion in the world, rewriting it as a representation of the same transcendental subjectivity given in the "sphere of my ownness." This perception that is no perception but the self-articulation of an undifferentiated, infinitely iterable voice, translates both the self-certainty of the perceiving subject and the intersubjectivity of the perceptual world into the register of the transcendental: the former, as the self-constituting transcendental ego, and the latter, in the presentation of the other as the same in transcendental reflection. At stake in this philosophical appropriation of visual perception are the "I" and the "we" of phenomenology, or rather, the "I" that is a "we." What authorizes this "we" and its "mature normal civilization" is the reduction of the embodied perceiver to the ideality of a linguistic operation. (See *OG*, p. 258.) It remains to be seen, however, whether this open "I" of a "univocal language" can altogether close itself to the perspectives and horizons of its sensuous "other."

Mobile Vision, or the Phenomenology of Perception

We start by taking an example. Keeping the table steadily in view as I go round it, changing my position in space all the time, I have continually the consciousness of the bodily presence out there of this one and self-same table, which itself remains unchanged throughout. But the perception of the table is one that changes continuously, it is a continuum of changing perceptions. I close my eyes. My other senses are inactive in relation to the table. I have no perception of it. I open my eyes, and the perception returns.

—Husserl, *Ideas*

Visual perception serves an exemplary function within phenomenological analysis in at least three senses. First, Husserl regularly relies on it as the epitome of acts of consciousness. The constitution of the visual thing in space is the "normal and basic instance of constitution" (*SGP*, 10). And what is said of perception "holds good, obviously, of those other experiences [recollections, "representations similar to recollections," and the "free play of fancy"], essentially different as they are" (*Ideas*, sec. 35). This is so because visual perception provides a paradigm of the synthetic activity through which the presentation of any objective sense is achieved. Second, visual perception exhibits a logic of parts and wholes that will be recapitulated in the register of the transcendental. Specifically, it demonstrates the capacity of a part to disclose the whole, a feature that will reappear as essential to time-consciousness, eidetic seeing, and transcendental self-perception. Finally, the evidence of visual perception, the immediacy of perception or the being before the object of the perceiver, supplies by analogy the criterion for the evidence of transcendental perception. *"Essential insight is a primordial dator act*, and as such *analogous to sensory perception*, and *not to imagination"* (*Ideas*, sec. 23). Both the evidence of visual perception and that of phenomenological perception are discovered to be "incomplete," and Husserl establishes the "apodicticity" of the latter precisely by distinguishing it from the ideal of "adequacy" that regulates the former's presentation of its object.

Husserl, like Kant, locates the essence of perception in the phenomena of perspective and synthesis.[4] Both consciousness and the thing are synthetic unities. Perception reveals two correlative unities, each of which results from a discernible constitutive synthesis: "A *single* perceptual thing appearing with ever-increasing completeness, from endlessly new points of view, and with ever-richer determinations ... which, in principle, can be given only as the unity of such ways of appearing" and "a singly intentional consciousness," which through its own active synthesizing continually reconstitutes itself as the same throughout the differentiated motions of visual perception (*Ideas*, p. 42).

As in Kant's analysis, however, these unities result not from what is presented to the senses but from the general synthetic activity of consciousness. In explicating "synthesis as the primal form of consciousness," Husserl remarks that in the perception of "for example ... this die" the " 'visual perspectives' change": we can view it from here or there, from one side or the other, or we can pay attention to this or that property, its color or shape or size; nevertheless, these aspects comprise the unity of "*this* identical" die (*CM*, p. 78). The thing is a "point of intersection belonging to my constitutive synthesis" (*CM*, p. 135). Anything that can become an object of consciousness, anything at all, is identified as a node in a complex network of syntheses. And the ability of the mobile perceiver to see in the partial presentation the objective unity of the thing itself provides a paradigm for all acts of consciousness.

In any given act of perception there is presented to the senses only one aspect or perspective of the object; yet the whole of the object is not merely implied but actually presented through this part:

When we view the table, we view it from some particular side, and this side is thereby what is genuinely seen. Yet the table has still other sides. It has an unseen back side, it has an unseen interior; and these are actually indexes for a variety of sides, a variety of complexes of possible visibility. That is a very curious situation peculiar to the matter. For belonging to the very sense of every perception is perception's perceived object as its objective [*gegenstandlicher*] sense, i.e., this thing, the table seen. But this thing is not [merely] the side genuinely seen in this moment; rather (according to the very sense of perception) the thing *is precisely the full-thing* that still has other sides, sides that are not brought to genuine perception in this perception, but that would be brought to genuine perception in other perceptions. (*SGP*, p. 2)

What is seen in perception, then, is more than what is actually given to the eyes. The given perspective does not merely represent or indicate the "full-thing"; it presents the thing itself, the table, for example. The whole is fully given in the part, even though some of its sides are not "genuinely" seen.

In conformity with Husserl's metaphorics, the system of (dis)analogies binding visual perception and transcendental reflection, this originally perceptual logic of parts and wholes reappears as essential to the self-constitution of the transcendental ego and at the same time provides the point of division between the perception of things and the self-perceptions of consciousness. On the one hand, consciousness presents a paradox, or rather several. It exists both as a part of the world and as the part that in transcendental reflection encompasses the whole. As time-consciousness, it is at once always now, occurring as an act in immanent time, and an act presenting the whole of the temporal field. And, in transcendental intersubjectivity the ego, though only one example among others, is "absolute." In each case the part-whole logic of perception reappears, though in another register.

On the other hand, it is precisely in this reappearance in another register of the perceptual logic of parts and wholes that Husserl reads the difference between the perceptual thing and consciousness. Neither consciousness, nor the thing, can be given-apprehended "all at once." Each is presented as a whole in the presentation of a part. Each is said to be "incomplete" in its evidence; however, the incompleteness of the evidence of perception turns out to be vicious, opening up the constant possibility of error, while the incompleteness of the evidence of "self-perception" proves benign. This establishes the radical difference between immanent and transcendent perception, and the necessity of elaborating an allergy between them.

In spite of its incompleteness, though it is qualified by an "indeterminately general presumptive horizon" that is said to be "like" the horizon of external perception (*CM*, p. 62), the ego's self-evidence is said to be "absolute" and "apodictic." "An experience casts no shadows" (*Ideas*, sec. 42). It has no other side that is withheld from the perceiver, and it does not show itself in "aspects," "perspectives," or "views" to an encircling perceiver. It is apprehended in its own "horizons," which are not those of the thing of actual perception.

"Enigmatically," consciousness is "interwoven [*verflochten*]" with a being that is "foreign" to it, with a "world that is alien to consciousness" (*Ideas*, sec. 39). While the thing and consciousness are "essentially related to each other, [they] are in principle and of necessity not really [*reell*] and essentially one and united" (*Ideas*, sec. 41). This difference between the thing and consciousness founds Husserlian phenomenology and marks the fundamental divisions of its epistemology and ontology.

Let us start with an example. In front of me, in the dim light, lies this white paper. I see it, touch it. This perceptual seeing and touching of the paper as the full concrete experience *of* the paper that lies here as given in truth precisely with this relative lack of clearness, with this imperfect definition, appearing to me from this particular angle—is a *cogitatio*, a conscious experience. The paper itself with its objective qualities, its extension in space, its objective position in regard to the spatial thing I call my body, is not *cogitatio*, but *cogitatum*, not perceptual experience, but something perceived. Now that which is perceived can itself very well be a conscious experience; but it is evident that an object such as a material thing, this paper, for instance, as given in perceptual experience, is in principle other than an experience, a being of a completely different kind. (*Ideas*, sec. 35)

This difference between the writer's seeing and his paper exemplifies "the most fundamental and pivotal difference between ways of being, that between Consciousness and Reality" (*Ideas*, sec. 42). A certain incompleteness qualifies the "essential nature of spatial thinghood": in the presentation of a visual thing what is "really presented" has "margins," and at them yields to "an outlying zone" of "vague indeterminacy." Here "foreign [*uneigentlicher*] co-data" are more or less clearly suggested but, strictly speaking, left unpresented: indeterminate but determinable: "For example, there belongs to every external perception its reference from the 'genuinely perceived' sides of the object of perception to the sides 'also meant'—not yet perceived, but only anticipated" (*CM*, pp. 82–83).

As the seeing subject circles around the perceptual thing or envelops it in his gaze, these determinacies are explored and filled out, but only in succession, never all at once. Having margins, the visual thing withholds itself in its presentation, casts shadows, and offers, in the distance, further, unexplicated evidence. "Being of this species can, in principle, be given in perceptions only by way of perspective manifestation" (*Ideas*, sec. 42). Perception is an infinite task requiring the constant motility of the body for the constitution of a world, and "a margin of determinable indeterminacy always remains over," however completely filled out the view of the thing may be.

This "incompleteness" of the visually given spatial thing constitutes a double disability. First, these margins prescribe their own explication so that the glance of the perceiver is not entirely free in unfolding the object, and, in fact, apprehends the object only as a synthetic unity, a continuum of perspectives, by following these prescriptions. The perception of the die prefigures what lies on and beyond the margin; what lies beyond the margin is "construed in advance." Thus, the "freedom" of consciousness to alter its orientation or adopt new modes of consciousness is constrained by or regulated by these "horizon intentionalities." The thing is never present in perception as a "finished datum." Every determination "leaves further particulars open." And this "leaving open ... is precisely what makes up the horizon"— open, but "predelineated" (*CM*, pp. 82–83).

Second, these prefigurings can deceive. We can err in our expectations or be surprised in our explication of the multiple presentations of the visual thing in space. In the distinction between "genuinely perceived" and "also meant" lie many possible misprisions. Thus, the evidence of the visual presentation of the spatial thing can only approach adequacy and can never be apodictic. The identity of the visually given spatial thing may be revisioned entirely in the filling out of its perspectives. (These texts on "margins," "indeterminacy," and "incompleteness" are, of course, other descriptions of what is represented so positively under the titles of "synthesis" and "constitution.")

The vision of the mobile perceiver operates responsively in relation to the call of things and must in order to succeed in its register be determined by that call: "In every moment of perceiving, the 'perceived' is what it is in its mode of appearance as

a system of indicating implications [*Verweisen*] with an appear-
ance-core on which appearances have their hold. And in this
indicating it calls out to us, as it were: 'there is still more to see
here'" (*SGP*, p. 3).

The incompleteness of the perceptual horizon "cannot be filled
up in just any manner." An actual perception includes indications [*Hinweisen*] of systems of possible appearances that would
confirm and develop the identity of the object perceived.[5] These
indications, though "presentations of the "full-thing," embody
only controvertible possibilities—possibilities that may be determined otherwise: "Every appearance draws with it a *plus ultra* in
the empty horizon. And since perception does indeed pretend to
give the object [completely] in the flesh in every appearance, it
in fact constantly pretends to accomplish more than, by its very
nature, it can accomplish" (*SGP*, p. 11). On the one hand, perception makes accessible the "full-thing," though only one of its
aspects is "genuinely seen." On the other, the integrity of the
perceived object remains suspect, for though perceptual consciousness "pretends otherwise," there remains always the possibility of a contradiction between what is implicated in the
indication and explicated in its unfolding.

Both the identity of the thing and the givenness of a world, a
"whole of interconnected possibilities," depend on the con-
sistency of actual perceptions with their previous indications.
Every perception appears to implicate an infinity of possible
determinate perceptions. Husserl often remarks that the horizon
of perception is indeterminate but determinable. In his account
it is also always explicitly drawn as an array of determinate possibilities of perception.

Precisely because the horizon of perception is traced by a
system of determinate anticipations, the evidence of literal or
"transcendent" perception is "imperfect." Perception operates
within a "multiform horizon of unfulfilled [but determinate]
anticipations." And no matter how assiduously the mobile perceiver explores this horizon, no synthesis will ever be adequate to
dispel it. Thus, "there always remains open the possibility that

the belief in being, which extends into the anticipation, will not be fulfilled, that what is appearing in the mode 'it itself' nevertheless does not exist or is different" (*CM*, pp. 96–97). The objective unity of the thing, as well as of the world, depends on the mobile perceiver's operating under the requirement of a "harmonious synthesis." To be is not merely to be perceived, but to be perceived again and again in a multiplicity of presentations as the same. Perception, of necessity, remains open to the reconstitution of its object. The mobile perceiver is led on indefinitely by the horizon of determinate anticipations, and in this explication of perspectives the object is either constantly reconfirmed or revealed to be something altogether other. Thus, the evidence of sensuous seeing, while "adequate" to the presentation of the object, can never be "apodictic."

This constraint and dubitability, however, adhere only to the perception of the thing in its specificity:

If a concrete object stands out for us in experience as something particular, and our attentively grasping glance [*Blick*] then becomes directed to it, it becomes appropriated in this simple grasping as an "undetermined object of empirical intuition." It becomes a determined object, and one undergoing further determination, in a continuation of the experience in the form of a determining experience, which at first unfolds only what is included in the object itself: a pure *explication*. In its articulated synthetic course, on the basis of the object given as self-identical in a continuous intuitive synthesis of identification, this pure explication unfolds, in a concatenation of particular intuitions the object's very own determinations, the "internal" determinations. These present themselves originaliter as determinations in which it, the Identical itself, is what it is and, moreover, exists in itself, "in and of itself"—determinations wherein its identical being becomes explicated as the particulars making up its ownness: what it is, specifically [*in Sonderheit*]. (*CM*, pp. 131–132)

That in perception which is dubitable and constraining is precisely that which constitutes the specificity of the thing, perceptual determinations and their indeterminate horizons of determinate possibilities. These indeterminate horizons of determinate anticipations prescribe a space within which the thing can be itself, boundaries whose violation would constitute a

change of identity. The grasping glance caught up in the explication of the thing operates out of a faith in what is anticipated,
while remaining forever vulnerable to its nonexistence.

Moreover, Husserl argues, it is precisely specificity that resists
phenomenology's loquacious gaze. Though "it is only the individual element which phenomenology ignores," even eidetic
singularities, the "lowest specific differences" in the system of
essences (red, for example, as a specification of color or two as a
specification of number), admit of no "conceptual and termino-
logical fixation," nor any "unambiguous determination ... in
our realm of description." With the "genera" or "more general" essences comprehending these singularities, "it is quite
otherwise." These prove to be thoroughly accessible to phenomenological analysis. They are "susceptible of stable distinction,
unbroken self-identity, and strict conceptual apprehension, likewise of being analyzed into component essences, and accordingly
they may very properly be made subject to the conditions of a
comprehensive scientific description" (*Ideas*, sec. 75; see also,
sec. 12, "Genus and species," and sec. 14, where the "individual" is clearly defined as a "this-here"). They can be said. The
phenomenologist's loquacious gaze can give voice only to what is
generalized, and it remains mute not only before the particular
thing, but also before its "distinguishing features" [*eigenwe-
sentliche Merkmale*]. The essences or general truths of phenomenology appear only in opposition to the specificity of its
exemplars: "Difference [of the examples in eidetic variation] is
that which ... does not make an essence appear" (*EJ*, sec. 87e).

Husserl necessarily invokes the concept of specificity in the
analysis of perception, for the glance of the mobile perceiver
encircles only this table and this paper or the like, not a "thing
in general." Yet it is just this specificity that he incessantly, assiduously attempts to eliminate from the domain of phenomenology, where everything that appears, including the ego itself, is
"only an example." Husserl insists that the examples of eidetic
variation are not intuited individuals given by experience, but
"arbitrary variations" produced "by an act of volition." The
"freedom" of the phenomenological imagination consists pre-

cisely in its being freed from the constraining contingency of experience (*EJ*, sec. 87a). Thus, through the reduction of the actual individual to the status of an "arbitrary example," Husserl endeavors to liberate the glance from the trajectory of determination implied in the thing's horizon. Disinterested, decathected, the glance is free to direct itself anywhere, to imagine and possibilize without the constraint of perception's "harmonious synthesis."

Given that the exemplars of eidetic variation are freed from the horizon of the life-world, it is not surprising that even Husserl's descriptions of actual perceptions are already theoretical reconstructions:

By viewing an object I am conscious of the position of my eyes and at the same time—in the form of a novel and systematic empty horizon—I am conscious of the entire system of possible eye positions that rest at my disposal. And now, what is seen in the given eye position is so enmeshed with the entire system that I can say with certainty that if I were to move my eyes in this or that direction, specific visual appearances would accordingly run their course in a definite order.... The system of lived-body movements is in fact characterized with respect to consciousness in a special way as a subjectively free system. I run through this system in the consciousness of the free "I can." It may happen that I unintentionally dwell upon something, that for instance my eyes turn this way or that. But at any time I can exercise my will and pursue such a line of movement or whatever line of movement I like. (*SGP*, p. 14)

Does this transparent, unhindered body exist, whose vision is never obscured, whose motion is never compromised? When I am "aware of my eye-positions," is it not because I fear to meet someone's gaze or am sneaking a peek, rather than being free to pursue "whatever line of movement I like"? Hasn't Husserl himself demonstrated the degree to which I can never "say with certainty" what will be discovered in the explication of the perceptual thing's horizons? Can the forces that determine the body in love or in addiction or in illness be altogether eliminated from a description of the perceiving body, if it is still to be a description of a "lived body"?

Mary C. Rawlinson

In actuality the gaze rarely roams freely. It is arrested by a beautiful face, lured by a roadside accident, fascinated by a glittering display of merchandise, dispersed in an anxious search, deflected or seduced by the foreign and forbidden. Husserl insists on this: not only does the mobile perceiver encounter the things themselves, persisting there on their own before and after my perception of them; but also these presentations necessarily include an element of valuation or interest. (See, e.g., *Ideas*, sec. 27: "This world is not there for me as a mere *world of facts and affairs*, but, **with the same immediacy**, as a *world of values*, and a *world of goods*, a *practical world*" [boldface added].) And Husserl's insistence on the unity of the percept as a synesthetic, kinesthetic whole hardly implies an isolated, disinterested, infinitely mobile vision. When the thing is something specific, the gaze is always already engaged and prescribed.

Husserl anticipates Maurice Merleau-Ponty's critique of any philosophy of reflection that substitutes for the concretely given a "second positivity."[6] In his criticism of the misguided tendency of natural science to identify its abstract thing with the thing of actual perception, Husserl argues that "the physical space of the thing of physical science cannot be the world of bodily perception" (*Ideas*, sec. 40). Otherwise, Berkeley would be right: there would be no difference between primary and secondary qualities, as these cannot be separated in experience.

Husserl's analysis distinguishes, in fact, three things, for the thing appearing in the theoretical space constituted by the phenomenological reductions is no more the thing of bodily perception than is the theoretically produced entity of natural science. It is precisely what is never perceived, the "thing in general." In Husserl's examples, a disinterested gaze wanders freely over an indifferent object, whose "call" has no tone of its own, whose voice offers no resistance. It calls only to offer itself, passively allowing itself to be unfolded, excavated: "Turn me so you can see all my sides, let your gaze run through me, draw closer to me, open me up, divide me up, keep on looking me over anew, turning me to see all sides. You will get to know me like this, all that I am, all my surface qualities, all my inner sensuous qualities, etc." (*SGP*, p. 3). In the theoretical space of phenomenology the thing—unlike the beloved or money or a small child—stands still, submissive, circumscribable, uncontested. Though distinct from the thing of science, the thing of phenomenological analysis is nonetheless an abstraction. (See *CM*, p. 126.) Phenomenology lights up the genus or type, the form of any possible object and a taxonomy of kinds.

The subject who entertains these abstractions is similarly abstracted from the world. By breaking the "natal bond with the world," Husserl constructs a position and a space of reflection wherein the gaze moves freely and the thing has been liberated from its specificity. Here the "predelineated horizons," rather than indicating determinate but dubitable anticipations of perception, inscribe the apodicticity of formal rules. Yet this apodicticity itself is modeled on visual perception. "Every perceiving consciousness," Husserl remarks, "has this peculiarity, that it is the consciousness of *the embodied* [*leibhaftigen*] *self-presence of an individual object*" (*Ideas*, sec. 38). This being before the object of the perceiver comes to define phenomenological evidence in general: "Self-evidence means nothing more than grasping an entity with the consciousness of its being itself there [*Selbstda*]" (*OG*, p. 257). Phenomenological evidence, then, takes the form of experience. (See, e.g., *CM*, p. 93.) And this experience is explicitly characterized as a seeing. "Evidence is, in an extremely broad sense, an '*experiencing*' of something that is, and is thus; it is precisely a mental seeing of something itself" (*CM*, p. 52). Both the analysis of essences and the self-analysis of the transcendental ego are defined by analogy to visual perception. In explicating evidence as "itself-givenness," Husserl remarks that for the transcendental ego, this implies "not aiming confusedly at something, with an empty expectant intention, but being with it itself, viewing, seeing, having insight into, it itself" (*CM*, p. 93). Similarly, in his account of eidetic analysis, Husserl identifies evidence with the being in the presence of the object characteristic of visual perception:

We speak of an essential "seeing" and, in general, of the seeing of generalities. This way of talking still requires justification. We use the expression "to see" here in the completely broad sense which implies nothing other than *the act of experiencing things oneself,* the fact of having seen things themselves, and, on the basis of this self-seeing, of having similarity before one's eyes, of accomplishing, on the strength of it, that mental overlapping in which the common, e.g., the red, the figure, etc., "itself" emerges—that is, attains intuitive apprehension.... With this we wish to indicate that we appropriate, directly and as itself, a common and general moment of as many examples as desired, seen one by one, in a manner wholly analogous to the way in which we appropriate an individual particular in sensuous seeing. (*EJ,* sec. 88)

The credibility of vision, then, the perceiver's inability to disbelieve what is before his eyes, supplies the model for the phenomenological method in general and for the apodicticity of its evidence. To proceed phenomenologically, one need only say what one sees.

The danger here, however, is that the evidence of phenomenological analysis will be infected by the "imperfections" to which the evidence of perception is subject in virtue of its incompleteness. Were the evidence of eidetic analysis and the transcendental ego's self-explication exactly analogous to the evidence of perception, the phenomenologist, like the perceiver, would find his judgments both dubitable and constrained. Thus, the employment of the metaphor of vision "still requires justification." Husserl asserts that "the extension of the expression 'seeing,' which not without reason is customary in ordinary language, is unavoidable." Yet in the same discussion of evidence, he insists on the nonperceptual character of this seeing: "We speak of an essential 'seeing.' ... This, naturally, does not mean a sensuous seeing" (*EJ,* sec. 88). The analogy, then, requires both an identification and an alienation between phenomenological analysis and the credibility of visual perception. Establishing the apodicticity of phenomenological evidence by appropriating the subject's immediate relation to the object in visual perception, Husserl must at the same time inoculate phenomenology against the "imperfections" of perception. Phenomenological method at once arrogates to itself the credibility of vision and exhibits an allergy to sensuous seeing.

Beyond the Horizon: The Volitionally Directed Glance and the Spectacle of the Other

Thus it is that each is biased by his own system. We see only what surrounds us, and we think we see everything: we are like children who imagine that when they come to the end of a plain, they shall be able to touch the sky with their hand.

—Etienne Bonnot de Condillac, *An Essay on the Origin of Human Knowledge*

While repeatedly criticizing the very analogies by which phenomenology lays claim to the immediacy and credibility of visual perception, Husserl renders both internal time-consciousness and the eidetic method as forms of self-perception, and, more specifically as forms of *seeing* or *glancing*.[7] Any act of consciousness can become the object of a "so-called 'inner perception'": "to its essence belongs in principle the possibility of a 'reflexive' directing of the mental glance toward itself" (*Ideas*, sec. 38). This turn from the visual thing to consciousness itself opens up the nonspatial space of the transcendental; here extension is purely temporal. The cogito is "not a being in space" (*CM*, sec. 15). (See also *Ideas*, sec. 41: "Experience is possible only as experience and not as something spatial.") While explicitly likening transcendental self-perception to the explication of perspectives in the perception of the visual thing in space (see, e.g., *CM*, p. 132), Husserl insists that "experience ... does not present itself. This implies that the perception of experience is plain insight into something which in perception is given ... as 'absolute,' and not as an identity uniting modes of appearance through perspective continua" (*Ideas*, sec. 44, "The Merely Phenomenal Being of the Transcendent and the Absolute Being of the Immanent"). The apodicticity of immanent perception depends (1) in time-consciousness, on a coincidence of the subject with itself that renders the horizonality of the now nonpernicious, (2) in eidetic seeing, on an absolute freedom from horizons that makes any actual individual "only an example," and (3) in the self-perception of the transcendental ego, on an alienation from the life-world and the body that absolutizes the ego as an example of transcendental life.

Husserl characterizes the self-temporalization of the *cogito* as a "self-alienation." Time-consciousness seems to involve necessarily the absent and nonpresent and to introduce difference into the self-coincidence of immanent perception: "Even an experience [*Erlebnis*] is not, and never is, perceived in its completeness, it cannot be grasped adequately in its full unity. It is essentially something that flows, and starting from the present moment we can swim after it, our gaze reflectively turned towards it, whilst the stretches we leave in our wake are lost to our perception" (*Ideas*, sec. 44). Though immanent perception is distinguished from transcendent perception by the fact that the intentional object belongs to the same stream of experience as the perceptual act itself, the "absoluteness" of its being and the apodicticity of evidence can be secured only if the flux includes a gaze, a *cogitatio*, capable of "lay[ing] hold of at a glance" the flux itself in its unity. Husserl argues that the "incompleteness or 'imperfection' which belongs to the essence of our perception of experience is fundamentally other than that which is of the essence of 'transcendent' perception, perception through a presentation that varies perspectively through such a thing as appearance." The horizonality of temporal differentiation can be so distinguished from that of perspective variation only because immanent perception always involves a "double intentionality": the swimming gaze grasps not only some specific *cogitatio* but also the unitary stream itself within which that *cogitatio* holds a place. Thus, "The flux of the immanent, temporally constitutive consciousness not only is, but is so remarkably and yet so intelligibly constituted that a self-appearance of the flux subsists in it. The self-appearance of the flux does not require a second flux, but qua phenomena it is constituted in itself" (*ITC*, sec. 39).

Only the empirical ego and its acts constitute mere parts of the flux. Self-constituting time-consciousness comprises at once a point of orientation within the flux and the unity of the flux itself. This is so because "the flow of the modes of consciousness is not itself a process, the *Now-consciousness is not itself now*" (*Ideas*, sec. 83). It is a "primal source-point," which "persists" spontaneously without "alteration" or "duration" or "generation," a "form that persists through a continuous change of content" (*Ideas*, sec. 81). Thus, if the concrete connections among experiences can never be given through "a single pure glance," nonetheless, the unity of the stream is apprehended by the "swimming gaze" as a certain " 'limitlessness in the progressive development' of immanent intuitions" (*Ideas*, sec. 83). This intuition first opens up that transcendental "space" within which the subject can, at will, direct and redirect its gaze from one empirical experience to the other. The formality of the intuition ensures that what is "not [yet] the object of a personally directed look" can be brought within the "focus of pure mental vision." If its content is never fully determined in a single glance, still the "Now-consciousness" prefigures that content, ensuring that it can only be more of the same, as a rule or law prefigures all its possible determinations. (See also *CM*, p. 84.)

Moreover, through the distinction between primary and secondary memory, Husserl identifies the horizonality of the now as precisely that which constitutes the unity of the temporal stream. Though secondary memory or recollection involves reproduction or a representation of what is, strictly speaking, absent, "primary remembrance," Husserl asserts, "is perception. For only in primary remembrance do we *see* what is past" (*ITC*, sec. 18). Husserl extends to "immanent retention" the same "absolute right," the same validity, that he extends to immanent perception (*Ideas*, sec. 78). In primary memory the experience is "retained," still immediately given, and every perception carries with it such a retentional fringe, so that experiences within the stream of time-consciousness are, in fact, not discrete, but nested one in the other, each implying or rather presentifying the others. Thus, the unity of the stream is described as a "joining of horizons" (*ITC*, sec. 40). Not only is the incompleteness characterizing immanent perception not pernicious, it is precisely what guarantees the apodicticity of this perception.[8]

The continuity of time-consciousness is a continuity of accessibilities. The horizon of the now marks the openness of the form of consciousness—the Now which is not itself now but constitutes the access of one now to the other. Like the theoretical appropriation of primary memory to perception, this purification of the now's horizon—rendering it purely formal in its implications—is a strategy aimed at securing in time-consciousness an apodictic self-presence. And here again the descriptive fidelity of phenomenology to experience resists the theoretical reconstruction that would secure its apodicticity. Husserl's own analyses reveal the indissoluble intertwining of this self-same I with the sensuous eye of the body. It is in the continuity of a tone, the history of a relationship, the progress of a work that the I discovers itself, and these local unities are rarely, if ever, synthesized in a single perception or univocal will. Every local unity, however, has its horizons and joins or resists or obscures the others. And these (in)accessibilities comprise the I.

The apodicticity of eidetic seeing, however, is guaranteed by the fact that it is unqualified by any horizon. Eidetic seeing accords to "free fancy" a certain "privilege" over perception. (See, e.g., *Ideas*, sec. 70.) By varying imaginatively that which is actually presented, eidetic seeing gains insight into the form of which the actual is only an instance:

Starting from this table-perception as an example, we vary the perceptual object, table, with a completely free optionalness, yet in such a manner that we keep perception fixed as perception of something, no matter what ... we change the fact of this perception into a pure possibility, one among other quite "optional" pure possibilities—but possibilities that are possible perceptions. We, so to speak, shift the actual perception into the realm of non-actualities, the realm of the as-if, which supplies us with "pure" possibilities, pure of everything that restricts to this fact or to any fact whatever ... we might have taken as our initial example a phantasying ourselves into a perceiving, with no relation to the rest of our de facto life. Perception, the universal type thus acquired, floats in the air, so to speak—in the atmosphere of pure phantasiableness. Thus removed from all factualness, it has become the pure eidos perception, whose "ideal" extension is made up of all ideally possible perceptions as purely phantasiable processes. (*CM*, pp. 104–105)

The eidos as a "pure possibility" anticipates or prefigures all of its possible determinations; however, these determinations are not prefigured as are those of the unexplicated perspectives in a visual perception where the exploring gaze is "constrained." The possible determinations prefigured in the eidos of eidetic seeing are presented with a pure optionality. We may realize in imagination now one and now the other. In the actual experience of an individual object, "horizons are prescribed for further possible experiences." The unity of the object, as well as the unity of the field of experience itself, requires a coherence or unanimity of presentations. In eidetic seeing, however, the examples supplant and contradict one another: "The sudden change is that of an individual into a second individual incompatible with it in coexistence.... If, for example, we envisage to ourselves an individual house now painted yellow, we can just as well think that it could be painted blue.... This house, the same, is thinkable as *a* and as *non-a* but, naturally, if as *a*, then, not *at the same time* as *non-a*" (*EJ*, sec. 87d).

In this series of mutually exclusive individuals, unqualified by the requirement of a "harmonious synthesis," which applies to all that can appear within the horizon of the actual world, something is perceived that is not itself an individual. Eidetic seeing is a seeing through this series to the essence, which appears "again and again." The arbitrary examples exhibit an "overlapping coincidence ... in which they all appear as modifications of one another and then as arbitrary sequences of particulars in which the same universal is isolated as an eidos" (*EJ*, sec. 87e). The glance of the phenomenologist disregards the determinate differences that distinguish the examples of the series. "Difference is that which, in the overlapping of the multiplicities, is not to be brought into the unity of the congruence making its appearance thereby, that which in consequence, does not make an eidos visible" (*EJ*, sec. 87e). Having blinded itself to the specific differences determining the examples, eidetic seeing grasps the essence as an "invariant what."

And just as eidetic seeing exhibits no attachment to the specificity of its examples, so too is it detached from the life-world. While admitting that the experienced world is the "universal field of all our activities," even eidetic seeing, Husserl insists that it is precisely this bond between the actual world and the domain of essences that must be suspended: "Only if we become conscious of this bond, putting it consciously out of play, and so also free this broadest surrounding horizon of variants from all connection to experience and experiential validity, do we achieve perfect purity. Then we find ourselves, so to speak, in a pure world of imagination, a world of absolutely pure possibility" (*EJ*, sec. 87e).

This domain of the essence, however, is not strictly a world. Each arbitrary example implies the whole of a world, which might be imaginatively unfolded, but these possible worlds mutually exclude one another and cannot be gathered within a single horizon. This "universe of free possibilities" lacks a "unity of context" and is not governed by the requirement of coherence. The "freedom" of eidetic seeing is constituted when "we have removed every bond to the factually valid historical world and have regarded this world itself as one of the conceptual possibilities" (*OG*, pp. 266–267). Through the "direction of our gaze upon the apodictic variant," we phenomenologists discover the "self-evidence of being able to repeat the invariant structure at will." This "volitionally directed gaze" empowers the phenomenologist's voice and makes accessible "what can be fixed in univocal language." Thus, phenomenology "achieves the possibility of creating a ground for itself through its own powers, namely, in mastering, through original self-reflection, the naive world" (*Crisis*, sec. 53, p. 181).

Not only the world but the ego itself is rendered a "pure possibility." Although "the beginning phenomenologist is bound involuntarily by the circumstance that he takes himself as his initial example," the transcendental reduction reveals that the de facto transcendental ego has the significance "merely" of an example of a pure generic type (*CM*, pp. 107, 110). Overcoming the "positivity" of this concrete beginning, the phenomenologist passes into the domain of "absolute phenomenology" and discovers the "transcendental ego, who indeed no longer has a horizon that could lead beyond the sphere of his transcendental being and thus relativize him" (*CM*, p. 107). Through a certain "splitting," the ego reestablishes himself "above the world" as the "non-participant on-looker":

If the Ego, as naturally immersed in the world, experiencingly and otherwise, is called *"interested" in the world*, then the phenomenologically altered—and, as so altered, continually maintained—attitude consists in a splitting of the Ego: in that the phenomenological Ego establishes himself as *"disinterested onlooker,"* above the naively interested Ego. That this takes place is then itself accessible by means of a new reflection, which as transcendental, likewise demands the very same attitude of looking on "disinterestedly"—the Ego's sole remaining interest being to see and to describe adequately what he sees, purely as seen, as what is seen and seen in such and such a manner. (*CM*, p. 73)

Having effected this split in the ego and the theoretical reconstruction of vision in the register of the transcendental, the ego no longer sees the world as a place of existential commitments. Objects are only the "intentional correlates of modes of consciousness of them," examples of forms considered disinterestedly. In fact, in virtue of the transcendental reduction, "the sense 'Objective' which belongs to everything worldly—as constituted intersubjectively, as experienceable by everyone—*vanishes completely*" (*CM*, p. 128). Moreover, the "blacking out" or "screening off" of what is other [*der Ablendung des Fremden*] leaves my transcendental ego "wholly unaffected."

Husserl deflects the charge of transcendental solipsism by arguing that "within myself, within the limits of my transcendentally reduced pure conscious life, I *experience* the world (including others) ... not as my *private* synthetic formation, but as other than mine alone" (*CM*, p. 123). Though the transcendentally reduced ego can "never reach the point of ascribing being" to the other, the other is nonetheless presented in the sphere of "my ownness" as a constituted sense. The "enigma" of intersubjectivity consists in the fact that "the sensuously seen body is experienced forthwith as the body of someone else and not merely as an indication [*Anzeige*] of someone else" (*CM*, p. 150). Husserl insists that "what I actually see" in a "perceiving [that] goes on exclusively in the sphere of my ownness" is "not a sign [*Zeichen*]," "not a mere analogue"; rather, "it is someone else" (*CM*, p. 153). While perception offers only dubitable "indications," the sensuous seeing of the other's body—when purified by phenomenological reflection—yields apodictic evidence of the other and secures the intersubjectivity of consciousness. Only through an appeal to the sensuous spectacle of the other's mobile body can Husserl escape transcendental solipsism; only by acknowledging the availability of the perceptual thing to other perceptions, other perceivers, can Husserl insist that the world is a world for "all of us."

The apodicticity of the evidence, however, can be established only if the phenomenologist blinds himself to these very features, thereby transforming perceptual indications of the other's body into an immanent sense. What he sees is not the sensuous other, but (the form of) himself. The spectacle of the other's body in motion in the world introduces nothing alien into the sphere of transcendental self-perception. Not only is the other given only as a constituted sense, but also the sight of the other's body has the effect of returning the gaze to itself. Thus, "The 'Other,' according to his own constituted sense, points to me myself; the other is a 'mirroring' of my own self" (*CM*, pp. 125–126). The other, who is "not a mere analogue," is nonetheless constituted analogically: "I apperceive him as having spatial modes of appearance like those I should have if I should go over there and be where he is" (*CM*, p. 146). The apperception, moreover, requires a displacement or transference of sense: a "shrouding" or "veiling" [*sichuberdecken*] of the other with the sense "like me" (see *CM*, pp. 142, 147). The other can be presented as another ego only insofar as he is "the same." The "transcendence" of the other is explicitly distinguished from the transcendence of perceptual things and compared to the self-alienation characteristic of time-consciousness. The difference from the other is an interior difference.

And just as the other can be given only in an analogical apperception emanating from the "zero-point" or "zero-body" of the transcendental ego, "the cultural world too is given 'orientedly' in relation to a zero member or a 'zero personality.'

Here I and my culture are primordial, over against every alien culture" (*CM*, p. 161). Every human being "has his fellow men": the others are "'my' others ... with whom I can enter into ... relations of empathy" (*OG*, p. 258). This community constitutes the "horizon of mature normal civilization (taking away the abnormal and children)," and it is to this horizon that "common language belongs" (*OG*, p. 258).

The ability of the phenomenologically reflecting consciousness to say what it sees depends, then, on the dream of a common language. Freed from the constraining horizons of actual perception while preserving in itself the self-certainty of immediacy, phenomenological reflection exhibits an intertwining of vision and voice, a loquacious gaze, which finds its voice by blinding itself to specific difference. Even the spectacle of the other is only a mirror of itself. In the end the transcendental ego sees only itself, but, thereby, it would see everything. This language in which the dream of a common language is articulated is, in fact, already marked: masculine, European. (See, e.g., "Universal Teleology," p. 337, where in the context of an analysis of sexuality, the position of the subject is clearly identified with the man, while the woman is cast as his object. Or recall the texts from *The Origin of Geometry* to the *Crisis* in which Husserl explicitly identifies his philosophical program as European.) Coupled with the invocation of "mature normal civilization," this pretension of the phenomenological "we" to give voice to any possible subject acquires the prescriptive tone of a language of mastery.

Husserl, however, does not develop this tone. In spite of the constant imperative to abstract and the laborious theoretical reconstruction of sensuous seeing as the apodictic insight of transcendental reflection, Husserl just as constantly reverts to the eloquent description of experience and to the themes of perception, horizonality, perspective, and specific difference. While insisting on the self-presence of the subject to itself, Husserlian phenomenology regularly reveals a being constituted by "horizons," "self-alienations," and "incompleteness," just as it employs the vocabulary of sensuous seeing to articulate its claim to a nonsensuous perception. On the other side of the purifications

Mary C. Rawlinson

and abstractions of phenomenology, the enigmas, paradoxes, and riddles of experience remain.

Acknowledgments

I thank David B. Allison and Edward S. Casey for their very helpful criticisms of an earlier draft of this chapter.

Notes

1. References to Husserl's works will be given using the following abbreviations:

Crisis = *The Crisis of European Sciences and Transcendental Phenomenology*

CM = *Cartesian Meditations*

EJ = *Experience and Judgement*

FTL = *Formal and Transcendental Logic*

Ideas = *Ideas* (Book I): *General Introduction to Pure Phenomenology*

ITC = *The Phenomenology of Internal Time-consciousness*

LI = *Logical Investigations*

OG = *Origin of Geometry*

UT = *Introduction to "Universal Teleology"*

SGP = "Self-Givenness in Perception"

2. In fabricating "above the world" the place of phenomenological analysis, Husserl evokes the subject of phenomenology by invoking as an alter ego the "man in the street." The "man in the street" shares with the "man of science" a faith in the givenness of the object: neither has yet opened his eyes to what the phenomenologist sees. Phenomenology requires, as the prerequisite for admission into its domain of illumination, the suspension of this perceptual faith and a "disconnection from the life-world." In this sphere not only the perceptual thing, but all that appears within the "horizon of mature, normal civilization" is presented again, re-presented, as a result, or as given only correlative to some constitutive synthesis. See, e.g., *Ideas*, sec. 39–40; *OG*, p. 258.

3. See *CM*, p. 131. A "screening off" or "blacking out" of what is "other" or "alien," not only the transcendent object of perception but also the eye that sees, is necessary to transcendental reflection.

4. Kant not only understands every objective presentation to be the result of synthetic activity but also, like Husserl, distinguishes the blindness of this power as it operates in actual perception, from the clear insight into itself achieved in transcendental reflection. See, e.g., *Critique of Pure Reason*, A78, B103. See also A141, B180 where the schematism in its application to appearances is said to be "an art concealed in the depths of the human soul, whose real modes of activity nature is hardly likely ever to allow us to discover, and to have open to our gaze."

5. Thus, while the "full-thing" is presented in any actualized perspective, its other possible presentations or perspectives are only *indicated* or implied.

6. See Maurice Merleau-Ponty, *The Visible and the Invisible*, chap. 1, "Reflection and Interrogation," especially, pp. 33–35, 44–46. In Husserl, Merleau-Ponty argues, reflection is "specular," a "gaze" that is transparent to itself. "It is a reflection that finally is not installed in an active constituting agent [*Auffassungsinhalt-Auffassung*], but finds at the origin of every reflection a massive presence to self, the Retention's *Noch im Griff*, and, through it, the *Urimpression*, and the absolute flux which animates them. It presupposes the reduction of nature to immanent unities. Yet the *Tonen* is not immanence—unless one understands immanence in the sense of ecstasy!—it utilizes the very structure of the flux." On the tone, see below.

7. The famous example of hearing a tone invoked by Husserl in his analysis of time-consciousness might seem to suggest otherwise, especially as Husserl explicitly prefers it to other visual experiences of duration (e.g., that of observing a bird in flight); however, the supposedly aural example of the tone is in fact elaborated by analogy to the mobile visual perception of a thing in space. "The same sound which is heard now is, from the point of view of the flux of consciousness which follows it, past, its duration expired. To my consciousness, points of temporal duration recede, as points of a stationary object in space recede when I 'go away from the object.' The object retains its place; even so does the sound retain its time. Its temporal point is unmoved, but the sound vanishes into the remoteness of consciousness; the distance from the generative now becomes ever greater" (*ITC*, sec. 8).

8. For an analysis of the difficulties Husserl encounters in attempting to interpret the horizonality of the now as consistent with the self-presence claimed for the self-constituting transcendental ego, see Jacques Derrida, *Speech and Phenomena*, especially chap. 5, "Signs and the Blink of an Eye." See also Robert Sokolowski, *Husserlian Meditations*, p. 143, where, in explicating Husserl on this point, Sokolowski describes the "profiles" of the elapsed now-phase as "what is absolutely present to inner consciousness."

Bibliography

Derrida, Jacques. *Speech and Phenomena*. Translated by David B. Allison. Evanston, Ill.: Northwestern University Press, 1973.

Husserl, Edmund, *Cartesian Meditations*. Translated by Dorion Cairns. The Hague: Nijhoff, 1960.

———. *The Crisis of European Sciences and Transcendental Philosophy*. Translated by David Carr. Evanston: Northwestern University, 1970.

———. *Experience and Judgment*. Translated by James S. Churchill and Karl Ameriks. Evanston: Northwestern University Press, 1973.

———. *Formal and Transcendental Logic*. Translated by Dorion Cairns. The Hague: Nijhoff, 1969.

———. *Ideas*. Translated by Boyce Gibson. New York: Collier, 1972.

———. *Logical Investigations*. Translated by J. N. Findlay. London: Routledge and Kegan Paul, 1970.

————. "The Origin of Geometry." Translated by David Carr. In *Husserl's Shorter Works*. Edited by Peter McCormick and Frederick Elliston. Notre Dame: University of Notre Dame Press, 1981.

————. *The Phenomenology of Internal Time-Consciousness*. Translated by J. S. Churchill. Bloomington: Indiana University Press, 1964.

————. "Self-Givenness in Perception." In *Genetic Phenomenology and the Lifeworld*. Edited by D. Welton. Dordrecht: Kluwer, 1966.

Merleau-Ponty, Maurice. *The Visible and the Invisible*. Translated by Alphonso Lingis. Evanston: Northwestern University Press, 1968.

Sokolowski, Robert. *Husserlian Meditations*. Evanston: Northwestern University Press, 1974.

9

Ducks and Rabbits: Visuality in Wittgenstein

William James Earle

It's notorious that with Wittgenstein you can hardly ever tell how to read the text. I don't propose to argue for my exegesis.
—Jerry A. Fodor, "*Déja vu* All Over Again: How Danto's Aesthetics Recapitulates the Philosophy of Mind"

It is one thing to see the interconnectedness of things, another to postulate that all aspects of a culture can be traced back to one key cause of which they are the manifestations.
—E. H. Gombrich, *In Search of Cultural History*

Ma purtroppo noi siamo fatti a zone: a zone specializzate. In alcune progrediamo, in altre restiamo fermi.
—Pier Paolo Pasolini, *I dialoghi*

Here the temptation to believe in a phenomenology, something midway between science and logic, is very great.
—Wittgenstein, *Remarks on Color*

Cultures are complex collections of people and artifacts that face off against environments of hazards and opportunities that their interactions (people-people, people-artifacts, artifacts-artifacts) perpetually diminish and augment. Nothing holds the whole thing together: no *Zeitgeist*, no World-Spirit, no *Weltanschauung*, no *episteme*, no Spirit of the Age, no Western Philosophical Tradition, no (as Gombrich puts it) "key cause." The scattered—or, more fashionably, "dispersed"—bits and pieces, to the extent that they are connected at all, are connected by real, empirical, and, probably always, causal influences. And any big culture splits into relatively autonomous spheres (Pasolini's *zone specializzate*), which we live in or visit or avoid like the plague, find appealing or appalling, or—in a great variety of strengths and degrees— are knowledgable about, ignorant of, fascinated by, bored by, or just indifferent to and/or uninterested in.[1]

All large-scale cultures include people, by definition relatively few people, whose personal systems of interest and aversion are statistically unusual or in mismatch with their neighbors. Wittgenstein, compared at least to standardly trained academic philosophers, is one such. This is description, not praise or blame. Wittgenstein is intensely interested in, actually obsessed by, a very small set of philosophical *topoi* and disgusted by (Wittgenstein's version of being indifferent to) all the rest. Wittgenstein never studied philosophy in any scholastic mode. For several years beginning in 1908, he was registered as a research student in the Engineering Department of Manchester University. He was interested in aeronautics and spent some of his time building kites, but according to Ray Monk, even during the Manchester period, his interest in philosophy began to dominate.[2]

We can only speculate on the effect that engineering drawings and diagrams may have had on Wittgenstein's conception of pictures and pictorial representationality. What we do know (this is still Monk's account) is the kind of philosophy he read: Gottlob Frege's *Grundgesetze* and Bertrand Russell's *Principles of Mathematics*. In Frege, he read, "Since the number one, being the same for everyone, stands apart from everyone in the same way, it can no more be researched by making psychological observations than can the moon."[3] In Russell, he read that "Philosophy asks of Mathematics: What does it mean? Mathematics in the past was unable to answer, and Philosophy answered by introducing the totally irrelevant notion of mind. But now Mathematics is able to answer, so far at least as to reduce the whole of its propositions to certain fundamental notions of logic."[4] There is here a single conception of philosophy as the analysis of concepts and propositions, especially those of logic and mathematics, cleansed of psychology in either its idealist or empiricist variant. And it is to this conception of philosophy that Wittgenstein remained committed. (Empiricism is just that partial[5]—and apparently seductive—"picture" of a world of highly informative visible objects that write retinal images on the eye, and then, a cause or two along the causal chain, impressions in the mind that form the indispensable substance of our cognitive lives; whereas Frege, referring to the *Grundgesetze*, writes, "Unpropitious for my book is the widespread inclination to acknowledge as existing only what can be perceived by the senses. That which cannot, people try to deny or else to ignore."[6])

Everything about Wittgenstein is, I suppose, up for discussion, which leads to the kind of exasperation Fodor evinced. I shall, in any case, here follow Dummett's view. Dummett writes in the introduction to his magisterial work on Frege (the philosopher who influenced Wittgenstein more than any other):

The most far-reaching part of Descartes's revolution was to make epistemology the most basic sector of the whole of philosophy: the whole subject had to start from the question "What do we know, and how?" It is this orientation which makes post-Cartesian philosophy so different from that of the scholastics, for whom epistemology, in so far as they considered it at all, was no more than a sidestream. Descartes's perspective continued to be that which dominated philosophy until this century, when it was overthrown by Wittgenstein, who in the *Tractatus* reinstated philosophical logic as the foundation of philosophy, and relegated epistemology to a peripheral position.[7]

Philosophical logic, or philosophical grammar, remains the dominant preoccupation, early and late, and along with a thoroughly Fregean antipsychologism, gives to Wittgenstein's work a unity at least as fundamental as the differences, from early to late, which Wittgenstein himself probably overemphasized.[8] In the next section I consider some passages in the *Tractatus*, including some that have to do with the famous picture-theory of propositions, where one might expect to find something about visuality. But the result of this examination is largely negative. In the main section of the chapter, I turn to the *Philosophical Investigations* and related materials where Wittgenstein discusses "seeing as" or "seeing an aspect." Here too I conclude that the remarks about seeing are made (at least, largely made) in the service of more general theses about language games and forms of life and are, as Ray Monk emphasizes, designed precisely to avoid "the very theory of sensory experience that is the target of Wittgenstein's philosophy of psychology—the phenomenalist notion that the objects of immediate experience are the private, shadowy entities empiricists call sense-data."[9]

There is, in fact, next to nothing about vision, the visual, or visibility in the *Tractatus*.[10] "Picture" or *Bild*, which sounds visual, always refers to representations or models viewed purely abstractly in terms of their isomorphism (or, in the case of false propositions, isomorphism failure) with the reality they purport to picture; in any case, as David Pears reminds us, "the German word *Bild* means not only 'picture' but also 'model.'"[11] "The *Tractatus* provided [this is P. M. S. Hacker's summary] a complex and non-trivial logico-metaphysical *explanation* of the pictoriality of thought by way of the doctrines of isomorphism and atomism. Agreement between thought and reality was held to be agreement in form, and an elaborate atomist logic and metaphysics was delineated to explain isomorphism."[12] "Pictoriality," in other words, does not mean more than "representationality."

A later—circa 1932–1933—comment by Wittgenstein is helpful: "Here instead of harmony or agreement of thought and reality one might say: the pictorial character of thought. But is the pictorial character an agreement? In the *Tractatus* I had said something like: it is an agreement of form."[13] Exactly how to understand the formality—or, as it may be, isomorphic potentiality—of pictoriality has exercised many commentators on the *Tractatus*. George Pitcher (commenting on 4.031, "In a proposition a situation is, as it were, constructed by way of experiment") says: "But perhaps the best way to state Wittgenstein's position is to say that the proposition is a projection (as the term is used, for example, in projective geometry) of the situation it describes."[14] Proposition 4.031 is itself related to a remark in Wittgenstein's *Notebooks: 1914–1916*: "In the proposition a world is as it were put together experimentally. (As in the law-court in Paris a motor-car accident is represented by means of dolls, etc.)."[15] One does, of course, look at the model of the accident, not because it shows what the accident looked like but rather because its items (dolls, toy cars, etc.) have the same cardinality and, according to some rule of projection, the same disposition as the ingredients of the accident. Like Pitcher, Rush Rhees suggests a mathematical analogy:

> The idea of *Abbildung* came into logic from the mathematicians' practice of finding a model for one system in another: finding a model for a non-euclidean geometry in Euclid, for instance, or a model for geometry in the arithmetic of real numbers—which in German was called an *Abbildung* of one system in the other. The method was used to show the consistency and validity of, say, Lobatchevsky's geometry. And I think Wittgenstein has it in mind when he speaks of the "Logik der Abbildung" (in 4.015, for instance) and even when he speaks of an "Abbildung der Wirklichkeit." We have to translate this by "picturing reality," but we lose much of the connotation when we do; and in particular we lose the reference to a rule.[16]

The idea of projection also finds its way into Robert J. Fogelin's account: "For depiction, the form of a fact must be projected on the logical space of states of affairs picturing the way a set of represented objects are supposed to stand to one another."[17] Probably the clearest account, certainly the most comprehensive, is given by Anthony Kenny. According to Kenny, what Wittgenstein meant by calling a proposition a picture "can be summed up in eight theses":

(1) A proposition is essentially composite.

(2) The elements which compose a proposition are correlated by human decision with elements of reality.

(3) The combination of such correlated elements into a proposition presents—without further human intervention—a possible state of affairs.

(4) A proposition stands in an internal relation to the possible state of affairs which it presents.

(5) This internal relationship can only be shown, it cannot be informatively stated.

(6) A proposition is true or false in virtue of being compared to reality.

(7) A proposition must be independent of the state of affairs which makes it true or makes it false.

(8) No proposition is *a priori* true.[18]

If Kenny's theses succeed in capturing Wittgenstein's picture-theory (as can plausibly be maintained), then Wittgensteinian pictures have no more to do with visual pictures than logical space has to do with the ordinary three-dimensional space we move around in.

Although the picture-theory of propositions and propositional meaning is deeply correspondentialist, it is hard to see how this shows the dominance, standard in the philosophical (or, pleonastically Western philosophical) tradition, of "seeing" in early Wittgenstein. Wittgenstein speaks of "the feelers of the picture's elements with which the picture touches reality" (2.1515). This is a vivid *tactile* image, but what is seriously meant is just "correlations of the picture's elements with things" (2.1514). Where structure counts, the medium does not matter: the musical phrase is "pictured," indifferently, by the phonographic grooves of the record and the conventional notation of the printed score (4.0141). What carries over from early to late Wittgenstein is a principled disinterest in experience (in just that "lived experience" dear to phenomenologists) and the correlative attempt to capture, perspicuously, the completely unprivate "logic of our language."[19]

Wittgenstein remarks "For the form of the visual field is surely not like this" (5.6331):

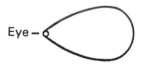

I take it that Wittgenstein is not concerned with the shape of the visual field. What makes the picture wrong is that "the eye" is within the visual field. This is not a contingent mistake dependent on the fact that one cannot see one's own eyes (but at best their mirror image). I can, for example, feel one of my hands with the other while it is feeling something else. And I suppose some insects can with one eye observe the other. None of this matters because Wittgenstein is not making a point about anatomy-based limitations. It is perhaps difficult to state the point he is making uncontroversially. It might be (and probably is) that what does the seeing—here "I," not "eye"—cannot be among the things I encounter in the world, the things that I can observe and describe. P. M. S. Hacker calls this "the non-encounterability of the self in experience" and gives it a Humean ancestry.[20] But Wittgenstein remarks immediately after the incorrect picture of the visual field: "This is connected with the fact that no part of our experience is at the same time *a priori*" (5.634). For Wittgenstein, the self does not disintegrate impressionistically. It is not infra- but supra-encounterable. What we experience—the a posteriori—could all have been different, but not the fact that it is *my* experience. Surely there is something experience-transcendent or a priori—if only the grammatical scaffolding indicated by reflexive pronouns and other syncategorematic bits and pieces of our language. In any case, it seems obvious that nothing here has a special connection with seeing or visual experience.

The nearest anticipation of later concerns occurs at 5.5423, where we are given the following drawing of a Neckar cube:

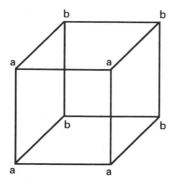

This remark surrounds the illustration: "To perceive a complex means to perceive that its constituents are related to one another in such and such a way. This no doubt also explains why there are two possible ways of seeing the figure as a cube; and all similar phenomena. For we really see two different facts." I accept Max Black's suggestion that "this may be directed against Russell's idea that we perceive a complex by standing in a complex relation to its several constituents."[21] Wittgenstein is here simply reaffirming the basic abstract architecture (a world of facts, not things) of the *Tractatus*. Indeed, as a remark about visual perception, 5.5423 is far-fetched. We do not see two facts; we see a single—ontologically stable—line drawing. What happens next, in the standard account, "is that alternative hypotheses of what the object is (or where its parts lie in space) are entertained in turn. This occurs when the sensory data do not particularly favor just one hypothesis."[22] The standard account—the words here are R. L. Gregory's—is, in an altogether familiar way, scientific: it explains by reference to the hidden.[23]

Wittgenstein famously eschews this approach in *Philosophical Investigations* and the associated manuscript (and now mainly published) material. It is easy to ask "why?" but less easy to supply an accurately complicated—and qualified—response. There is a vast literature on "Wittgenstein's conception of philosophy." A plausible brief account might run as follows: Philosophy is whatever we can use in the "battle against the bewitchment of our intelligence by means of language."[24] Philosophy clears away misunderstandings, assembles reminders for particular clarificatory purposes, generates perspicuity or *Ubersichtlichkeit*, and its methods are like therapies, its treatments of questions like the treatments of illnesses.[25] One can accept this conception and still have a complaint. Wittgenstein ought to have seen that philosophy, as a therapeutic activity, intervening in the multiform—and exogenously generated—muddles, confusions, and opacities of everyday life (including ordinary, averagely careless intellectual life) was just about the last thing to have a fixed essence, just about the last thing, in other words, not to be family resemblant about. Who can say what will be helpful? How do we know ahead of time what will coax the fly out of its bottle?[26] Most telling, why should therapy exclude theory? Even medicine—indeed even psychoanalysis—is supposed to be a science or at least to be science based. I agree with Dummett that "the idea—if it *is* Wittgenstein's idea—that no systematic theory of meaning is possible is not merely one which is, at the present stage of enquiry, defeatist, but one that runs counter to obvious facts."[27] It is nevertheless possible that Wittgenstein, working within self-imposed and indeed arbitrary and indefensible limits, produces genuine illumination.[28] I think this is the case. I hope to show that it is the case in the remainder of this chapter.

The main source for the following is part II of *Philosophical Investigations*, especially section xi. This is where Wittgenstein struggles with "seeing as" or "noticing an aspect." Here is a typical example from the beginning of that discussion: "I contemplate a face, and then suddenly notice its likeness to another. I *see* that it has not changed; and yet I see it differently. I call this experience 'noticing an aspect.'[29] This passage raises a number of questions. First, what kind of suddenness is involved in "sudden noticing"? How does this compare to the suddenness of, for example, "Suddenly he pulled a gun"? Second, in what sense is this an "experience" (*Erfarhrung*)? What does it mean to assert or deny, or what exactly turns on asserting or denying, that something—for example, thinking, calculating, undergoing anesthesia, sleeping, hoping, believing, talking, walking— is an experience? These are questions that occupy Wittgenstein throughout the discussion. Initially, however, Wittgenstein uses the example to indicate the kind of interest—philosophical rather than scientific—that operates in his discussion: "Its *causes* are of interest to psychologists" and then in a separate paragraph: "We are interested in the concept and its place among the concepts of experience."[30]

The basic pattern, for Wittgenstein, is always as follows. Initially, there has to be something that perplexes us—that is in some way troubling. Otherwise philosophy will have nothing to do. It is worth thinking about the status of this perplexity as

Wittgenstein conceives it. Although the perplexity is supposed to disappear as we get clearer about concepts and their relations to each other, and although this process is not supposed to involve anything that could properly be called a discovery, Wittgenstein would not have been happy with people immune from birth to conceptual inquietude. For example, some students, exposed to the noticing-an-aspect examples, ask, "What's the problem?" They are not star pupils of philosophy by anyone's, including Wittgenstein's, standards. After all, Wittgenstein in passage after passage himself generates, rather than quotes or alludes to, the conceptually problematical examples that ultimate perspicuity will disarm.[31] You cannot read the *Investigations* without feeling the much more than dutiful interest Wittgenstein takes in the matters under discussion.[32] Again, although there is no question of discovery—the German *Entdeckung* is just as obviously connected, etymologically, with "uncovering the hidden" as "discovery" is—there is nevertheless something that is sought: "What I am looking for [Wittgenstein writes in the course of a related discussion] is the grammatical difference."[33] This is something that can be missed (fudged, conflated, confused) and that, accordingly, credit is due for finding and isolating crisply.

The relevant grammatical difference here is between two kinds of seeing or two ways we use the verb "to see" (or *sehen*).[34] Not surprisingly, this is not a matter of our becoming aware of a difference in our visual experience. Scrutinizing our experience will always, in Wittgenstein's book, get us nowhere. Context is what counts, and "The contexts of a sentence are best portrayed in a play."[35] The one use of "see" is in the context of the question, "What do you see there?" asked by someone who cannot, perhaps because of location, see what you are seeing. "The other: 'I see a likeness between these two faces'—let the man I tell this to be seeing the faces as clearly as I do myself."[36] The man is seeing$_1$ the same thing (faces) I am seeing$_1$, but not seeing$_2$ what I am seeing$_2$ (a resemblance). Seeing$_1$ is, I think, what Wittgenstein also calls observing, which happens when a person "puts himself in a favorable position to receive certain impressions in order (for example) to describe what they tell him."[37]

The connoisseur and the philistine, walking the same route through the Clyfford Still room at the Metropolitan Museum of Art, observe (in any case, can observe) the same paintings, but no matter what spatial positions he takes, the philistine will not be able to see$_2$ those aesthetic features—indeed excellences—prized by the connoisseur. The aesthetic excellences of paintings must be visible$_2$ but are never visible$_1$. You can make something more visible$_1$ by increasing illumination, but this has no effect on visibility$_2$. Seeing$_1$ is mainly a matter of where you are and what is there; seeing$_2$ is not. Leading a horse to water is like seeing$_1$. Making him drink is like seeing$_2$.

Does the connoisseur see$_1$ and see$_2$ simultaneously? Does he perhaps, on the model of perlocutions, see$_2$ by seeing$_1$? Both questions suggest a Wittgenstein-inadmissible introjection. We should be counting neither inner psychic acts nor kinds of experiences. The connoisseur can play games of question and answer that the philistine cannot. (He can play a scene from a different play.) We might even say, if there were any point to it, that the philistine has qualitatively identical experiences but does not know how to use them. A nonphysicist—this example is essentially Norwood Russell Hanson's—has (could have plenty of) visual experiences of the laboratory, but he cannot use them to provide an inventory of its scientific apparatus: "Would Sir Lawrence Bragg and an Eskimo baby see the same thing when looking at an X-ray tube?"[38] Hanson answers, "Yes, and no": yes for seeing$_1$, no for seeing$_2$.

"Seeing [Hanson writes] is not just the having of a visual experience; it is also the way in which the visual experience is had."[39] These are analytically distinguishable but not countably separate: "Is the physicist doing more than just seeing? No; he does nothing over and above what the layman does when he sees an X-ray tube."[40] But it is still correct to say that "the layman must learn physics before he can see what the physicist sees."[41] Hanson (his student and my colleague Douglas Lackey tells me) described *Patterns of Discovery*, from which I have have been quoting, as "theory, observation, and the cloven hoof of Wittgenstein." Certainly Hanson was greatly influenced by Wittgenstein, but his examples from philosophy of science, though closely related to the kinds of examples considered by Wittgenstein, are easier to understand. What makes them easier is that they involve two observers who can be credited with different background knowledge, conceptual preparedness, theoretical sophistication —a difference perfectly straightforwardly illustrated by the microscopist who sees coelenterate mesoglea, and his new student who "sees only a gooey, formless stuff."[42]

The Eskimo baby has a single, stable visual take on the X-ray tube. Sir Lawrence Bragg has a different, but equally singulary and stable, visual take. Neither baby nor Bragg is subject to sudden shifts or labilities. The cases that interest Wittgenstein most are those in which there are shifts, ordinarily quite sudden, for one observer. Perhaps the most famous of these is the so-called duck-rabbit picture:

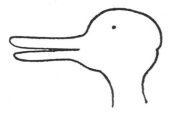

"It can be seen [says Wittgenstein] as a rabbit's head or as a duck's."[43] This has to be short for "rabbit's-head-picture" and "duck's head picture." Though Wittgenstein speaks of a picture-man and a picture-animal, this is the same ontologically non-committal mode of expression used by Nelson Goodman who speaks of man-pictures, animal-pictures, unicorn-pictures, and the like.[44] There is the question, discussed inadequately by Goodman,[45] and not so much as mentioned by Wittgenstein, of the relation between our ability to recognize X's and our ability to recognize X-pictures. I should, in any case, suppose that were there duck-rabbits in the animal kingdom, we should see the above image without the instability; it would be no more problematical—no more remarkable—than dog-pictures in our world or dog-cat-pictures in a world with dog-cats among its denizens.

Someone shown the duck-rabbit picture and asked what he is seeing has available to him a response in terms of seeing$_1$. He simply produces the following drawing:

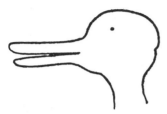

Admittedly, this may seem an evasion—as when X, asked what Y said, answers, "Oggi è venerdì" (a faithful rendition or accurate acoustic image of what X heard, a slavish quotation of what Y said) when what is wanted is "Today is Friday."[46] "Hearing" is perhaps seldom, outside the office of the audiologist, used in parallel to seeing$_1$. "What have you heard?" would rarely be a request for merely acoustic information though this, as usual, depends on context, on circumambient interest. In normal circumstances, of course, we do not hear accoustically—that would be more or less hearing$_1$—and then add layers of interpretation or translation. The acoustic image, when we attend to it at all, is either an artifact of special, isolating, often technical, attention or a by-product of frustrated efforts at more substantive understanding.

As used here, *acoustic image* is the correlative of hearing$_1$. In parallel, one might use *optical picture* as the correlative of seeing$_1$. This usage is Malcolm Budd's, as in the following: "When we 'see something different'—when there is an apparent change in colour or shape—the 'optical picture' changes, but when we experience a change of aspect the 'optical picture' does not need to undergo a comparable change."[47] Corresponding to the duck-rabbit-picture is presumably a single optical picture in Budd's sense. Yet the duck-rabbit-picture can be seen as a rabbit or seen as a duck. Some people who first see it as a rabbit will suddenly see it as a duck. Some people who first see it as a duck will suddenly see it as a rabbit. After a while, everybody (or at least all parties to the psychological and/or philosophical discussion) will see it as a duck-rabbit-picture, and that is that.[48]

There are other possibilities. "The picture [Wittgenstein writes] might have been shewn to me, and I never have seen anything but a rabbit in it."[49] Wittgenstein makes two (connected) points about cases like this. First, I would not say, because it would not make sense for me to say, "*Now* I am seeing it *as* a rabbit."[50] Second, when I say (perhaps naively), "It's a rabbit" or "It's a rabbit picture," "I should simply have described my perception: just as if I had said 'I see a red circle over there.'"[51] Wittgenstein also speaks of "reporting my perception." The "describing" or "reporting" mode is a variety of language-game, comparable to accrual (as opposed to cash) basis accounting. We should resist the temptation to construe it as the only case of "really" seeing, coordinate with some special— phenomenologically distinctive and internally recognizable— form of immediacy. Again, like seeing$_1$, it fits into some but not other narrative contexts. Wittgenstein emphasizes the flexibility (Budd calls this the "polymorphous character")[52] of the concept of seeing, which covers, impartially, the philistine and the connoisseur, the baby and Bragg.[53] Immediacy (and correlative economies of reportage) should be thought of as matters of speed and smoothness within a social world, within a *Lebensform*.

Wittgenstein, though almost obsessively interested, is not interested in the duck-rabbit-picture *qua* perceptual anomaly. Cases like the duck-rabbit ones where we would "naturally" say, "*Now* I am seeing X *as* Y," are meant to be contrastive.[54] If I am observing an ordinary knife and fork in the ordinary circumstances of ordinary life, I do not say:

"Now I am see this as a knife and fork." This expression would not be understood.—Any more than: "Now it's a fork" or "It can be a fork too."
    One doesn't "*take*" what one knows as the cutlery at a meal *for* cutlery; anymore than one ordinarily tries to move one's mouth as one eats, or aims at moving it."[55]

This is, of course, a place where some "theory of meaning" might come in handy. Because on some theories, it certainly makes sense to say (and would even express a true proposition) of any fork at any time: "Now it's a fork." Wittgenstein is perhaps a trifle unclear about the difference between a remark that is meaningless and a remark that is pointless. (Only by grasping its meaning can we judge it pointless.) And we may want to scold Wittgenstein along the following lines. I take this from a lecture by Dummett to an Italian audience:

No doubt Italy is different from England in this respect; but if we were to attend to what people in England do say about dogs, we should find that it consisted principally of remarks like, "He understands every word you say." Plainly such a remark, however frequently made, has no authority: we need to distinguish between what is customarily said and what the conventions governing our use of language require or entitle us to say. Now, however, it appears rather less a matter of assembling reminders of what everyone knows than Wittgenstein liked to make out: to draw such a distinction requires some theoretical apparatus.[56]

Dummett rightly regrets the absence of explicit apparatus. In philosophy, explicit display is, after all, everything. Nevertheless, Wittgenstein can be exonerated from the charge of providing a mere description of what is commonly said, of offering a mere transcription of the vulgate. There is, in all the late work, a latent theorization of the *Lebensform*, and the primacy (or, perhaps more accurately, finality) of practice does not preclude, though it renders finite, a space of justification.[57] Even if everyone, including learned psychologists, thought of seeing the cutlery on the table as involving a perceptual core and an interpretation and expressed themselves accordingly, Wittgenstein would still count this devoid of justification. People can be, at various levels of education, confused and filled with wrong ideas. This is nicely illustrated by the following comment of Joachim Schulte: "In Wittgenstein's view, the idea that an utterance of the sentence 'Now I am seeing it as a rabbit' is a description of an experience is due to an illusion similar to the one which can make us believe that 'I am in pain' is the description of an experience and not its utterance."[58] A vulgar illusion is still an illusion. How many people actually think, "I am in pain," is more exclamative than declarative? For Wittgenstein, the obvious answer has no philosophical significance. This is precisely because Wittgenstein does have something, as Dummett wishes, amounting to a distinction between "what is customarily said and what the conventions governing our use of language require or entitle us to say."

Gombrich, who in *Art and Illusion* makes much of the duck-rabbit-picture (his own version is a shaded rather than simple line-drawn version), uses it to make the following general point: "AMBIGUITY—rabbit or duck?—is clearly the key to the whole problem of image reading. For as we have seen, it allows us to test the idea that such interpretation involves a tentative projection which transforms the image if it turns out to be a hit. It is just because we are so well trained in this game and miss so rarely that we are not often aware of this act of interpretation."[59] For Wittgenstein, too, being well trained within a given form of life (or, alternatively, knowing the local language-games) is what produces a stable, broadly consensual visual world. But this is not, according to Wittgenstein, because there is agreement in interpretation. It is because interpretation, construed as a series of moves in a special game, does not come up. Again, as Schulte puts it, it is like this: "Whenever I look around the room I am in, I shall simply see things; I do not normally see them as this or that. I see things on my desk, I recognize them, I notice details about them, but that is far from being a peculiar experience."[60] Interpretation is missing from this scene, not because the world itself is unproblematically given but because an interpretation can only arise as one member of a set of rival interpretations.

Where our training suffices (as it does not in the case of the duck-rabbit-picture), we simply see. If someone can invent a challenge, plausible within the *Lebensform*, to our description or perceptual report, our simple seeing is transformed—by a kind of Cambridge change—into seeing as, and our report, correspondingly, becomes a more-or-less successfully defensible interpretation.

Do philosophical stories have detachable morals? Do examples yield *dicta*? These would, I suppose, be the philosophical theses

Wittgenstein disowns. Yet it is, on balance, reasonable to think he has some. In treating the difference between seeing$_1$ and seeing$_2$ as a grammatical difference, a creature of circumstance rather than intrinsic (or perhaps "lived") experience, I am honoring one of them. Call this the "thesis of the primacy of grammar." The sense of "grammar" here is—is just—the sense in which *Philosophical Investigations* is a grammatical investigation. This is not quite the famous "linguistic turn." For one thing, the domain of the conceptual, what actually gives definite shape to our or any other form of life, is more extensive than the narrowly linguistic. So Wittgenstein argues that samples—color chips, for example—should be counted "among the instruments of language."[61] We therefore have sentences, but also sample sentences, sample dogs and cats, sample storms, masterpieces, fiascos, beautiful girls, rainbows, and trouble in the making. Our "natural history [*Naturgeschicte*]" has to include not only what we say, but what we talk about, live among, point to, and gesture in the general direction of.[62]

The primacy of grammar thesis will strike Cartesians and neo-Cartesians (for example, the Husserl of *Cartesian Meditations*) as a shift, deflationary and disappointing, away from the real problems of philosophy in the direction of the superficial, the arbitrary, and the ethnographic. Indeed we move with Wittgenstein into a world of surveyable practice, though not a world—as the density of real ethnography and the correlative "thickness" of its descriptions serves to remind us—of either the easily or the already surveyed. What needs to be said about practice, it is obvious enough, is seldom obvious. This is precisely what the duck-rabbit case illustrates. There is the temptation to say one of two wrong things: either that inner experience, having been ducky becomes rabbitty, or the reverse, or else that interpretation, always latent in perception, is in this kind of case overt.

The latter is Gombrich's mistake in *Art and Illusion*. Unusual cases, like the duck-rabbit, are striking but do not generalize. It is important, for Wittgenstein, that such cases are rare or, as Monk puts it, that "we do not see everything as something."[63] Relying on ordinary linguistic competence, we can easily compose sentences that outrun our capacity to understand them—there is no guarantee that artifacts, verbal or other, be transparent to their makers—and the duck-rabbit is just a drawn, or drawing-relative, analogy. Nothing is intrinsically recognizable, labeled by nature for immediate cognitive consumption. We learn, and are sometimes explicitly trained, to recognize things. We learn, and are sometimes explicitly trained, to recognize pictures. And, as usual, there is "interanimation" between types of training (or resultant capacities) as in recognizing pictures of things from things and things from their pictures. Here as elsewhere, training is indefinitely, but not infinitely, expansible, projectible. The duck-rabbit drawing, in the final analysis, presents a comparatively trivial conceptual emergency that leaves us momentarily puzzled about what to call something, but which we finally, and stably, call the duck-rabbit drawing, one more easily recognizable artifact.

Notes

1. Perhaps the best theorization of these "relatively autonomous spheres" is that given by Pierre Bourdieu under the heading *field* or *champ*. See *La Distinction: critique sociale du jugement* (Paris: Minuit, 1979), translated by Richard Nice as *Distinction: A Social Critique of the Judgment of Taste* (Cambridge: Harvard University Press, 1984). A useful collection of Bourdieu's essays related to this concept is *The Field of Cultural Production: Essays on Art and Literature*, ed. Randal Johnson (New York: Columbia University Press, 1993).

2. Ray Monk, *Ludwig Wittgenstein: The Duty of Genius* (New York: Free Press, 1990), pp. 28–35.

3. Gottlob Frege, *The Basic Laws of Arithmetic*, trans. Montgomery Furth (Los Angeles: University of California Press, 1967), p. 16.

4. Bertrand Russell, *The Principles of Mathematics*, 2d ed. (London: Allen & Unwin, 1972 [originally, 1903]), p. 4.

5. In the sense in which psychoanalysts speak of partialisms whereby (certain) organs of the body receive excessive, or at least unusual or supplemental, cathexis.

6. Frege, *Basic Laws of Arithmetic*, p. 10.

7. Michael Dummett, *Frege: Philosophy of Language* (London: Duckworth, 1973), p. xv.

8. See Anthony Kenny, *Wittgenstein* (Cambridge: Harvard University Press, 1973), p. 232: "It is possible that Wittgenstein himself somewhat exaggerated the the difference between his earlier and his later philosophy: this would not be surprising since in the decades between them his attention had been concentrated on the problems which divide them. But as we move further in time from the writings of the *Investigations* we can see that the likenesses to the *Tractatus* are as important as the unlikenesses."

9. Monk, *Ludwig Wittgenstein*, p. 508.

10. References given in the text are to Ludwig Wittgentein, *Tractatus Logico-Philosophicus*, 2nd impression, trans. D. F. Pears and B. F. McGuinness (London: Routledge & Kegan Paul, 1963).

11. David Pears, *Ludwig Wittgenstein* (New York: Viking Press, 1970), p. 76.

12. P. M. S. Hacker, "The Rise and Fall of the Picture Theory," in *Perspectives on the Philosophy of Wittgenstein*, ed. Irving Block (Cambridge: MIT Press, 1981), p. 195.

13. Ludwig Wittgenstein, *Philosophical Grammar*, trans. Anthony Kenny (Oxford: Blackwell, 1974), p. 163. The key phrase in German is "eine Ubereinstimmung der Form," and *Form*, in German, does not mean, any more than "form" in English, "silhouette" or "visual profile." *Philosophische Grammatik* (New York: Barnes & Noble, 1969), p. 163.

14. George Pitcher, *The Philosophy of Wittgenstein* (Englewood Cliffs N.J.: Prentice-Hall, 1964), p. 80.

15. Ludwig Wittgenstein, *Notebooks: 1914–1916*, trans. G. E. M. Anscombe (Oxford: Blackwell, 1961), p. 7e.

16. Rush Rhees, *Discussions of Wittgenstein* (New York: Schocken Books, 1970), p. 4.

17. Robert J. Fogelin, *Wittgenstein* (London: Routledge & Kegan Paul, 1976), p. 21.

18. Kenny, *Wittgenstein*, pp. 62–63.

19. The full sentence, from the Preface to the *Tractatus*, reads, "This book deals with the problems of philosophy, and shows, I believe, that the reason why these problems are posed is that the logic of our language is misunderstood" (p. 3).

20. P. M. S. Hacker, *Insight and Illusion* (Oxford: Clarendon Press, 1972), p. 59.

21. Max Black, *A Companion to Wittgenstein's Tractus* (Ithaca N.Y.: Cornell University Press, 1964), p. 302.

22. R. L. Gregory, "Illusions" in *The Oxford Companion to the Mind*, ed. R. L. Gregory (Oxford: Oxford University Press, 1987), p. 339.

23. Gregory's account does involve the hidden because "are entertained" does not mean the same as "I entertain." The later phrase is for conscious entertainment (something I do), the former for subpersonal, modular, or homuncular processing (something that happens inside me).

24. Ludwig Wittgenstein, *Philosophical Investigations*, trans. G. E. M. Anscombe (New York: Macmillan, 1958), p. 47e.

25. The phrases in this sentence refer to passages in ibid. that occur on pp. 43e, 50e, 49e, 51e, and 91e, respectively.

26. Ibid., p. 103e: "What is your aim in philosophy? To show the fly the way out of the fly-bottle."

27. Michael Dummett, "Can Analytic Philosophy Be Systematic, and Ought It to Be?" in *Truth and Other Enigmas* (Cambridge: Harvard University Press, 1978), p. 451.

28. Wittgenstein's antitheoretical animus is not aimed, in the present context, so much against a possible theory of meaning as against psychological theory about which the following, from *Remarks on the Foundations of Psychology*, 2:12e, is typical: "Psychological concepts are just everyday concepts. They are not concepts newly fashioned by science for its own purpose, as are the concepts of physics and chemistry. Psychological concepts are related to those of the exact sciences as the concepts of the science of medicine are to those of old women who spend their time nursing the sick."

29. Wittgenstein, *Philosophical Investigations*, p. 193e.

30. Ibid.

31. "Ultimate" does not refer to some mythical "final analysis," but indicates only "last" in the sense of "latest" or "*pro tem* best" or "best so far."

32. This, from a 1912 letter to Russell, seems never to have entirely disappeared: "There is nothing more wonderful in the world than the *true* problems of Philosophy." Wittgenstein, *Letters to Russell, Keynes and Moore*, ed. G. H. von Wright (Ithaca N.Y.: Cornell University Press, 1974), p. 14.

33. Wittgenstein, *Philosophical Investigations*, p. 185e. The identical remark occurs in *Last Writings on the Philosophy of Psychology*, ed. G. H. von Wright and Heikki Nyman, trans. C. G. Luckhardt and M. A. E. Aue (Chicago: University of Chicago Press, 1990), 1:54e.

34. Wittgenstein, *Philosophical Investigations*, p. 193e–g.

35. Wittgenstein, *Last Writings on the Philosophy of Psychology*, 1:6e. Wittgenstein adds, though this is not the practice he anywhere literally employs: "Therefore the best example for a sentence with a particular meaning is a quotation from a play" (pp. 6–7).

36. Wittgenstein, *Philosophical Investigations*, p. 193e.

37. Ibid., p. 187e.

38. Norwood Russell Hanson, *Patterns of Discovery* (Cambridge: Cambridge University Press, 1965 [originally, 1958]), p. 15.

39. Ibid.

40. Ibid., 16.

41. Ibid.

42. Ibid., 17.

43. Wittgenstein, *Philosophical Investigations*, p. 194e.

44. Nelson Goodman, *Languages of Art* (Indianapolis: Bobbs-Merrill, 1968) pp. 21–22.

45. Ibid., pp. 24–25. Goodman, however, does make the unimpeachable point that we cannot have learned to recognize unicorn pictures by first having learned to recognize unicorns.

46. "Image," here, is not used in relation to imagination and not as Wittgenstein uses it in *Remarks on the Philosophy of Psychology*, ed. G. H. von Wright and Heikki Nyman, trans. C. G. Luckhart and M. A. E. Aue (Chicago: University of Chicago Press, 1980), 2:13e: "Images are subject to the will" or "One would like to say: The imaged is in a different *space* from the heard sound."

47. Malcolm Budd, *Wittgenstein's Philosophy of Psychology* (London: Routledge, 1989), p. 97.

48. This is not to disagree with Ernst Gombrich, who writes of the duck-rabbit-picture, in *Art and Illusion*, 2nd ed. (Princeton N.J.: Princeton University Press, 1961), pp. 5–6: "We can switch from one reading to another with increasing rapidity; we will also 'remember' the rabbit while we see the duck, but the more closely we watch ourselves, the more certainly we will discover that we cannot experience alternative readings at the same time. Illusion, we will find, is hard to describe or analyze, for though we may be intellectually aware of the fact that any given experience *must* be an illusion, we cannot, strictly speaking, watch ourselves having an illusion." To see the duck-rabbit-picture as such is not, accordingly, to see it as representing both a rabbit and a duck but to see it as representing neither.

49. Wittgenstein, *Philosophical Investigations*, p. 194e.

50. Ibid., pp. 194e–198e.

51. Ibid., pp. 194e–195e.

52. Budd, *Wittgenstein's Philosophy of Mind*, p. 99.

53. Wittgenstein, *Philosophical Investigations*, p. 198e: "The concept of a representation of what is seen, like that of a copy, is very elastic, and so *together with it*

is the concept of what is seen." Or, p. 200e: "The concept of 'seeing' makes a tangled impression. Well, it is tangled."

54. *Naturally* is an adverb meant to mark (certainly *not* to approve) those *Lebensform*-relative, and relatively spontaneous and facile, judgments made by adroit players within a social world, those Husserl described as "naturally immersed in the world" or "turned toward the world." See *Cartesian Meditations*, trans. Dorion Cairns (The Hague: Martinus Nijhoff, 1960), p. 35.

55. Wittgenstein, *Philosophical Investigations*, p. 195e.

56. Michael Dummett, *Origins of Analytical Philosophy* (Cambridge: Harvard University Press, 1993), p. 165.

57. People are fond of saying that, according to Wittgenstein, justification comes to an end without seeming to notice that justification could not end without having gotten started.

58. Joachim Schulte, *Experience and Expression: Wittgenstein's Philosophy of Psychology* (Oxford: Clarendon Press, 1993), p. 56.

59. Gombrich, *Art and Illusion*, p. 238.

60. Schulte, *Experience and Expression*, p. 56.

61. Wittgenstein, *Philosophical Investigations*, p. 7e.

62. Ibid., p. 125e: "What we are supplying are really remarks on the natural history of human beings [Naturgeschicte des Menschen]; we are not contributing curiosities however, but observations which no one has doubted, but which have escaped remark only because they are always before our eyes."

63. Monk, *Ludwig Wittgenstein*, p. 508.

10

Dewey's Critique of Democratic Visual Culture and Its Political Implications

Yaron Ezrahi

John Dewey's critique of the Enlightenment "spectator theory of knowledge" contributed to and anticipated the emergence, later in the twentieth century, of an alternative view of the cultural chemistry of democracy. Discarding the "scopic paradigm" of democratic politics, the presupposition that public actions and their consequences can be transparent to critical, democratic citizens, would involve a radical recasting of the very nature of authority, action, and accountability in modern democracy.[1]

It is easy to miss Dewey's move because his vocabulary is still rooted in classical Enlightenment metaphors and because in some respects the shift is less than complete. In fact his writings occasionally show a tendency to romanticize the Enlightenment ideal of a government fully visible to the public. I would like to suggest, however, that the significance of Dewey's shift away from spectatorial democratic politics and the force of his revisionist approach have only increased over time. His concerns about the "eclipse of the public" as an observing agency become especially relevant in the context of the spreading late-twentieth-century distrust of the earlier Enlightenment faith in the possibility of visually manifest rationality in public affairs.[2] Dewey's work sheds light on recent debates over such issues as whether democracy can be upheld in a polity in which the gestural, theatrical, and aesthetic aspects of politics emerge as no less, and often more, relevant to the reputations of political actors than indicators of the factual-instrumental success of their actions or whether political power can be publicly accountable in a polity in which at least some of the important connections between public actions and their consequences are invisible to the public. Dewey's critique raises the question of what checks on the abuses of political power or what means of exposing arbitrary actions can replace earlier Enlightenment notions of "reality" or observable facts as public standards for distinguishing between acceptable and unacceptable descriptions of the world or between instrumentally rational and irrational actions.

The dimensions of Dewey's break with the established spectatorial model of democratic politics can be appreciated particularly when juxtaposed with Tocqueville's influential articulation of the place of sight in the American democracy nearly a hundred years earlier. "It is on their own testimony," Tocqueville said with regard to democratic citizens, "that [they] are accustomed to rely.... They like to discern the object which engages their attention with extreme clearness [and] they, therefore, strip off as much as possible all that covers it; they rid themselves of whatever conceals it from sight, in order to view it more closely and in the broad light of the day. This disposition of mind soon leads them to condemn forms which they regard as useless or inconvenient veils placed between them and the truth."[3]

Stripping off the veils of power is an idea, to use Thomas Paine's language, of a democratic government whose "excellences or its defects ... are visible to all."[4] Both Paine and Tocqueville present democracy as a system of government that depends on a belief in the power of sight to uphold the relations between governments and their citizens. It was this feature that was supposed to distinguish the "honest" politics of democracy, the utterances and actions that are transparent in the open world of public facts, from the dishonest theatrical politics of the monarchy and the aristocracy, a political universe in which the "real" is concealed behind the contrived pomp and splendor of outward forms. According to this view, democratization is largely a process through which the accountability, and therefore the legitimacy, of the government depend on the increasing transparency of government policies and actions to an ever-growing number of citizens. In the democratic polity, the government is obliged to reveal itself, to expose its considerations and actions, to the citizens, and the citizens are expected in turn to observe, witness, and judge the government.[5] Considering that the role of sight in modern democratic political theory and practice was affected by the rationalization of observation and inspection as sources of knowledge in the experimental scientific tradition,[6] Dewey's references to the decline of both the spectator's conception of scientific knowledge and the spectator's notion of politics are not unrelated. His revisionist conception of democratic politics seems to be influenced by his appreciation of the profound changes in the science of his time and their wider cultural implications. William James noted as early as 1909 that Dewey's views were originally influenced by "changes in current notions of truth."[7] "There are so many geometries," observes James, "so many logics, so many physical and chemical hypotheses, so many classifications, each one of them good for so much and yet not good for everything that the notion that even the truest formula may be a human device and not a literal manuscript has *dawned upon us*—we hear scientific laws now treated as so much 'conceptual shorthand,' true so far as they are useful but no farther." "Truth we conceive to mean everywhere ... not the constructing of inner *copies of* already complete realities but rather the *collaborating with realities* so as to bring about a clearer result"[8] (emphasis added).

In his *Quest for Certainty* (1929), Dewey is very specific in describing the "spectator theory of knowledge," which he rejects. According to this theory, the knower "must be outside what is known, so as not to interact in any way with the object to be known." It is a theory of knowing "modeled after ... the act of vision.... The real object is the object so fixed in its regal aloofness that it is a King to any beholding mind that may gaze upon it."[9] In place of that conception of science, Dewey discerns the emergence of an alternative conception. "Science in becoming experimental has itself become a mode of directed practical doing ... of substituting [the] search for security by practical

means for [the] quest of absolute certainty by cognitive means."
"If we see that knowing is not the act of [an] outside spectator but of a participator inside the natural and social scene, then the true object of knowledge resides in the consequences of directed action"[10] (emphasis added). Dewey links this change, among other things, with a shift from focusing on the properties of objects to focusing on relations between events, which he in turn associates with the shift from Newtonian to Einsteinian physics.[11] Although Dewey discerns the move from the "outside spectator" to the inside "participator" in both the natural and the social sciences, the most significant connections between the two seem often more implicit than explicit in his writings.

A growing sense that the spectator conception of democratic politics is not working well was, of course, not uncommon in the period between the two world wars. Walter Lippmann, perhaps the other most prominent contemporary critic of the notion that citizens can function as spectators according to the principles of democratic government, gave special attention to this theme in his influential book *The Phantom Public* (1925).[12] He held that because of the gulf between "insiders"—by whom he meant those who have an inside view of the government of which they are a part—and "outsiders," who are distant from the field of government action, the inner workings of the political process are not transparent to the latter. At best, outsiders can try to infer the true inside process of government by sampling the external visible aspects of the behavior of the insiders. This, of course, falls short of the requirement that the governors be fully visible to the citizens. In the final analysis, Lippmann's skepticism with regard to the capacity of both the public and the press to know and understand the governmental process leads him to emphasize the significance of experts. Dewey's own analysis of this failure to realize the ideals of spectatorial democracy, his deep concern for *The Public and Its Problems* (1927), seems at times to suggest that he thought the decline of the gazing democratic public to be correctable.[13] He observed, for instance, that while "it is not necessary that the many should have the knowledge and skill to carry on the needed investigations, what is required is that they have the ability to judge of the bearing of the knowledge supplied by others upon common concerns. [But] until secrecy, prejudice, bias, misrepresentation, and propaganda as well as sheer ignorance are replaced by inquiry and publicity, we have no way of telling how apt for judgment of social policies the existence of intelligence of the masses may be. It could certainly go much further than at present."[14]

Despite this cautious optimism, in the final analysis the weight of Dewey's readiness to opt for an alternative cultural paradigm of democratic politics seems greater than the weight of his hopes for saving the citizens as competent spectators. He does not seem really to believe in the possibility of reversing "the eclipse of the public," which he attributes, in part, to the fact that many of the consequences of collective actions remain invisible to laypersons.[15] I shall try to support this claim by examining more closely three distinct, albeit related, arguments with which Dewey tried to challenge and transcend the spectatorial paradigm of democratic politics: that the relations between the causes and the consequences of public actions in the modern industrial society are increasingly more complex and therefore commensurably less visible to the wider public; that seeing or observing is not a passive recording of external objects but a series of acts of engaging, selecting, and organizing visual experience; and finally that hearing is more influential on the formation of public opinion and in substantiating sociopolitical participation than seeing.

The Increasing Complexity and Invisibility of the Causes and Effects of Collective Actions

Dewey held that the classical liberal "idea of a natural individual in his isolation ... is ... a fiction in psychology." According to this fiction, he suggests, "desire and pleasure were both *open* and *above-board* affairs. The mind was seen as if always in the *bright-sunlight*, having *no hidden* recesses, *no unexplorable* nooks, *nothing underground*. Its operations were like the moves in a *fair game* of chess. They are in the *open*, the players have nothing up their sleeves; the changes of position take place by express intent and *in plain light*; they take place according to rules all of which are, known in advance.... Mind was consciousness, and the latter was a *clear, transparent, self-revealing* medium in which wants, efforts and purposes were *exposed* without distortion"[16] (emphasis added). I deliberately quote this citation at length in order to underscore the many terms Dewey uses to describe the dependency of what he regards as anachronistic, classical rationalistic economic liberalism on faith in the powers of sight and the visibility of human motives and actions. Dewey suggests that "today it is generally admitted that conduct proceeds from conditions which are largely out of focal attention, and which can be discovered and brought to light only by inquiries more exacting than those which teach us the concealed relationships involved in gross physical phenomena."[17] In other words, the ability to account for human behavior requires expert social science research and depends on knowledge not naturally or widely accessible. While classical liberals believed that human conduct is the outcome of simple, visible, natural, and rational motives, Dewey insists that it is the product of underlying social conditions. Human choices are not entirely natural. "They mirror a state of civilization."[18] Consistent with early-twentieth-century American orientations, which legitimated sociology as a scientific study of human behavior, Dewey suggests a more complex account of human conduct that is thoroughly at odds with the earlier model. The fact that human conduct is shaped in part by "artificial" rather than natural conditions weakens, in his opinion, the grounds of the belief in the transparency of individual behavior and its consequences. Dewey goes further to suggest that because of the evolution in modern society of new forms of collective action influenced by massive organizations and by large technological systems, individual actors are constantly confronted by the adverse experience of unintended and unanticipated consequences. Because of these structural factors, the links between deliberate actions, consciously intended to bring about certain desired results, and the actual results that ensue are disrupted. Dewey thought that a glaring disparity between the secondary results of the industrial revolution and the conscious intentions of those who were engaged in it provides a compelling illustration of the point.[19]

The operation of vast, impersonal, not easily recognizable causes leads to a state of affairs in which "persons are joined together not because they have voluntarily chosen to be united in these forms, but because vast currents are running which bring men together."[20] Such new forms of combined action do not uphold the earlier model of liberal-democratic politics according to which conduct is in principle transparent and the governors can become publicly accountable by virtue of the visibility of the grounds of their actions and their consequences. In the light of these considerations, Dewey was led to wonder whether the public was a "myth."[21] The elusiveness of both the causes of human actions and their consequences, undermining the very objects of public judgment and action, in fact leads, in his opinion, to the disintegration of the public as an active agency; it subverts collective action as a progressive, experimental learning process in the course of which actions are constantly readjusted as means to obtain desirable consequences. The invisibility of the consequences of collective actions is then the principal reason for the "eclipse of the public." While a few experts may be able to inquire into the relevant facts, "the public and its organization for political ends [becomes] ... a ghost which walks and talks, and obscures, confuses and misleads governmental action in a disastrous way."[22] Such a public, unable to check the uses of arbitrary power, is in itself a blind and dangerous force. It lacks the means to organize its "inchoate and amorphous estate" into "effective political opportunities."[23] Dewey offers here a harsh diagnosis of the destructive consequences of the public loss of the ability to shape its own life. Under such conditions, agencies that can "channel the streams of social action" are absent, and the public becomes "inarticulate" and "scattered."[24] Obviously the sense of sight does not function here as it did in the classical liberal system, where it mediated between a gazing, judging, and, according to Dewey, an active public on the one hand and a transparent and responsive government on the other. In the absence of publicly visible relations between social processes or human actions and their consequences, public instruments of collective action and accountability disintegrate.

Seeing Regarded Not as Outside Beholding But in Fact as Participatory and Constructive

Underlying Dewey's skepticism concerning the validity of the spectatorial conception of democratic political accountability lies a more radical revisionist theory of vision according to which seeing is always, at least in part, an act of producing what is seen, not just a passive reception of what is given. This shift reflects, according to Dewey, a move from the conception of mind as engaging in "knowing as an outside beholding to knowing as an active participation in the drama of an on-moving world."[25] Accordingly, seeing is always an aspect of acting and interacting, of coping with problems and trying to adapt and improve rather than just contemplate, mirror, or record. Modern science, according to this analysis, does not try to find fixed forms behind phenomena but to break down apparent fixities and to induce changes. "The world or any part of it as it presents itself at any given time is accepted or acquiesced in only as material change. It is accepted precisely as the carpenter, say, accepts things as he finds them."[26] Knowing, according to Dewey, is not achieved through contemplation but through "intelligently conducted doing."[27] This shift from a spectator to what can be called an actor theory of knowledge is, in Dewey's system, a process in which the human quest of certainty is achieved through intervening, acting, and changing rather than through the mental possession of a sense of immutable reality. "Knowing is one kind of interaction which goes on within the world."[28] By uniting the traditionally separated functions of inspecting with acting, theoretical with experimental-practical knowledge, Dewey discards the distinction between spectators and performers—between those who know from afar and those who act. Integrating the eye with a deeply democratic conception of knowledge as an aspect of action, a process of continually shaping and reshaping experience, Dewey advances a concept of knowledge as something produced through social interaction.

At least by implication, then, Dewey replaces the classical Enlightenment notion that arbitrary human power and authority can be checked and humbled by decisive references to a publicly given, objective, factual reality with a more open-ended, socially interactive conception of reality as something evolving from a never-ending series of encounters and adaptations, of individuals and groups engaging in experimenting, learning, and improving. For the ideal of a closure fixed by immutable reality that rewards rational and penalizes irrational actors, he substitutes the ideal of an infinite process of piecemeal improvement. If in the former a given accessible, objective world is thought of as externally guaranteeing that human claims can be divided between valid and false and actions into instrumental and noninstrumental, in the latter, claims and actions are thought of as checked by the inherent limits and tentativeness of any given state of knowledge or action, the absence of a privileged, comprehensive knowledge of the world, and the inescapable partiality of every perspective. If in the spectatorial model human ambition is humbled by publicly established truths, in the other model it seems tempered by both universally acknowledged uncertainties and a learning through constant experimentation. Since perceiving is a constitutive act, the diversity of perspectives on experience is commensurate with the diversity of observing subjects. Recognition is "a perception arrested before it has a chance to develop freely."[29] By contrast with simply recognizing, seeing as making and producing is in each case a particular, individual form of acting and experiencing. If the theocratic society postulates a total knowledge, a total God's-eye view of the world, and if the monarchy transfers the privileged synoptic view from above to the king, then modern science secularizes and depersonalizes the comprehensive view of the world as a cooperative enterprise of rational inquirers. While Dewey often uses the language of the proponents of the spectatorial view, he is clearly predisposed to a version of liberal-democratic epistemological individualism according to which the views of various individuals are inherently partial and diverse. Consistent with such an approach, Dewey emphasizes that "knowledge does not encompass the world as a whole."[30] The way to expand one's view is not to add up partial views to a comprehensive-total picture but to subject the views relevant to one's place and condition to the test of experience and interaction with the world. Democratic perceptual and intellectual processes do not produce authoritative synoptic conceptions of reality but infinitely diverse experiences of trying to redirect life through individual and social interactions with the environment.

Seeing, moreover, is not just doing. It is also undergoing. We are not only participating in creating what we see but are also transformed by our experience of seeing. One's eye is not fundamentally different from the eye of the artist or the scientist, which is remade in each act of making. One's eye is guided by one's position, interests, and feelings to select, simplify, clarify, abridge, and organize the materials of visual experience in particular ways.[31] These visual experiences in turn shape the future expectations, orientations, and selections of the observing eye. There is no seeing without acts of not seeing, of ignoring, as well as of abstracting and extracting, of arranging the initially scattered, chaotic visual materials encountered.

Dewey's theory of vision as an aspect of acting or of shaping experience therefore has a strong aesthetic component. Seeing consists of imposing patterns or organizing raw, disorderly external stimuli. It is always a series of interactions that evolve in the course of time. "Perception and its object are built up and completed in one and the same continuing operation."[32] By temporalizing the experience of seeing, Dewey injects the inherent open-endedness of the flow of time as a means of discarding the possibility of spatial, visual closure and of seeing as contacting immutable truths. He thus questions claims of privileged knowledge that can end disputes. Dewey thus "Heraclitizes" a Platonic-Cartesian tradition of knowledge as aiming at seeing eternal truths. Furthermore, by insisting on the inescapable mediative role of the imagination in the formation of all experience, he denies the self, the individual spectator, as a fixed

archemedian point from the perspective of which experience
can be solidly founded. This is a part of Dewey's antifoundation-
alist notion of knowledge as involving dynamic shifting of orientations toward experience. Each spectator is in fact embedded
in a particular culture, tradition, and acquired skills, all of which
shape his or her visual experience as part of a comprehensive,
but never totally complete, experience. "It requires apprentice-
ship to see through a microscope or telescope, or to see a landscape as the geologist sees it."[33]

Dewey's most direct attack on the foundations of the spectatorial view of politics as a process mediated by detached intellectually disciplined visual perception is his insistence that the
operations of the eye, like those of all other sensual organs, are
not distinct and compartmentalized but rather connected to the
other senses. They are, in addition, deeply embedded in human
emotional responses to the world. "In seeing a picture," he writes
in *Art as Experience*, "it is not true that visual qualities are as such,
or consciously, central, and other qualities arranged about them
in an accessory or associated fashion. Nothing could be further
from the truth. It is no more true of seeing a picture than it is of
reading a poem or a treatise on philosophy in which we are not
aware in any distinct way of the visual form of letters and words.
These are stimuli to which we respond with emotional, imaginative, and intellectual values drawn from ourselves."[34] This
means that even such a genre of visual experience as the documentary film or text is not free of our emotional and aesthetic
responses.[35] Furthermore, since in this view sense itself blends
with relations, Dewey could regard a difference such as the one
between the aesthetics of the decorative and the expressive as
merely a matter of emphasis.[36] In the final analysis, "nothing is
perceived except when different senses work in relation with one
another."[37]

Ultimately Privileging Hearing over Seeing

"The connections of the ear with the vital and outgoing thought
and emotions are immensely closer and more varied," observes

Dewey, "than those of the eye."[38] While "through vision we are
connected with what is distant ... [and although sounds] come
from outside the body, ... sound itself is near, intimate; it is an
excitation of the organism. We feel the clash of vibrations
throughout our whole body.... Because of the connections of
hearing with all parts of the organism, sound has more reverber-
ations and resonances than any other sense."[39] While such rever-
berations and resonances are what renders the ear less reliable
than the distancing and intellectually more controllable eye that
operates in the spectatorial regime of the Enlightenment model
of democratic politics, for Dewey it is precisely because hearing is
more diffused and interconnected with other senses, precisely
because "the ear is the emotional sense" while "what is seen stirs
emotion indirectly, through interpretation,"[40] that the ear is the
better instrument for cementing public opinion and associative,
social responses to experience. It is precisely the particularly
intense "connections of the ear with vital and out-going thought
and emotion" that render it the more reliable mediator of social
interaction and communication. "There is no limit to the liberal
expansion and confirmation of limited personal intellectual
endowment which may proceed from the flow of social intelligence [observes Dewey] when that circulates by word of mouth
from one to another in the communications of the local community. *That and that only gives reality to public opinion*" (emphasis
added).[41]

In the final analysis this is Dewey's remedy for what he and
Lippmann regarded as the deterioration of the democratic public into just a "phantom public." His reliance on the sense of
hearing is, in part, why to Dewey the appeal of music can be
much more widespread, much more inclusive than that of any
other art. Dewey reverses here the Enlightenment move to rely
on the eye rather than on the spoken word as a strategy of cool-
ing off politics, of separating the style of political from the style
of religious discourse.[42] It is because of the special links between
sounds, music, immediate emotions, and religious enthusiasm
that liberal democratic thinkers and ideologues, more often than
not, tended to prefer the eye and "attestive visual orientations"

as a medium of social and political interaction.[43] But Dewey seems to be satisfied that sound shaped and disciplined by language, that speech in live conversation rather than in written form, is the most important means to actualize public opinion and integrate it into ongoing communal political action.

If Dewey refers here to the crucial role of conversation and persuasion in the formation of public opinion and the evolution of "collective intelligence," he does not reckon with the problem of how meaningful conversation can take place in the larger society beyond the boundaries of local communities in which individuals can engage in ongoing face-to-face relationships. After all, it was the spectatorial model of democratic politics, in which the few who can act are held accountable by virtue of the visibility of their actions to the many who can only observe, that was the preferred, if by no means perfect, solution to the need to secure government accountability in mass societies in which direct democracy was not a practical possibility. While Dewey does not seem effectively to answer this challenge directly, the shift from a concept of public opinion founded on seeing to one based on hearing and speaking does not leave his position entirely defenseless on this point. The strength of his approach lies in the special affinity, to which I have already alluded, between sound and temporality as a never-ending flow resisting all forms of closure. One can argue from Dewey's position that public opinion is a dynamic, ever changing product of a continual process of conversing and interacting with the social and the natural environments, an experience that resists the very idea of an end. As a process, public opinion formation need not be at any point actually inclusive in order to deny exclusiveness. A diffused, decentralized process of shaping and drawing on experience does not privilege any individual or group as a representative spokesman of public opinion. Nevertheless, the difficulties of evolving and maintaining a clear and focused public discourse in modern mass society seem to diminish the probability that such a society can generate unambiguous mandates for public action. How can the public guide government policies through such a diffuse network of conversations? The uses and impact of modern mass communications technology seem to suggest that there is no technical solution to the problem posed by the inability of public discourse to provide clear guidelines for the governors. This, however, is conceived as a problem fatal to a democratic regime only when one expects the government to function as an agent of clear and decisive collective choices and programs. But such expectations derive from the Enlightenment spectatorial model that Dewey, at least implicitly, discards. The relevance of Dewey's thought to late-twentieth-century democracies, such as the North American, lies precisely in the fact that such expectations are anachronistic in the context of modern democratic political practice and that decisions, policies, and actions in these democracies usually appear to be eclectic, patched up, and internally contradictory, that they seem more the outcomes of constantly shifting political compromises than of decisive preferences expressed by clear majorities.

In such a context, the meanings of both the nature of and the interactions between public opinion and public action are radically transformed. Although Dewey notes in his diagnosis of contemporary democracy that the new conditions seem to eclipse the public and give rise to the influence of experts, his ideas about social learning and public action seem to have anticipated some of the most sophisticated and perceptive late-twentieth-century accounts of democracy as a system in which policies are generated by "pluralistic probing" rather than by decisive public majorities. Charles E. Lindblom's *Inquiry and Change* (1990) is illustrative.[44] Lindblom stresses the "never-ending" inconclusiveness of probing as a process of learning and acting. Unlike the scientific process, probing is more manifestly open, flexible, inconclusive, and inclusive.[45] Like Dewey, Lindblom discards the notion that decisions can be grounded in clear and distinct collective preferences and truths. Action is the result of much humbler processes. "No one can dis- or uncover a volition; and instead people form, choose, decide upon, or will. This they do through a mixture of empirical, prudential, aesthetic and moral probes." The acknowledged impossibility of anyone's ever achieving a full grasp of the relevant complexities of society compels action under conditions of at least partial ignorance. This approach, according to Lindblom, counts on strategies like trial and error, in which the trial serves not simply as an attempted solution but as a means to produce information useful for subsequent attempts.[46] This more decentralized model of acting and interacting downgrades elites and centralized power.[47] In this very Deweyian account, problems are not solved but are coped, or reckoned, with. It discards holistic views of collective decisions and actions and enhances the intimacy between citizens, social scientists, and governors.[48] In contrast to what Lindblom describes as the highly "unilateral exercises of influence and power," processes of self-government conceived as a bundle of decentralized multilateral and uncertain adjustments do not lend themselves to the notion of politics as a view in which the transparency and clarity of the actions of the governors allow the citizens to exercise their rights and powers as the legitimators or delegitimators of the incumbent government.[49] In such a polity, speaking, persuading, and bargaining are not less but more important than viewing and visually knowing.

Conclusion

While the transparency of the process of government as well as the status of the public gaze are, according to John Dewey, questionable, seeing and being seen remain important aspects of interaction and social communication. Hence by comparison with antiocularcentrism in modern French thought, for example, Dewey's critique of the role of sight in politics and society is much more moderate. Insofar as his antiocularcentrism is embedded in a deeply American liberal theory of action as interaction, the denigration of vision is not reinforced, as it is in twentieth-century French thought, by the propensity to associate seeing with social invasion into the private sphere of the self.[50] This tendency has developed in France as part of deeply rooted traditions of conceiving the individual as an entity much more sharply distinct and separated from society, and locating freedom in the internal sphere of the private self away from the public, the more formal and coercive sphere of social interaction.

Juxtaposed with Dewey's critique of the eye as an instrument of communication and interaction, Martin Jay's illuminating discussion of the positions of modern French thinkers and writers like Henri Bergson, Georges Bataille, André Breton, Jean-Paul Sartre, Maurice Merleau-Ponty, Iouis Althusser, and Michel Foucault indicates, at first sight, some obvious continuities.[51] Also in the French case one can discern doubts about the Enlightenment trust in dispassionate visual cognition from a distance, an appreciation for the interaction of the eye with the other elements of the human body, a recognition of the temporal dimension of the experience of seeing, a shift from stressing visual perception in the context of representation to stressing its role in the context of action, a critique of the notion that truths are visually manifest on the surface layers of our experience, and doubts concerning the belief that objects, and particularly persons, can be known through seeing. Also in the French case one can find reference to music as liberating one from the chains of the visual, a perspective from which knowledge is perceived as the outcome of an elaborate process of production not as mirroring—and a French-Marxist variant of the shift from knowledge as contemplation to knowledge as an aspect of action.[52] Such similarities between American and European tendencies to discard what Jay calls "the fetish of opticality in traditional modernist theory"[53] and with it the political forms and practices that were upheld by this fetish[54] indicate the depth and comprehensiveness of early-twentieth-century criticism of Enlightenment models of culture and politics in the West, criticism that contributed eventually to postmodernist tendencies to denigrate vision and its psychological, social, and political implications on both sides of the Atlantic Ocean. Nevertheless, the differences between continental, particularly French, and American criticisms of the role of the eye are at least as instructive. In the French case, the critique of sight is in part an element in a long local tradition identifying the gaze with social domination and control of the individual, a threat to his or her freedom and autonomy. Because for so many French thinkers and writers individual freedom and autonomy do not arise in, but away from, the sociopolitical context, and are therefore more internally intellectual, psychological, spiritual, and cultural, the eye of the other is often regarded more as a threat—the confining and controlling agent of the social gaze, not the means of reciprocal, equal interaction. As a polity with a long tradition of centralized power associated with the legacy of the absolutist monarchy and the omnipresence of a controlling bureaucracy, France encouraged the evolution of a particular variant of individualism more insular and atomistic than its Anglo-Saxon and especially its American counterpart. French individualism seem less tempered by the degree to which voluntary associations are relied on to uphold the sociopolitical order.[55] In the French context, the true reality of the individual is presumed to be hidden and inaccessible to the eye. Visible behavior is characteristically regarded as social and therefore a less authentic form of behavior.[56] True communication, in this view may require "mutual opacity" rather than reciprocal transparency.[57] In addition to Dewey's commitment to social-interactive rather than French-style insular individualism, his more restricted critique of vision reflects his more moderate rejection of the Enlightenment paradigm of culture and politics. Dewey's thought reveals a deeply American commitment to the master narrative of progress and to the remaining significance of science as a force of social improvement. Despite his criticism of, and ambivalence toward, technology, Dewey basically regards technology as a progressive force for social change nourished by human cooperation and collective learning. Walter Benjamin captured an important feature of European individualism and its implications when he observed that "the average European has not succeeded in uniting his life with technology because he has clung to the fetish of creative existence."[58] Dewey's trust in the operation of a social intelligence that improves both individual and collective actions commits him to a much more socially interactive view of creative individualism—one that can accommodate at least some elements of the classical liberal democratic theory of action according to which social learning and the public acknowledgment of facts constitute a constraint on human hierarchies, dependencies, and arbitrary behavior.

Dewey's importance as a twentieth-century democratic thinker resides, however, in the degree to which he has gone beyond this classical vocabulary of the democratic discourse on culture and politics. I have tried to allude to his critique of vision as a useful clue to his importance in anticipating the more comprehensive and socially or culturally thoroughgoing late-twentieth-century challenges to the Enlightenment paradigm of democratic politics. Particularly noteworthy are Dewey's moves to replace the citizens as spectators with the citizens as interactors and to redefine public opinion as the outcome of ongoing social speech, a network of social conversations rather than of a comprehensive gaze.

Modern mass society has posed the dilemma of how the imperative of inclusive citizen participation, a necessary condition of self-government, can be realized in the larger social context, beyond the boundaries of the local community, where face-to-face relationships are an impractical basis for generating guidelines for collective actions. The Enlightenment cult of the eye opened the way to the modern solution of substituting universal accountability by means of the transparency of the government to the public eye, for the unachievable ideal of direct democracy. What was regarded as unavoidable practical constraints on the perfect decentralization of power seemed balanced or at least mitigated by an inclusive conception of the citizens as "attestive witnesses" capable of legitimating or delegitimating the government. Dewey was one of the first and most prominent Western, and especially American, thinkers to challenge this solution and point in the direction of a possible alternative based on reinstating a variant of participatory democracy as a highly decentralized, continual, open-ended process of interactive pragmatic shaping and reshaping of collective social and political life. His position and the position of his followers remain, of course, vulnerable on several key points. If indeed "the flow of social intelligence when it circulates by word of mouth from one to another in the communications of the local community . . . [is what] gives reality to public opinion," isn't it just as vulnerable and limited as visual communication has been at the level of the larger society?[59] If the complexity of the causal links between social actions and their consequences makes them at least partly invisible to the public, and if the public, lacking the ability to examine key aspects of the political process, tends to disintegrate, how does the dynamic of a word-of-mouth communication correct the situation? Can't speech degenerate into forms of imperfect and even distorted communications just as sight has, according to Dewey? Don't words lend themselves like pictures to becoming, as Hobbes put it, the "coins of fools" and persuade by evoking aesthetic and emotional responses, devoid of disciplined cognitive contents? Can't sounds be just as centrally manipulated and deceptive as words? Doesn't the human imagination that Dewey celebrates as a mediator of all experience (and that Rousseau feared as the engine of political decay) often serve more as the means to escape social interaction and politics than to join in order to cope effectively and pragmatically with shared problems? These are only some of the questions raised by Dewey's remedy for the inadequacies and anachronisms of the Enlightenment's democratic optics and the discrediting of sight in mediating democratic politics in advanced societies. And yet so much of what Dewey suggested seems to have survived and continues to make sense in the context of contemporary debates.

By temporalizing, localizing, and individuating the experience of seeing, Dewey disempowered the eye as both an instrument of control and a privileged means to establish and communicate truths authoritatively. The strained, analytically detached, focused, and cognitively ambitious eye of the Enlightenment democrat has been replaced by the more relaxed, exploratory, yet far more playful and occasionally reflexive eye of the late-twentieth-century democratic citizen. Vision has become a part of new conceptions of politics and citizenship tempered by a deeper and more widely shared sense of limits.

Dewey astutely recognized the dilemmas created by the propensity to rely on public opinion in the modern industrial society.

He was also more attuned than most of his contemporaries to the tendency to replace monumental political engineering in the style of the Enlightenment by a practical, ad hoc series of local probings and adjustments. Dewey understood that neither the detached nor the elevated eye can be democratic; that claiming to see too much or with finality is incompatible with the inherent underdeterminism of the democratic experience of the real. In the final analysis, Dewey's critique of the scopic paradigm of democracy that Tocqueville enunciated so clearly is just another step in the emancipation of democratic politics from the grip of hierarchical cultural forms inherited from the predemocratic era.[60]

Notes

1. Yaron Ezrahi, *The Descent of Icarus: Science and the Transformation of Contemporary Democracy* (Cambridge, Mass.: Harvard University Press, 1990).

2. John Dewey, *The Public and Its Problems* (Chicago: Swallow Press, 1954).

3. Alexis de Tocqueville, *Democracy in America*, ed. P. Bradley (New York: Vintage Books, 1945), 2:4–5.

4. Thomas Paine, *The Rights of Man*, cited in W. J. T. Mitchell, *Iconology* (Chicago: University of Chicago Press, 1986), p. 147.

5. Ezrahi, *The Descent of Icarus*.

6. Ibid.

7. William James, *Pragmatism* (New York: New American Library, 1909), p. 233.

8. Ibid., p. 234.

9. John Dewey, *The Quest for Certainty* (New York: Capricorn Books, 1960), p. 23.

10. Ibid., pp. 245, 196.

11. Ibid., pp. 144–145.

12. Walter Lippmann, *The Phantom Public* (New York: Harcourt Brace, 1925).

13. Dewey, *The Public and Its Problems*.

14. Ibid., p. 209.

15. Ibid.

16. Ibid., pp. 102–103.

17. Ibid., p. 103.

18. Ibid., pp. 103–104.

19. Ibid., pp. 106–107.

20. Ibid., p. 107.

21. Ibid., p. 123.

22. Ibid., p. 125.

23. Ibid.

24. Ibid., pp. 131–132.

25. Dewey, *The Quest for Certainty*, p. 291.

26. John Dewey, *Reconstruction in Philosophy* (New York: Mentor Books, 1950).

27. Ibid., p. 106.

28. Dewey, *The Quest for Certainty*, pp. 204–205.

29. John Dewey, *Art as Experience* (New York: Capricorn Books, 1958).

30. Dewey, *The Quest for Certainty*, p. 296.

31. Joseph Ratner, ed., *Intelligence in the Modern World: John Dewey's Philosophy* (New York: Modern Library, 1939), pp. 973, 971, 975, 977.

32. Dewey, *Art as Experience*, p. 177.

33. Ibid., p. 53.

34. Ibid., p. 123.

35. On the aesthetic of the documentary, see Susan Sontag, *On Photography* (New York: Dell Publications, 1977).

36. Dewey, *Art as Experience*, p. 126.

37. Ibid., p. 175.

38. Dewey, *The Public and Its Problems*, pp. 218–219.

39. Dewey, *Art as Experience*, pp. 237, 238.

40. Ibid., p. 257.

41. Ibid., p. 219.

42. See on oral discourse and religion in Walter J. Ong, *The Presence of the Word* (New Haven: Yale University Press, 1967).

43. Ezrahi, *The Descent of Icarus*, pp. 67–96; See also Michael Heyd, *"Be Sober and Reasonable": The Critique of Enthusiasm in the Seventeenth and Early Eighteenth Centuries* (Leiden: E. J. Brill, 1995).

44. Charles E. Lindblom, *Inquiry and Change* (New Haven: Yale University Press, 1990).

45. Ibid., p. 216.

46. Ibid., pp. 216, 219.

47. Ibid., pp. 219–220.

48. Ibid., p. 226.

49. Ibid., p. 240.

50. Ezrahi, *The Descent of Icarus*, pp. 197–208.

51. Martin Jay, *Downcast Eyes: The Denigration of Vision in Twentieth-Century French Thought* (Berkeley: University of California Press, 1993).

52. Ibid., esp. pp. 146, 152, 197, 230, 281, 374–375.

53. Ibid., p. 407.

54. Ezrahi, *The Descent of Icarus*.

55. Ibid., pp. 197–208.

56. Ibid., p. 200; also Louis Dumont, *German Ideology* (Chicago: University of Chicago Press, 1994).

57. Jay, *Downcast Eyes*, p. 407; Ezrahi, *The Descent of Icarus*, pp. 67–96.

58. Walter Benjamin, *Reflections* (New York: Harcourt Brace Jovanovich, 1978), p. 272.

59. Dewey, *The Public and Its Problems*, p. 219.

60. See Yaron Ezrahi, "Modes of Reasoning and the Politics of Authority in the Modern State," in David R. Olson and Nancy Torrance, eds., *Modes of Thought* (Cambridge: Cambridge University Press, 1996).

11

Materialist Mutations of the *Bilderverbot*

Rebecca Comay

Why should only idealists be permitted to walk a tightrope, while materialist tightrope walking is prohibited?
—Walter Benjamin, in Gershom Scholem, *Walter Benjamin: Story of a Friendship*

I Secularizations

No idealist, but only a materialist deliverance from myth
—Walter Benjamin, "Karl Kraus"

What could be at work in the Marxist rendition of the theological prohibition of images? In *Negative Dialectics*, Theodor Adorno explicitly binds the by now familiar critique of representation (mediation, mediatization, the society-of-the-spectacle) to the secular imperative to "grasp the object" itself in its corporeal truth. Such a "grasp" [*Begriff*] would seem to reinflect the theological longing for redemption along decidedly atheological lines: "It is only in the absence of images that the full object could be conceived. Such absence concurs with the theological ban on images. Materialism brought that ban into secular form by not permitting Utopia to be positively pictured; this is the substance of its negativity. At its most materialistic, materialism comes to agree with theology. Its great desire would be the resurrection of the flesh, a desire utterly foreign to idealism, the realm of the absolute spirit" (ND207/207). Setting aside, for the moment, the apparent appeal to immediacy implicit in this citation, I propose to use this startling passage—a formulation that seems to announce nothing less than the recoil of the ascetic ideal upon itself—as a starting point to reexamine the well-rehearsed debate between Adorno and Benjamin.

How does "theology" here become not only allied with but essentially identified with "materialism"? Whatever the nature of the negotiation, it will in any case be more than a question of finding vague parallels or surreptitious borrowings—an easy dig at Marxism as chiliastic "creed" or "dogma," a familiar nod toward the Jewish return to history—not a question of compatibility or complicity, but rather an "agreement" forged precisely where the antithesis would seem most intractable. For according to such a refunctioning of the monotheistic prohibition, the apparent mortification of the senses would come to signal not the familiar payoff of supersensuous fulfillment—the sublime passage from physical blindness to spiritual insight (Oedipus, Teiresias)—but rather the vindication of the body itself at the very point of its most irreparable disfiguration. At its limit, then, materialism is said to absorb or reinscribe theology precisely in speaking of a restitution beyond every idealizing compensation and in this sense intransigently unconsoling.

Why does the iconoclastic imperative get attached here to the promise of resurrection? And how would each (apart or together) withstand the pressure of otherworldliness? If the prospect of redeeming the suffering body precludes any representation of its singularity, this would imply a kind of return outside the restricted economy of a salvation effected through the spiritual metamorphosis of a body raised to divine immortality, rationality, and *apatheia*, and would thus indicate the persistence of matter precisely in its utterly unreconciled alterity.

Such redemption would therefore suggest something other than the *theiosis* of the perfected individual formed in the image of the incorruptible divine. This latter notion would inevitably substitute for the banished idol the essentialized image of an incorporeal God. Spiritual insight would redeem the blindness of corporeal vision.[1] "Image of the invisible" (Colossians I:15), the apparition of Christ would present the possibility of a vision ultimately purified of sensuous immediacy and thus the very promise of spirit's victory over dead matter. The transfiguration of the Pauline grain of wheat—"sown in humiliation, raised in glory" (1 Corinthians 15:44)—presupposes the divine *oikonomia* of a redemption mimetologically secured through the figure of Christ as *imago Dei* and thus guaranteed to humanity precisely as bearer of the heavenly "stamp," "seal," or imprint.[2]

What would it mean to articulate the *Bilderverbot* without recourse to the sublimated mimetology of idealism? And what would a nontransfiguring resurrection begin to look like? It would be tempting but misleading to confront a "Christian" with a "Jewish" eschatology—Ezekiel's dry bones pitted against the spiritual body of St. Paul, the mended pot of the Sanhedrin[3] pitted against Augustine's recast statue—in order to mark the essential terms of opposition. If it would be overly hasty simply to oppose here a Jewish emphasis on the body to a Christian otherworldliness (historical considerations alone make it impossible to draw a clean divide between two interlocked traditions), the philosophical challenge of thinking a nonreconciling restitution remains nonetheless pressing.

"Redemption," as Benjamin writes (the allusion is here to Kafka), "is no reward or recompense for existence but the last way out [*die Erlösung ist keine Prämie auf das Dasein, sondern die letzte Ausflucht*]" (II.2.423; ILL 125): not the return of spiritual commensuration but rather a rupture all the more radical in being premised on an imperceptible difference—a "slight adjustment [*eine Geringes zurechtstellen*]" (II.2.432; ILL 134)—between this world and the next. Whatever the "weakness" of the Messianic power (I.2.694; ILL 254)—the angel of history cannot linger, cannot awaken the dead, cannot make whole what has been smashed, and so on (I.2.697 ff.; ILL 257)—the very identification of the Messianic with the domain of transience or "downgoing" (II.1.205; R 313) (the Nietzschean overtone is unmistakable) would suggest that redemption cannot be thought beyond or apart from the eternal return of bodily remnants or remainders, without totalizing compensation. If the dead cannot be revived, this is no doubt for the same reason that they cannot be said properly or securely to die: "Even the dead are not safe from the enemy if he wins" (I.2.695; ILL 255).[4] Our permanent assignation with "past generations" (I.2.694; ILL 254) indicates precisely the tenacity of dead matter as that which haunts the plenitude of the living present. "Living on [*Überleben*]" becomes thus the perpetual obsolescence that at once both defines and subverts tradition.

Adorno will evoke Kafka somewhat similarly. If the theory of the "unsuccessful death" (Odradek, Gracchus) "is the sole promise of immortality ... permit[ted] to survive the ban on images" (P 286/270 ff.), the very possibility of redemption would hinge precisely on the fact that it inevitably comes too late. Thus the famous litany of missed opportunities—philosophy's failure to have sublated itself in practice (*Negative Dialectics*), the bourgeoisie's inability to "find a successor" (P 273/260), the necrology of art announced in the *Aesthetic Theory*—a guilty longevity testifying to an imperative all the more urgent for being announced too late. "The resurrection of the dead would have to take place in the auto graveyards" (P 273/260).

Benjamin's Dilemma

In the notorious preface to the *Trauerspielbuch*, Benjamin identifies the regime of vision—*Schau, Anschauung*, the phenomenological projection of horizons—as the acquisitive or "possessive" operation of the subject seeking confirmation in what it knows (I.1.215; OGT 35). Famously, truth is said to resist this. Nonintentional and nonrelational, truth, according to Benjamin's familiar formula (which in this respect resembles that of Levinas), "is not an unveiling [*Enthüllung*] that destroys the mystery but a revelation [*Offenbarung*] which does it justice" (I.1.211; OGT 31).[5] It has become somewhat conventional to read here a continuation and radicalization of a certain tendency within both orthodox and heterodox Judaism toward an attenuation of any positive concept of revelation: the rabbinic emphasis on aurality (the "voice from Sinai"), the kabbalistic emphasis on the divine name: the hermeneutic excess of interpretation over meaning, and thus the demystification of every authoritative disclosure.

The predominance of language over vision, according to such a convention, would suggest a certain privilege of symbolic over imaginary and thus the foreclosure of every fantasy of fusion. Visualization invites identification and thus inevitably the spectre of idolatrous confusion. The heterogeneity of the absolute requires a denunciation of *schöne Schein* as the renunciation of the appropriative order of the Same.

Benjamin will speak indeed of sacrifice. Beauty is to be immolated—but equally seeks "refuge"—on the "altar of truth" (I.1.211; OGT 31). The priority of "truth" to "beauty" in this context (Hermann Cohen is never distant) will elsewhere provoke an extended invocation of a certain sublime (I.1.181): Kant, Novalis, the familiar "fable" of the "veiled image" of Isis, whose unveiling is said to be fatal—shattering, even castrating (*zusammenbrechend*)—for the inquirer (I.1.216; OGT 37).[6]

The prohibition at work here is by no means a simple one. If Benjamin will invoke a traditional enough trope of truth-as-woman—inaccessible, invisible, inexpressible object of an impossible desire—this is not to reinstate mystery cults under the rubric of iconoclasm. That would be to reduce the *Bilderverbot* to a simple esotericism—"some enigmatic cruelty in actual meaning" (I.1.216; OGT 36)—and thus ultimately to reify the lost object as simple positivity.

For the exposure of the truth here—the object neither "veiled [*verhüllt*]" nor "unveiled [*enthüllt*]" but rather precisely "the object itself in its being-veiled" (I.1.195)—implies simultaneously a "surrender [*Preisgabe*]" (I.1.184) and an "intensification [*Steigerung*] of Schein in a final and most extreme form" (I.1.186). The loss in representational or intentional mediacy would involve in this sense a corresponding gain in "presentational [*darstellende*]" effectiveness: a sacrifice—Benjamin speaks in a related context of Proust's sacrifice of character, plot, "play of the imagination" (II.1.314; ILL 204)—counterbalanced by the expansion of a certain "image sphere [*Bildraum*]" in which language itself comes to the fore.

And herein precisely will lie the entire kernel of the dispute. Such a "sublime" sacrifice might well appear to involve a compensatory logic familiar at least since Kant and Hegel: less is more, *qui perd gagne*, the slave logic of recuperative self-denial. The issue will be to redeem such a sacrifice from the rationalist calculus identified by Adorno and Horkheimer as the dialectic of *Aufklärung*—the mythic circle of renunciation and reward. What will prevent Benjamin's version of the saving of the phenomena from collapsing into a simple legitimation of the existent? *This precisely will be Adorno's final question to Benjamin.*

II Before the Law

In breaking a statue one risks becoming a statue.
—Jean Cocteau, *Le Sang d'un poète*

How can a materialist prohibition against images be enunciated? Is there not something profoundly contradictory about the very representation of the law forbidding representations of the future? Would not the law inevitably transgress itself in its own pronouncement? Would it not, indeed, stimulate the very iconophilia that it prohibits—this according to the irreducible imbrication of law with desire, proscription with enjoyment—and thus undermine itself in its own enactment?

The issue here involves somewhat more than the double bind attendant on every law in its self-universalizing force and promise. Hegel had already identified that initial problem, a formal one, in his chapter on "Force and the Understanding": the paradox of a law rendered vacuous by its inherent repeatability and binding power. It involves more, too, than the performative self-contradiction of a pronouncement delegitimating itself by virtue of its own legality: to pronounce the *Bilderverbot* is itself to assume legislative authority—thus to identify with the origin of the law even if only in order to speak of it and on its behalf—in this sense committing self-idolatry precisely in order to prohibit it in others, contaminating transcendence in the very effort to protect its purity, assuming the essential guilt it would deter. Follow me/ do not follow me. Is not the *Bilderverbot* in this respect the most self-transgressive of all laws? Destined to be forgotten, invoked in order to be violated, does it not exemplify the ultimate impossibility of the law as such? There is, however, more than one way of responding to such an impossibility.

The issue here is not only the familiar psychoanalytic point (regarding the return of the repressed as neurotic symptom), nor only the Foucauldian one (concerning the positive productivity of the law in its very negativity). One might remark with equal cogency—indeed this will be my essential argument—that if every prohibition both incites and requires a corresponding transgression, it is also conversely the case that through its apparent self-infraction, the law only binds us closer (although to what remains undetermined). In this case the law's very inability to authorize itself may testify equally to an even deeper, if perhaps ultimately inscrutable, prohibition—but perhaps equally to the claim of an unspeakable desire.

Perhaps something more than dialectical reciprocity is at work in such a chiasmus of law and transgression. Perhaps in this doubly contaminating movement of self-deregulating regulation and self-regulating deregulation, another relationship to both the law and the image may begin to announce itself.

Since Kant, if not indeed since Longinus, it has become habitual to remark on the "meta-sublime" nature of the very law announcing the essential incommensurability between law and manifestation—the Second Commandment here taken to be not only the paradigmatic statement about the sublime but the very paradigm of a "sublime utterance"[7]—suggesting the ultimate aporia of a law exemplifying itself precisely in pronouncing the impossibility of every example. Thus the biblical warning regarding every possible (inevitable) reification of the law. Moses' smashing and rewriting of the tablets at Sinai expresses precisely the necessity of the second-degree iconoclasm necessary to sustain the law by mitigating its eidetic self-evidence, thus marking its origins in a prior event of self-erasure and hence its irreducible

inscription within the domain of history. The replacement set—
no longer identified as "God's handiwork" (Exodus 32:16) but
inexorably marked as substitute or simulacrum, writing rather
than "engraving"—as such signifies the impossibility of any
immediate relation to the original. This announces the originary
doubling of the law as the permanent imbrication of law and
interpretation. "It is from an already destroyed word that man
learns the demand that must speak to him."[8]

But if the law thus incorporates its own infraction as the very
condition of its own articulation, it follows equally that every
adherence is marked by a corresponding violation. The smashing
of the tablets anticipates the pulverizing of the golden calf,
which in turn in its literalizing aggressivity only confirms the
charismatic power of the idol. The accusation of idolatry in this
sense typically presupposes (as Hegel already points out in his
analysis of Enlightenment's crusade against superstition) a "not
very enlightened"[9] assumption regarding the relationship between finite being and the absolute, and for this reason mystifies
the very act of demystification as a "new serpent of wisdom
raised on high for adoration."[10]

And so on. The point is not simply a formal or logical one, nor
is the issue quaintly theological. It exposes a risk that affects every
radical politics. For the very renunciation of images threatens
precisely once more to determine the future as a tabula rasa or
blank slate receptive to the arbitrary projections of the present
day. "Homogeneous empty time" would be reinstated. The old
"geometrical conception of the future"—Bataille's expression—
would be reestablished. Even setting aside the familiar paradoxes
accompanying the notion of a utopia determined essentially as
the very absence of determination—the conventional picture of
a world without pictures—the danger of abstraction remains
ineluctable.

How to avoid an idealist relapse into indeterminate negativity
and thus immediacy? Does not every *Bilderverbot* presuppose the
familiar Platonic series of bifurcations—essence-appearance,
original-copy, truth-ideology—and hence a prolongation of the
ascetic ideal? Politically: how to resist positing negativity itself

Materialist Mutations of the *Bilderverbot*

as the very consolation to be denied? Theologically: how to avoid invoking negative theology as the symmetrical obverse of dogmatic fundamentalism?

We will not yet be able to name the law under which we stand.
—Benjamin, "Gedanken über Gerhart Hauptmanns Festspiel"

There are mythical and nonmythical articulations of the dilemma. That is, the inevitable circle of law and transgression can be entered in a variety of fashions. If, to introduce Benjamin's terms, the regime of fate is defined by the compulsive circle of guilt-retribution-guilt, which turns the "guilt context of the living" (I.1.138) into the nightmare of a "never ending trial" (II.2.412; ILL 114)—from the tragic cycles of Greek drama to the protracted vertigo of Kafka's *Prozeß*—such a regime also harbors an essential "ambiguity [*Zweideutigkeit*]" (II.1.199; R 296), which may conceal unexpected resources.

According to the terms of the "Critique of Violence," the mythical origin of the law (cf. II.1.154; R 328) suggests "the ultimate undecidability of all legal problems" (II.1.196; R 293) and eventually points to the inability of the law itself to determine practice. Thus Kafka's "new attorney" no longer practices but only "studies" law (II.2.437; ILL 139)—an impasse that will eventually receive its starkest formulation in Kafka's notion of a trial in which guilt is perpetuated even or especially in the judgment that would delimit or contain it. "Does it not turn the judge into the defendant?" (II.2.427; ILL 128 ff.). If this suggests (to Scholem's unease)[11] a final indeterminacy regarding the status of the law in its "purest" or most paradigmatic form as a Last Judgment (now indefinitely protracted and hence definalized owing to its complicity with its object), perhaps no firm distinction can be sustained (at least by way of any tribunal of judgment or "critical" discrimination) between the mythic cycle of retribution and the divine justice which would "only expiate" (II.1.199; R 297).

Adorno has rehearsed the problem with irritating rigor. The inescapable imbrication of myth and enlightenment implies the

persistence of superstition in the very "taboo" that would eliminate it and as such the inevitable relapse of every demytholog-
ization into yet another demonology. The "blank" purity of a
world from which idols have been eliminated not only "assumes
the numinous character" of a reality still governed by fear
and trembling (DA 45; DE 28), but moreover represses the
mimetic impulse without which happiness as such remains un-
thinkable. Thus the inevitable inscription of the very law forbidding representation within the logic of self-preservation (cf.
Exodus 33:20). In this sense absence itself can become a defense or fetish. "The destruction of illusion does not produce
truth but only one more piece of ignorance, an extension of our
'empty space,' an increase of our desert" (Nietzsche).[12]

Every move from here can be predicted. Every abstract or
undialectical *Bilderverbot* assumes and stimulates prudish fantasies
of purity that serve to reinforce the mystification under contest-
ation while providing the familiar comforts of self-mortification.
The mistakes of others in this regard are, as usual, instructive
for Adorno. From Kierkegaard to, yes, finally, Schönberg, a slavish adherence to the law satisfies a priggish need for punish-
ment while releasing a stream of phantasmagorical productions.
Thus Adorno's infamous diagnoses. Kierkegaard's longing for
"imageless presence" expresses the (class-based) asceticism that
would—in its eagerness to repudiate every finite semblance ob-
structing the "infinite good of happiness"—only reinscribe the
latter within a sacrificial calculus of "goods" or acquisitions, and
would in this way mistake the "emptiness of the concept" for the
desired gratification (K 190ff/134 ff.). Thorstein Veblen's desire
for a clean slate is found to be a variation on this. The "splen-
didly misanthropic" invective against the regime of kitsch or
spectacle (P 77/79)—history's transformation into a "world's
fair"—presupposes as the price of its insight a Platonizing
blindness with respect to the world of "deceptive appearances,"
which can only reproduce the puritanical fantasy of a fresh start
regulated by the bourgeois "idol" of production (P 83/83).
Ditto (mutatis mutandis) the curmudgeonly abjection—resentful,

crypto-Christian—of an Aldous Huxley. "His anger at false happiness sacrifices the idea of true happiness as well" (P 105/103). Not even Adorno's Schönberg in the end will be exempted. Schönberg's "entanglement in the aporia of false transition" (P 170/164) will symptomatically betray itself, in *Moses and Aaron*, in a neo-Strindbergian, neo-Wagnerian, ultimately even neoclassicist monumentalism, which will eventually elide the caesura between myth and monotheism and thus undermine the opera's own iconoclastic momentum: "Moses and the Dance around the Golden Calf speak a single language" (QF 241).

And so on. It is not my interest here either to reprimand Adorno for his unkindness or to rehearse the familiar litany of counteraccusations regarding Adorno's own malingerings in the "grand hotel abyss" of abstract negation. If there is something painfully self-revealing about Adorno's portrait of the raging penitent rubbing himself raw against the prison bars of self-denial—the description of Huxley's lavishly elaborated "vicious circles" (P 115/111) evokes both the terms and the pathos of Nietzsche's *Genealogy*—the point is less to procure from Adorno a corresponding autocritique (such confessions are not hard to extract and tend in any case to neutralize themselves) than to consider the specific demand here placed on thought. Adorno himself formulates the dilemma with precision: "How is potentiality to be conceived if it is not to be abstract and arbitrary, like the utopias dialectical philosophers proscribed? Conversely, how can the next step assume direction and aim without the subject knowing more than what is already given? If one chose to reformulate Kant's question, one could ask today: *how is anything new possible at all?*" (P 95/93).

It is precisely on this point that relations between Adorno and Benjamin will eventually become a little tense. Adorno will finally force the question on Benjamin. Will Benjamin's version of Messianism evade the dilemma here presented as being quite irresistible? Will the dialectical image ultimately escape the antithesis between abstract negativity and the idolatry of the given? The question will also in the end be Horkheimer's. Does Benjamin's "atheological theology" overcome the antinomy between positivism and otherworldliness? Is every image of the past condemned to confirm the present precisely by insisting on the possibility of redemption?

Both Adorno and Horkheimer will finally charge Benjamin with utopianism. Horkheimer convicts Benjamin of "idealism": to form a dialectical image of the past is to occlude its "closure"—"the slain are really slain"—and thus to smuggle in some kind of eschatological horizon of consolation (II.3.1332 ff.). Adorno charges positivism: to form any image of the future is inevitably to reify the present and thus to garnish the status quo with its ultimate apologia. Each will therefore come to diagnose Benjamin's problem as that of "insufficient dialectics." Too much theology on the one hand, not enough on the other—the symmetrical accusations typify what will indeed soon enough become the standard chorus of reproaches. "Janus-faced," "two tracked,"[13] Benjamin's project will be found to fall "between two stools"[14]—a graft as awkward as the stitching of a "monk's cowl" onto the withered body of historical materialism.[15]

III Illusion of a Future

A prophet facing backwards
—Friedrich Schlegel, *Athenaeum*

An early text of Benjamin presents the problem "figuratively [*in einem Bilde*]" (II.1.203; R 312). If the disjunction between theology and materialism implies simultaneously a reciprocity, this means, at once, both a foreclosure of every progressivist, secular eschatology and a vindication of its deepest claims. "Nothing historical can relate itself on its own to anything Messianic." Such a notion relates not only to the apocalyptic mystical strand of Judaism (as glossed by Scholem) but equally (this is typically overlooked by Benjamin's readers) to a certain rationalist tradition running from the Babylonian Talmud through Maimonides and beyond.[16] This means that a cataclysmic rupture divides the profane order of history (*olam hazeh*) from the kingdom of God (*olam haba*).

"From the standpoint of history," the Kingdom of God— redemption—"is not the goal [*Ziel*], but the end [*Ende*]" (II.1.203; R 312). Every teleological determination of history reduces to a narrowly instrumentalist or reformist series of improvements and adjustments—the opposition between a Lenin and a Bernstein in this sense immediately collapses—only sanctioning the hegemony of the present day.

Thus the familiar catalog of renunciations: the historian as the prophet facing backward (Friedrich Schlegel), the modern Orpheus who now stands to relose his Eurydice by looking ahead (Jean Paul). "Accursed is the rider who is chained to his nag because he has set himself a goal for the future" (Kafka's bucket rider) (II.2.436; ILL 138). The angel of history catches not even a glimpse of the future to which his back is turned (I.2.697 ff.; ILL 257). The "destructive character" who "clears away" without a constructive "vision" of the future leaves "for a moment, at least, empty space [*leere Raum*] in which 'ways' or 'crossroads' might open up" (IV.1.397 ff.; R 301 ff.). No image, similarly, inspires the revolutionary: neither "the ideal of liberated grandchildren" nor the utopia "painted in the heads" of the Social Democrats (I.2.700; ILL 260). The long view of historicist prognostication must thus contract to the lightning flash of historical materialist intervention.

Benjamin explicitly links such a renunciation to the iconoclastic imperative of Judaism: "We know that the Jews were prohibited from investigating the future" (I.2.704; ILL 264). The messianic moment—"Messianic power" in the "weak" sense (I.2.694; ILL 254)—remains as inscrutable as ultraviolet rays. "Whoever wants to know how a 'redeemed humanity' would be constituted, under what conditions it would be constituted, and when one can count on it, poses questions to which there is no answer. He might as well ask about the color of ultraviolet rays" (I.3.1232).

Rebecca Comay

Kant avec Marx

The image (yes) presented by Benjamin's first thesis on history indicates the complexity of the issue. Whatever the nature of the entanglement between "theological" dwarf and "historical materialist" puppet—collusion, codependence, unsublatable contradiction—the figure itself invokes the very spectre of idolatry, if only in order to demystify it. The automaton is in any case considerably less automatic than the animated images of Daedalus. To celebrate the unfettered progress of the "apparatus"— Social Democracy from one side, Stalinism from the other—is in itself to fall prey to the transcendental illusion that would hypostatize the absolute as already there.

Kant and Marx awkwardly join forces. The error of utopian socialism would be precisely to blur the critical border between the "realm of necessity" and the "realm of freedom"—the vocabularies of Kant and Marx curiously coincide here—thereby contaminating the very ideal of communism with the empirical categories of the present day. Every effort to write "recipes for the cookshops of the future" is guilty of this.[17] Hegel saw this clearly in the preface to the *Philosophy of Right* when he rejected the popular demand to "give instruction [*Belehren*]"—to construct the world "as it ought to be"—as presupposing an undialectical collapse of the critical gap between *Sein* and *Sollen*, constative and performative, thus introducing the spectre of unmediated abstraction.[18]

For Marx such a collapse marked the secret complicity between ideology and utopia. The "chimerical game" of painting "fancy pictures of the future structure of society"[19] could only whitewash the existent precisely by "leaving out the shadows."[20] For Kant such a collapse would introduce the logical contradiction of a theoretical noumenology. To the "magic lantern of phantoms" projected by natural theology[21] corresponds the commandeering gaze, which would "behold" or "prove"[22] what should remain properly conjectural: accomplished insight (*Einsichtsfähigkeit*) would usurp the place of the "weak glimpse [*schwache Blick*]" of reason.[23] The reduction of the law to the conditions of phenomenality would reduce action to the "lifeless" gesticulations of a "puppet" governed by fear and trembling: hypertrophic enlightenment would in this way come to signify nothing but the tutelage of a mortified nature.

In either case the result is fetishism: to depict redemption as a logical extension or continuation of the present is effectively to confuse possibility with actuality and thus only to confirm one's own immersion in the imaginary. Every "ideal of liberated grandchildren" cannot fail, in this sense, to function ideologically.[24] The very faith in a better future secretly prolongs and sanctifies the given, offering placating pictures that would only distract the viewer from the most urgent imperatives of the day. Thus idolatry: the substitution of the finite for the infinite, the existent for the ideal. To honor the false god of progress is precisely to fall victim to the "system of mirrors" creating the optical illusion of "transparency," Enlightenment, or clear sight. If theology today "has to keep out of sight" (dwarfish, "small and ugly") (I.2.693; ILL 253), this is ultimately because its promise contains the still unredeemed possibility of a happiness unrepresentable within the perspective of the present day.

Everything Benjamin writes, from the earliest reflections on the youth movement through to the final "Theses on the Philosophy of History"—thus the entire uneasy trajectory from hyperidealism to Messianism—will reiterate this basic point.

The Kantian commitments of the early writings establish the essential problematic. If the task of "youth" is to keep open the critical "abyss [*Kluft*]" (II.1.31) between the absolute and the apparent, any premature sighting of the Idea is tantamount to the "deadly sin" (II.1.32) of naturalizing *Geist* by hypostatizing its incarnation as already or even foreseeably accomplished. This would be the theological hubris of the "great seer [*der große Schauender*]" (II.1.32). Benjamin will target under an identical censure the otherwise contradictory conciliations proposed variously by German classicism, by the *Wandervogel*, and by the instrumentalism haunting Weimar, from the academic *Berufsgeist* to the progressivist optimism of *Der Anfang*, each of which will in turn be convicted of a veritable "idolatry of *Geist*" (III.1.320) in its sterile affirmation of the existent. Nietzsche had already identified the modern military state as the newest idol: a "horse of death" masquerading in the name of life itself, and thereby "clattering in the finery of divine honors."[25] Thus, for the young Benjamin (already traumatized from the outset), the degradation of the Idea into the "spirit of 1914" and the harnessing of the youth movement to the patriotic ratification of the status quo.

A certain optical conceit would indeed seem from beginning to end to mark the ideology of "life" as that which prolongs by dissimulating the mortified condition of a fallen nature. Every gaze into the "blue distance" (II.2.620)—from the Romantic *Fernsicht* to the *schauendes Bewußtsein* of a Jung or a Klages— would placate the viewer with the consolation of unattainable ideals all the more enticing for being "eternal" and thus present in their very absence.

Will not such an illusionistic distance be precisely the "urbanistic ideal" (V.56; CB 173) of the Second Empire?[26] Haussmann's boulevards would entice the spectator with the long perspectival vistas promising an infinitely deferred gratification (while at the same time effectively forestalling insurrection by preventing the building of barricades). The Eiffel Tower would offer a secure vantage point from which the spectator could admire his progress, reiterating the general point underlying the architecture of all the nineteenth-century world expositions ("modern festivals" [V.267] enabling the workers to gape at the very machinery that is rendering them superfluous), thereby confirming the Saint-Simonian "fairy-tale that *progrès* is the prospect of the very near future" (V.716). The glass architecture of the arcades would foster the illusion of the outside on the inside, promising a visual exteriority while in fact reinforcing the immanence of the exterior (meanwhile new technologies of artificial lighting would be turning the street itself into a domestic *intérieur*),[27] and in this way would mollify the demand for transcendence by providing the gratification of a good view. The crowds making their daily "pilgrimage" (V.86) to these "enchanted grottoes" (V.1045) of consumerism would enjoy the spectacle of goods whose very appearance of availability only underscores the scopophilic regime of private property—"look, don't touch" (V.267)—while the peepshow panoramas provide the visual sensation of a progressive movement securely contained and oriented within the private confines of a box.

It is no coincidence that the cruciform structure of the arcades will be observed by Benjamin to resemble church architecture (V.105). If the arcades are seen to preserve perspectival space with the same tenacity as cathedrals (V.1049), this is ultimately because the phantasmagoria of progress here will involve nothing less than a generalized fantasy of resurrection. Dead things promise to come alive within these enchanted "temples" (V.86). Vision would seek to confirm itself through the specular return of a gaze emanating from a universe packaged as merchandise, whose inviting glances exemplify the "theological caprices" of which Marx speaks. Thus Benjamin's rearticulation of the classic chapter on commodity fetishism: "things" acquire speech, glance, personality—the anthropomorphic features stripped from a by now thoroughly reified humanity—in a chiastic transfer whereby the transfer of "life" as such passes essentially by way of the eyes. Hence the multiplication of optical devices designed to prop up the subject's faltering sense of sight. "The opticians' shops were besieged" (V.830 ff.). The phantasmagoric gaze of the object becomes one more prosthetic extension designed to confirm the eidetic powers of the subject,[28] whose own ocular anxieties meanwhile betray themselves in obsessive fantasies of an uncanny nonreciprocity and nonsimultaneity, as in Baudelaire's images of jewel-eyed statues, blank-eyed prostitutes, eyes gleaming as vacantly as mirrors (V.1049) or as shop windows—"tes yeux illuminés ainsi que des boutiques" (I.2.649; CB 150). "Jugendstil sees in every woman not Helena but Olympia" (V.694).

Vision falsely promises here to fulfill the ego's fantasy of an immanence that would elide the temporal gap or nonidentity at work in all experience. This is the ideological aspect of the idealist "apotheosis of existence" (I.1.337; OGT 160), exemplified by Weimar classicism and theorized as the reconciliation of finite and infinite in the visual plasticity of the symbol, interpreted, as always, Hegelian-wise, as the "sensuous embodiment of the idea" (I.1.341; OGT 164). If such an incarnation of the noumenal involves a spiritual animation of nature and specifically the latter's self-representation, delimitation, and perfection in the human—henceforth securely installed (*eingestellt*) along the sacral course of *Heilsgeschichte* (I.1.337; OGT 160)—such a logic of substitution (*Stellvertretung*) (I.1.341; OGT 165) involves a fundamental distortion (*Entstellung*) (I.1.337; OGT 160) underwritten by a politics of "domination" and "usurpation" (I.1.336; OGT 159) whereby not only allegorical distance is occluded but with it the radical transience and suffering of a finite nature (I.1.343; OGT 166).

Such an occlusion would severely restrict the potential space of every action. In its "seamless transition" from phenomenal to noumenal (the "limitless immanence of the ethical world in the world of beauty"), the humanist apotheosis of the perfected individual would constrict the "radius of action" to a mere "radius of culture [*Bildungsradius*]" (I.1.337; OGT 160), would misconstrue particularity (*das Einzelne*) (I.1.343; OGT 166) as abstract inwardness or individuality (*Individuum*) (I.1.337; OGT 160)—would, in short, condemn the ethical subject to the "unmanly" posturings of the beautiful soul. The beautiful images or "constructions [*Gebilde*]" of the symbolic would efface the (Kantian) "abyss [*Abgrund*]" dividing "visual being [*bildliche Sein*] from meaning" (I.1.342; OGT 165)—phenomenon from noumenon—and would thereby erase the "jagged line of demarcation" that etches the traits of nature's untransfigured countenance as "untimely, sorrowful, unsuccessful" (I.1.343; OGT 166): the line of death.

In such a consoling vision of a transfigured nature, the "enigmatic question [*Rätselfrage*]" is suppressed regarding human "nature" both generally and in its historic specificity as tied inexorably to a fallen nature (I.1.343; OGT 166). Such occlusion will ultimately define the barbarism underwriting every "document of civilization" (I.2.696; ILL 256)—the secret link between humanism and militarism, "the unity between Weimar and Sedan" (III.1.258).

The seven-headed hydra of the *Geisteswissenschaften* ("creativity, empathy, timelessness, re-creation, *Miterleben*," etc.), with its vitalist identifications and its "lecherous urge for the big picture" (III.1.286)—historicism's "bordello" (I.2.702; ILL 262)—would institutionalize itself in the sacred groves of "timeless poets" (III.1.289) and "eternal values" (III.1.286), in a fanatic "exorcism of history" (III.1.289) that would entrench the hegemony of "Western man" under the cover of a universality posited as already there. It is in this sense that classicism is said to culminate in the "Germanic soteriology" (III.1.254) whose "'Rettung'" (III.1.257) (Benjamin's scarequotes) of the dead as *Vorbilder* (III.1.255)—objects of empathic identification—adds up to the *sauve qui peut* of a triumphant nationalism that would occlude the persistence of inherited power relations through an appeal to the presumed continuities of race or caste.

It is no coincidence here that such a soteriology is said to be orchestrated by "seers whose visions appear over dead bodies" (III.259). This is the empathic gaze that would find spiritual return in a past reanimated as ancestral prototype or precursor—so too Benjamin's eventual definition of aura as the inanimate object's ability to return the gaze[29]—an idealizing revival of the dead which inevitably accrues to the profit of the survivors in their triumphal march through the continuum of time.

IV Bilderflucht: Critical Resuscitations

Re(sus)citations

Which is not to exclude the possibility of another gaze, another resurrection. In the face of the "blooming, blazing vision [*blumenhaft flammende Blick*]" of neoclassicist revival, Benjamin opposes the (yes, still fertile) gaze of a *theoria* that would again summon back the dead—this time not for adulation but for interrogation.

We must stand ... by the inconspicuous [*unansehnlichen*] truth, the laconism of the seed, of fruitfulness, and thus of theory, which leaves behind the spell of vision [*Schau*]. If there are timeless images, there are certainly no timeless theories. Not tradition, but only originality [*Ursprünglichkeit*], can decide this. The genuine image may be old, but the genuine thought is new. It is of today. This today may be derelict, granted. But be that as it may, one must seize it firmly by the horns, if one is to be able to pose questions of the past. It is the bull whose blood must fill the pit, if the spirits of the departed are to appear [*erscheinen*] at its edge. (III.1.259)

What exactly is the distinction here between "vision" and "theory"? A temporal one, to begin with. Whatever the apparent continuities between flower and seed, between "image" and "appearance," there is (to be) a fundamental opposition between mythic violence, which would efface time by occluding the position of the present (thereby surreptitiously securing it), and the sacrifice that would vindicate the present precisely by exposing the latter's vulnerability and responsibility to—its "secret rendez-vous" with (I.2.694; ILL 254)—the past.[30]

On this distinction rests the difference between "tradition" and "originality." The former, we might gloss, aims at re-sur-rection: the spiritual transfiguration, exaltation, and uplifting of the dead as "cultural treasures" (I.2.696; ILL 256) within the homogeneous continuum of mythic time. The latter aims at re-sus-citation: the solicitation or summoning of the dead as *Abhub* or unsublatable remainder within the fractured discontinuum of a history brought to a caesura or Messianic standstill. The measure of "originality" is thus not the abstractness of a new beginning staked out within the linearity of tradition as a historicist "stream of becoming" (I.1.226; OGT 45). It will express itself rather according to the diphasic "rhythm" of a finite repetition whereby the past is restored or cited as radically "imperfect" and "incomplete" (cf. I.1.226; OGT 45).

"Vision" thus sees a face: the specular return-to-self of the viewing subject as it narcissistically constructs itself through the consoling tête-à-tête with the beautified or transfigured other. "Theory" sees a mask: the stain of the death's head whose vacant stare marks the radical alterity or noncoincidence of viewer and viewed, look and gaze (the Lacanian framework would seem productive here),[31] and as such the annihilation or traumatic wounding of the self-conscious subject hostage to the claim of an immemorial past. Such noncoincidence marks the scene of history as *facies hippocratica*, nonrecuperable alterity, the one-way street of irredeemable transience and suffering.[32] "It is as something incomplete and imperfect that objects stare out [*starren*] from the allegorical structure" (I.1.362; OGT 186).

Symbolic resurrection—"vision"—thus recalls the dead as object of consumption: the mourned object devoured or introjected as host or food for thought. Allegorical resuscitation—"theory"—recalls the dead as indigestible remainder and untimely reminder, the persistent demand of unsublimated matter. Thus the appearance of the returning spirits as vampires feeding at the present's trough.

Resurrection, as we read in the essay on Leskov, is in this sense to be conceived less as an idealizing transfiguration than as a radical disenchantment (*Entzauberung*): humanity's liberation from the "nightmare" of mythic immanence (II.2.458; ILL 102 ff.). Such a demystification does not and cannot assume a (mythic) opposition between myth and enlightenment. The operative distinction would seem to work rather within the interstices of myth itself, at the point where myth overturns itself and points toward its own exterior. These are the little "tricks" folded into the apparently seamless fabric of mythic identity— the "liberating magic" of the fairy tale's reassuring happy ending—Kafka's "proof that inadequate, even childish measures may serve to rescue one" (II.2.415; ILL 117).

Theaters of Redemption

The only break from the spell of the imaginary is thus by way of a thoroughgoing immersion. If, as Adorno has insisted, every abstract foreclosure of images elicits a hallucinatory return (as symptom or delirium), it is perhaps conversely the case (this is now what we must consider) that a certain intensification of images may open a breach or rupture within the seamless continuum of mythic *immanence*, and thus indeed point precisely to the *imminence* of what is radically unforeseen. To wit: the apparent violation of the *Bilderverbot* may indeed attest to its most productive power.

Iconophilia itself (or its appearance) may indeed thus come to assume iconoclastic proportions. Writing of the baroque extravaganza—the *folie du voir*[33] of a culture outdoing "even the Egyptians" (I.1.350; OGT 174) in effects of spectacularity—Benjamin perceives in the "eruption of images" of the stage-world a style nothing short of "sublime" (I.1.349; OGT 173). The allegorical detachment of appearance from signification—the "abyss separating visual being from meaning" (I.1.342; OGT 165)—intensifies ocular possibilities so as to heighten the eschatological tension between immanence and transcendence, thereby "securing for the latter the greatest conceivable rigor, exclusivity, and relentlessness" (I.1.359; OGT 183). It is the very profusion of images that will here block any fantasy of premature reconciliation.

If it is part of the very logic of modernity to convert every prohibition of images into yet another image of prohibition—thus the dazzle of negative signposts cluttering the urban landscape of *One-Way Street* ("Post no bills!" "Caution: Steps!" "No Vagrants!" "Protect these Plantings!")—it will take "heroic" (cf. I.2.577; CB 74) measures to negotiate the aporia of such a specularity without term.

One-Way Street presents the by now familiar aporia vividly. If the "imperial panorama" of progress masks the claustrophobia of the interior—"mirages of a glorious cultural future" projected against "folds of dark drapery"—not even the most sublime landmarks would remain intact: mountain tops would be shrouded while "a heavy curtain shuts off Germany's sky" (IV.1.98 ff.; OWS 58). It would be clearly no escape here to appeal to the presumed innocence or neutrality of a "critical standpoint," "prospect," or "perspective" (IV.1.132; OWS 89). Such a perspective would only smuggle in the optical illusion of the panorama, would intensify the phantasmagoria in the very effort to see through it, would therefore reinforce immanence precisely in the claim to externality or transcendence. This is the nightmare of total theater—Proust's aquarium,[34] indeed Aragon's[35]—the no-exit or "dead end" (as *One-Way Street* was originally baptized) of our spectacular modernity: "It is as though one were trapped in a theater and had to follow the events on stage whether one wanted to or not, had to make them again and again, willingly or unwillingly, the subject of one's thought and speech" (IV.1.98; OWS 57). The "way out" here can be figured, indeed properly staged, only as a dramatic pause within the phantasmagoria of total vision. If every premature attempt to quit the circle secretly prolongs what it would abandon (cf. IV.1.85 ff.; OWS 46), any rupture will require a certain collaboration with mythic forces and will thus assume an infinitely ambiguous guise. "Costume Wardrobe" presents the scene of redemption as nothing more and nothing less than a theatrical occurrence:

Again and again, in Shakespeare, in Calderón, battles fill the act, and kings, princes, attendants and followers "enter, fleeing." The moment [*Augenblick*] in which they become visible to spectators brings them to a standstill. The flight of the *dramatis personae* is arrested by the stage. Their entry into the visual field [*Blickraum*] of non-participating and truly impartial persons allows the harassed [*Preisgegeben*] to draw breath, bathes them in new air. The appearance on stage of those who enter "fleeing" takes from this its hidden meaning. Our reading of this formula is imbued with expectation of a place, a light, a footlight glare [*Rampenlicht*], in which our own flight through life may be likewise sheltered in the presence of onlooking strangers. (IV.1.143; OWS 100)

Redemption—here, as always, breath—is here figured within the *Blickraum* or *Bildraum* of consummated visibility. The decentering of the gaze (the transformation of spectator to potential spectacle) is here presented as a reversal without empathic reciprocity or symmetry. A Brechtian distance characterizes the position of both viewing subject and object viewed.

This is the "cunning" (V.1213)—"teleological"—whereby the dream, intensifying itself, pushes forward toward its own awakening.

There will, then, "still be a sphere of images [*Bildraum*], and, more concretely"—for this very reason—"of bodies [*Leibraum*]"

(II.1.309; R 192). If the modern epoch (despite or because of its hypertrophic specularity) represents the ultimate laming or maiming of the imagination (I.2.611; ILL 159), it is the image alone that will come to redeem a body and a body politic fractured irreparably by the force of time.

This is not the project of aesthetic *Bildung*. If to "organize pessimism" means necessarily to "work at important locations in [the] sphere of images" (II.1.309; R 191)—"wherever these may dwell" (III.1.196)—this is precisely so as to protect the desire for revolution from degenerating into the cheeriness of a "bad poem on springtime" (II.1.308; R 190). The expulsion of "moral metaphor from politics" (II.1.309; R 191)—the elimination of the social-democratic *gradus ad parnassum* (II.1.308; R 190)— requires precisely the "opening" or elaboration of a competing image sphere through which alone the body reconfigures itself in time. In this version of a materialist last judgment, the suffering body submits to a "dialectical justice" (Benjamin's rewriting of the Hegelian Bacchanalian revel) according to which "no member remains unrent [*unzerissen*]" (II.1.309; R 192). The reconstitution of a new *physis* (II.1.310; R 192) or "new body" (IV.1.148; OWS 104) for the corporeal collective (*leibliche Kollektivum*) (II.3.1041) involves the shattering of every harmony and specifically of every fantasy of aesthetic immanence. If Benjamin here announces the onset of a veritable "slave revolt of technology" (III.1.238), this is not to be confused with the ascetic consolation that would (as in futurism) vitalistically sublate the mortified conditions of a damaged life. This is not the resurrection of a body or a body politic spiritualized within the eternal community of mankind. If it is a fissured, epileptic (IV.1.148; OWS 104) body that is to enter the final court of judgment, this is precisely so as to repel every mythic solidarity suggested by the "idol" of a "harmoniously and perfectly formed humanity"— the "phantom of the unpolitical or 'natural' man" (II.1.364; R 270). "The subject of history: not mankind [*die Menschheit*] but the oppressed" (I.3.1244).

It could indeed be argued that Benjamin's familiar series of salvage operations (romanticism, surrealism, Proust, Baudelaire,

Brecht, Kafka, film, photography, and so on) will be directed precisely toward that kernel in the imaginary that defies idealization and thus negotiates an opening to the unforeseen. The biblical *Bilderverbot* is thus refunctioned as a *Bilderflucht* (V.410): a flight from the mythical image to the dialectical image divested of all consoling force. Benjamin's "dialectical optic" will pit image against image.

Whatever else may be at work in brushing cultural history against the grain of historicist (self)-misunderstanding—Goethe against Friedrich Gundolf, romanticism against *Sturm und Drang*, Kafka against Max Brod, cinema against Leni Riefenstahl, Mickey Mouse against Disney, surrealism against the musty "spiritualism" that would collapse the visionary impulse into the occultism of "tapping on windowpanes" (II.1.298; R 180) or the presumptuousness of "advance celebrations [*Vorfeier*]" (II.1.307; R 189)—whatever the force and legitimacy of Benjamin's specific rewritings, it will in each case be a question of a reinscription rather than a repression of ocular possibilities, and as such the vindication of an imaginary burdened by the essential "ambiguity" that announces the very "law" of the refurbished dialectic (V.55; CB 171).

If it is within the world theater that Kafka's "hope for the hopeless" is to be realized (II.2.415; ILL 100)—fake sky, paper wings: Adorno will indeed come to suspect this (II.3.1177 ff.)—this is precisely because the only "way out" (as in the *Report to an Academy*) is by recapturing the last vestige of a repressed mimetic impulse (II.2.423; ILL 125). "The mimetic and the critical faculties can no longer be distinguished" (II.3.1050). If Proust's frenetic search for images will involve the "vice" ("one is tempted to say, theological") of obsequious curiosity—the convergence of "*voir*" and "*désirer imiter*" (II.1.318; ILL 209) will extend to Proust's eventual stage management of his own illness (II.1.322; ILL 213)—this will indeed imply the entanglement of every image of redemption within the "enchanted forest [*Bannwald*]" (II.1.313; ILL 204) of mythic guilt.

All of which will lead soon enough to the predictable charges: bewitchment, cooptation, identification with the aggressor.

Rebecca Comay

V Bilderstreit: Adorno contra Benjamin

Mosaics

It is with the abortive *Passagenwerk*—"the theater of all my conflicts and all my ideas" (Br 506; C 359)—that the issues first come to a head. Benjamin will be observed playing sorcerer's apprentice, mesmerized by what he would subvert. Specifically: if it is the ocular regime of modernity that presents the face of history as sheer monstrosity—not only an "oversized head" (V.1011) but indeed (as Marx also observed)[36] a "Medusa head" (I.2.682)—Benjamin will be found petrified by what he sees.

By 1935 Adorno will indeed accuse him of capitulating to the force of capital and indeed to the logic of capitalization. Panoramatic representations of the panorama, kaleidoscopic representations of the kaleidoscope—the montage technique is here found not only to mime that of surrealism but effectively to adopt what will be for Adorno the latter's irremediably conciliatory position. A cryptic affirmation, *Behauptung*, would be detected in the physiognomic determination of Paris as *Hauptstadt der neunzehnten Jahrhunderts*, head or capital of the nineteenth century (a title "privately" translated into French by Benjamin[37] and eventually discarded), which would be thus transfigured as nothing less than the proscribed figure of utopia. Paris, decapitated site of missed revolutionary opportunities,[38] would be reinstated to center stage so as indeed to provide the alluring scene or spectacle of redemption. *Caput mortuum* would be thus figured or transfigured as—precisely, face.

It is not simply that Benjamin will aggressively rely on images to tell a story (cf. V.596); or just that what begins as an "album" (V.1324) will soon collapse under its own weight into a "rubble field" (Br 556; C 396) of Bouvard-and-Pécuchet-esque proportions; or even that the specific images to be culled here—the familiar shopping list: arcades, ragpickers, balconies, and the rest—will for Adorno bear an irredeemably consumerist stamp.

Nor is it only (although this is not irrelevant) a question of the respective commitments of Adorno and Benjamin as cultural critics: high culture versus mass culture, music versus photography, aural versus visual, and all the rest. If Adorno's complaint will come eventually to crystallize in the notorious assault on film culture as mass hypnosis—passive, magical, consoling—it is perhaps less the specific example of the medium that is significant here than the actual logic underlying the attack. If Benjamin will be rebuked, following the artwork essay, for the "romantic anarchism" (I.3.1003) that would hypostatize the "actually existing consciousness of actually existing workers" (I.3.1005) and thereby preempt revolution precisely by prefiguring it—the charge essentially reproduces Lenin's reproach to Luxembourg—it is important to consider the specific assumptions here at work. Underpinning what will be an otherwise conventional jeremiad linking media culture to mass idolatry (from Baudelaire's 1859 Salon[39] to Jacques Ellul) is a confrontation over the nature of memory and the specific temporality of the historical imagination.

The very conception of the dialectical image is here at stake. Benjamin's "stereoscopic" (cf. V.571) glance into the untimely constellation of an unrealized past and a regressive present will be condemned as doubly affirmative insofar as it would symmetrically entrench both, according to Adorno, within a shared horizon of conciliation. In short: any image of a "redeemed humanity" glimpsed from within the phantasmagoric dream sleep of modernity could only transgress the *Bilderverbot* and thereby inevitably recycle ideology as utopia.

Benjamin's citation of Michelet ("*Avenir! Avenir!*") is here decisive: "*Chaque époque rêve la suivante*" (V.46; CB 159). Benjamin reads here the crucial ambiguity of every image—the "law of dialectic at a standstill" (V.55; CB 171)—the inextricability of regression and utopia visibly at work in every time. "In the dream in which every epoch sees in images the epoch which is to succeed it, the latter appears coupled with elements of prehistory—that is to say, of a classless society" (V.46; CB 159). Adorno reads in such a coupling the monstrous simultaneity of nostalgia and otherworldliness (Klages married to Fourier): a linear relationship to the future spun from the cocoon of collective consciousness, a hallucinatory wish fulfillment destined only to accommodate the present by posing "undialectically" as the truth (Br 672; C 495). In short: in succumbing to the "spell of bourgeois psychology" (Br 674; C 497) Benjamin will not only divert psychoanalysis along Jungian lines but indeed disregard Freud's emphatic denial of all prophetic significance to the work of dream.[40] "Every epoch not only dreams the next" but in so doing presses "dialectically" (V.59; CB 176) and with "cunning" (V.1213) toward its own awakening: this is Benjamin's Proustian refunctioning of Hegel's *List der Vernunft*, the "Trojan horse" (V.495) installed within the dream sleep of nineteenth-century mass culture. Adorno, perhaps the better Freudian here, would see the essential purpose of the dream to prolong our dogmatic slumbers, and thus reads Benjamin as apologist of continuity or consummated "immanence" (Br 672 ff.; C 495 ff.). The dialectical image would in this way forfeit its "objective liberating power" and so resign itself to the sterile reproduction of *das Nächste*.

Adorno will be neither the first nor the last to accuse Benjamin of idolatry. By 1938, the montage effect will represent the ultimate disintegration of the Mosaic imperative into the concatenations of sheer mosaic—a "superstitious enumeration of materials" (Br 787; C 583) which in its "ascetic" abstention from conceptual elaboration would "demonically" (Br 783; C 580) restrict itself to a pious "incantation [*Beschwörung*]" of the bare facts (Br 786; C 582).

The status of "theory" as such is on the line. From the beginning it will have been a question of refunctioning the "tender empiricism" of a Goethe (I.1.60). "Everything factual is already theory" (Br 443; C 313).[41] This will come to apply, *mutatis mutandis*, to the neo-Platonic saving of the phenomena proposed in the preface to the *Trauerspielbuch* ("The value of fragments of thought is all the more decisive the less immediate their relationship is to the underlying idea" [I.1.208; OGT 29]); to the artless art of the vanished storyteller ("it is half the art of storytelling to keep a story free from explanation" [II.1.445; ILL 89]); and to the "technique" presented by the *Passagenwerk* ("Method of this work: literary montage. I need say nothing. Only show" [V.574]). Whatever the shift—Benjamin describes it as nothing short of "total revolution [*vollkommenen Umwälzung*]" (Br 659; C 486)—between the earlier "metaphysical" (ibid.) problematic and the cultural materialist agenda of the late work, the micrological commitment to the object would persistently forswear both the claims of a panoptic theory and thus any stable or consistent totalization of what appears. If the "saving of the phenomena" coincides here (as always) with the "presentation of ideas" (I.1.215; OGT 35) this is precisely because the phenomena are to be divested of any self-subsistent or "integral" unity or intactness, and submitted to the fracturing, dispersive and reintegrative, but also constantly self-revising, combinatorial of thought (I.1.213; OGT 33). This marks the fundamental continuity, whatever Adorno suspected, between the philosophical mosaic of the *Trauerspielbuch* and the much-maligned (by Adorno) "surrealist method."

Nothing less than life itself turns out to be at stake here. The issue ultimately concerns the very possibility of resuscitation. A "hopeless fidelity to things" (I.333; OGT 156) will require nothing less than a descent to the "ashes," a turn to the most recalcitrant or "heavy" remnant of unsublimated matter (I.334; OGT 157). If Benjamin's version of "theory in the strictest sense" (Br 586; C 586) risks the appearance of a certain empiricism, this is precisely out of a theological ambition to "let what is 'creaturely' speak for itself" (Br 442; C 313): that is, to restore precisely by abstaining from ventriloquizing or anthropomorphically representing the voice of a fallen nature and thus indeed of a history-now-mortified-as-second-nature.[42] This is the critical alchemy (I.1.126) or "philosopher's stone" promised by the "constructive" method (Br 687; L 507)—hope for the hopeless (cf. I.1.201)—the allegorical gaze directed toward that which in its very transience and ruination figures precisely as the cipher of resurrection (cf. I.1.405 ff.; OGT 232). *Tu m'as donné ta boue et j'en fait de l'or.* "In the monad," writes Benjamin, "everything that was mythically paralyzed [*in mythischer Starre lag*] as textual evidence comes alive" (Br 794; C 588).

Benjamin's rewriting of Goethe is crucial.[43] If Benjamin will insist for his presentation on a sense of "heightened visuality [*gesteigerte Anschaulichkeit*]" (V.574) exceeding both the "shabbiness" of Marxist historiography and the "cheapness" of the bourgeois kind (V.1217), the ultimate model for such a pictorial method is said to be provided by Goethe's morphological studies (V.1033). As with the *Urpflanze,* the revelation of the general in the detail involves a certain "unfolding"—"like a leaf," writes Benjamin (V.577)—in this case, of the specific temporal constellation (never stable) within which every "small individual moment" (V.574) is to be inscribed.

But what is announced here as a "transposition" or "translation" [*Übertragung*] of the morphological principle of observation from the "pagan context of nature into the Jewish contexts"—plural—"of history" (V.577) would seem to obey a familiar enough Benjaminian logic of translation according to which the original (and indeed the original concept of the originary) will by no means remain intact. Whatever else is at work in Benjamin's "transfer" of attention from an organic nature to a nature-history stripped of all immanent fulfillment, it becomes clear that the concepts of both nature and history will have been radically transformed.

Goethe's "genial synthesis"[44] of essence and appearance would not only involve the "ideal symbol" (VI.38)—timeless, total, instantaneous—but would indeed privilege the domain of biological "life" as the specific object of "irreducible perception" (VI.38). Benjamin's montage principle will not only introduce allegorical distance or nonsimultaneity into the "wooded interior" (I.1.342; OGT 165) of the monad but will, moreover, force a fundamental revision of the very concept of "life" itself.

If the micrological embrace of lumpen particularity involves as its "truly problematic" assumption the desire to "give nothing up" (V.578), to consider nothing irredeemably lost or beneath consideration, this is precisely out of a conviction, nothing less than theological, regarding the "indestructibility of the highest life in all things" (V.573). Such an appeal to life will preempt any fixed antithesis between living and dead, positive and negative, forward and backward, or, for that matter, between destruction and construction ("and so on *in infinitum*") (V.573), just as it will preclude any organicist—"vulgar naturalist" (V.575)—the-odicy whether along progressive-evolutionary or regressive Spenglerian lines ("the prophets of decline [*Verfall*]" [V.573]).

The familiar figures of cameraman and surgeon again converge here (as in the artwork essay)[45] to initiate the caesura or cut to be inflicted on the historical corpus as living corpse.[46] Whatever the nature of the historical materialist "operation"— freezing the image, choosing the angle, adjusting the lighting, clicking the shutter (I.3.1165)—it is only within the "darkroom of the lived moment" (II.3.1064) (equally the camera obscura of ideology)[47] that the full "development" of the image is to be achieved. This is in any case to be distinguished from the "bourgeois" gape [*Schauen*] enraptured by the spectacle of history as a display of "colorful images" (I.3.1165). A constant shift in perspective (*Verschiebung des Gesichtswinkels*) (V.573) eventually presents every negative as positive according to a theology of "historical *apokatastasis*"—the heretical source is Origen (cf. II.2.458; ILL 103)—until at the "high noon of history [*Mittag der Geschichte*]" (V.603) and out of the "dialectical nuances" (V.573) of the messianic optic—"light for shade, shade for light" (I.3.1165)—"life springs anew" (V.573). "As flowers turn their heads towards the sun, so by dint of a secret kind of heliotropism the past strives to turn towards that sun which is rising in the sky of history. The historical materialist must understand this most inconspicuous of all transformations" (I.2.695; ILL 255).

Adorno, notwithstanding, will suspect here an unsublimated naturalist residue, if not, in fact, something like the "neopaganism" parodied by Baudelaire. If the constructive method will be attacked as a version of philosophical empiricism (thus a betrayal or collapse of the precarious dialectic of concept and intuition, rationality and mimesis, universal and particular), this will ultimately bear the secret stain of a reason that would mask its own domination over the object it would claim to let speak. Underpinning the theoretical modesty that abstains from conceptual intervention would be the unacknowledged hubris of a rationality intent on mastering the very nature that it would redeem.

This is Odysseus, strapped to the mast, entranced by a siren song whose ultimate charm will amount to nothing more than the self-seduction of the controlling ego. Thus the "philosopher's stone" would cloak arrogance as humility. It will indeed be Benjamin's own project that will stand ultimately convicted of self-sanctification: "Gretel once joked that you lived in the cavelike depths of your *Arcades* and therefore shrank in horror from completing the work because you feared having to leave what you built. So let us encourage you to allow us into the holy of holies. I believe you have no reason to be concerned for the stability of the shrine, or any reason to fear that it will be profaned" (Br 788; C 583).

I want to love and perish that an image not remain a mere image.
—Nietzsche, *Thus Spoke Zarathustra*

It is perhaps unnecessary here to recite at length the familiar chorus of defenses: what is "dialectical" about the image is, for Benjamin, precisely what should preclude its complete assimilation into the homogeneous continuum of mythic time. The specific historicity of the image would exclude equally both nostalgia and prognostication and would as such undermine any evidential or pictorial relation to what might come. As already effectively past, or on the verge of disappearing (I.2.590; CB 87)—the model of monetary inflation is never distant (cf. II.2.620)—the image disturbs all contemplative reconstruction and so too every consoling blueprint of what might be. Jung and Fourier would here be symmetrically deflected.

As the memory of a lost future and the anticipation of a future absence—"sadness for what was and hopelessness towards what is to come" (I.2.586; CB 82)—the image in fact expresses the rigorously traumatic structure of all experience. The logic of latency would introduce a fundamental anachrony to the image such that any and every anticipation of redemption—the "classless society"—would appear as at once not only radically precipitate but indeed properly legible only posthumously, if not, indeed, too late. If the much-trumpeted *Auseinandersetzung*

(V.1160) with Jung, Klages, and company never properly as such transpires (indeed it is tempting to blame Adorno himself as much as anyone for this deferral), it becomes clear that any image of *Urgeschichte* could point only to an "origin" fractured by a retroactivity that would preempt all retrieval and thus equally every secure vision of a future or consummated end. If in the dialectical image the mutual illumination between past and present is typically characterized as both "flashlike" (V.576) and "explosive" (V.1032), this is because what is ruptured here is both the immanence of every epoch and the immanence of subjectivity, whether of an individual or of a phantom collectivity hypostatized in Jungian garb.

"The place where one encounters them is language" (V.577). If the "authentic image [*das echte Bild*]" is the "read image [*das gelesene Bild*]" (V.578 ff.)—the familiar Barthesian problematic opens up here[48]—this is precisely because the "point [*Punktum*]" of legibility involves the recognition of the now-time of reading or interpretation in its most "critical, dangerous" responsibility toward the past (V.578). Such punctuality would indeed shatter or "burst [*zerspringen*]" any timeless plenitude of truth just as it would rupture any contemplative relationship to what appears.

The temporal structure of the image converts seeing into reading, image into text. If what is in the end essential about the image is that it is "not seen before being remembered" (I.3.1064), every prophesy would ultimately become the guilty prophesy of a present that can only come too late (cf. V.598). "Hell is nothing that awaits us but this life here" (Strindberg) (V.592). This will in effect define the shape of Benjamin's iconoclasm. "To worship the image of divine justice in language ... that is the genuinely Jewish somersault" by which the mythic spell is to be broken (II.1.367; R 254).

Conjurations

Nor need we now rehearse the inevitable ripostes and rejoinders. If Adorno's somewhat hysterical rhetoric of exorcism follows a predictable enough logic of conjuration—demonology-counter-demonology—it will not take much to expose Adorno's own secret reliance on the phantasmagoria he would seek to "liquidate" (Br 784; C 580). Thus the frantic appeal to "mediation" as the magic wand that is to "break the spell" (Br 786; C 582) of a "satanic" (Br 783; C 579) positivity.

The charges are by now familiar: Adorno the "devil" (Lyotard), Adorno the "witch" (Agamben), Adorno the drunk, hooked on the "mysticism of the dialectical reversal" (Bürger).[49] Does not the invocation of the "total process [Gesamtprozeß]" (Br 785; C 582), to "development [Durchführung]" (Br 783; C 580), to "more dialectic"—more thoroughgoing, indeed perhaps more continuous dialectic, durchdialektisieren—does not this demand for mediation threaten precisely to reinstate a historicist continuity of the most orthodox Hegelian sort?[50] Does not the demand for theoretical elaboration threaten to reinvest the "contents of consciousness" with the occult properties which are specifically to be avoided? "Restoration of theology" (Adorno's request) (Br 676; C 498) as so much more German ideology?

More to the point: does not the very accusation of apologetics presuppose a linear temporality of the noch nicht? Would not the charge of premature reconciliation arrogate to itself the very standard of fulfillment that it would thereby withhold? Such that the very allegation of positivism could only indict itself in appealing to the proscribed standpoint of totality?

Things are complicated. It is indeed possible to argue here (as Benjamin almost does) that Adorno's own version of "theory"—whether as the esoteric redemption of the phenomena (Ideologiekritik) or as the bootstrapping of a philosophical Münchhausen—itself assumes the angelic standpoint (or "waxen wings" [Br 793; C 587]) of the detached observer. If there is, to be sure, a certain vanguardist conceit in Adorno's "carpings" (Br 683; C 503) (most clearly marked in his response to the artwork essay),[51] Adorno himself is the first to insist that the price of theoretical success would be not only practical failure but indeed a theoretical blind spot premised precisely on the repression of that original guilt.

If there is a willful stupidity here—Adorno stubbornly mistakes the dream-image for the dialectical image thereby inviting all the inevitable refutations and rejoinders—the misprision is revealing in that it points to a specific antinomy not yet properly addressed.

It may indeed be that Adorno's suspicions in the end (and despite everything) nonetheless retain a certain cogency. Perhaps both Benjamin and Adorno risk a certain fantasy of premature reconciliation. Perhaps such a fantasy is a necessary one. Suspended between the "desert" of the nineteenth century (V.366) and the "icy desert of abstraction" (NL 571/224), the struggle between Moses and Aaron would seem unbearably long. Does Benjamin's commitment to a fracturing of totality inevitably reinstate it at a higher level? If there is something resembling historicism in the indiscriminacy of the montage, this is precisely insofar as it would risk arrogating to itself the divine perspective—the "equal value" of Leopold von Ranke's *unmittelbar zu Gott,* Hermann Lotze's "miraculous vision"—from which alone redemption in the strict sense is to be thought.[52] Does *Rettung* here confuse itself with *Erlösung*? If the determination to give nothing up is, as Benjamin himself concedes, "truly problematic" (V.578), this is perhaps not automatically due to a simple empiricism or intuitionism but rather (which may however in the end not be so very different) to the secret hubris that would anticipate the perspective of a memory accessible exclusively to God (cf. IV.1.10; ILL 70). Is the heap or aggregate of images structured by the regulative ideal of the totality? If, "to be sure [*freilich*]"—strange concession—"it is only to a redeemed humanity that the past becomes citable in each and every one of its moments [*in jeder ihrer Momente*: admittedly, not "all" but "each and every" in its singularity]" (I.2.694; ILL 254), does the historian here turn into the chronicler who would assume the very reconciliation that it would by that very token render void? Does the "weak Messianic power" secretly claim an omnipotence that would subvert even a partial intervention into the past? Whatever the distinction between the consoling universal history of historicism and the "esperanto" proper to the Messianic (I.3.1239), does not the historical materialist risk both, and precisely in the same measure, insofar as he would surreptitiously occlude and thus hypostatize the present conditions of both thought and deed? If "every second" becomes "the narrow gate through which the Messiah might enter" (I.2.704; ILL 264)—yes, "the" Messiah—how is this different from the homogenizing abstractness that would efface the absolute singularity of the revolutionary event?

And if to make such a charge (as Adorno arguably could have done) is in itself equally to risk being tarred with the brush of a complacent historicism—to charge premature reconciliation is in itself to assume it, and so on—this in itself points to the inextricable interlocking of two "torn halves of a freedom" (as Adorno himself was famously to characterize the standoff in another context) to which "they do not, however, add up" (I.3.1003). Is Adorno guilty of the abstract negativity that would inevitably (Hegel) embrace the present in the exquisite gratification of its own despair? Is this the interminable standoff between the beautiful soul and its naive adversary?

It is perhaps not a question of decision here. However one is to (mis)construe the terms of the *Auseinandersetzung*—autonomous art versus mass culture, concept versus intuition, transcendence versus immanence, consciousness raising versus redemptive criticism, scientific versus utopian socialism, rationalism versus romanticism, Moses versus Aaron, Jeremiah versus Ezekiel (the oppositions are not unrelated, but by no means identical)—the very persistence of the antinomy in itself points to something irresolvable for thought.

Whatever the differences, in the end, between negative dialectics and dialectics at a standstill, the very entanglement indicates a permanent antinomy facing thought. If both Adorno and Benjamin inevitably transgress the *Bilderverbot* in their most strenuous efforts to honor it, this attests to an impatience founded in the radical nonsynchronicity of every time. Perhaps prematurity as such defines the permanent *Unmündigkeit* of every age. The logic of latency could mean nothing other than the risky venture of an image that cannot fail to come "too early" (but equally "too late"). There is in this sense always a little Fourier mixed into every imagination. It may indeed be (as Franz Rosenzweig insisted) that false Messianism inevitably comes to define not only the obstacle but equally the very possibility of redemption.[53] Shooting the clock-towers (cf. I.2.702; ILL 262) would at the very least shatter any illusion that either redemption or its image could ever come on time. That should equally preclude any easy ontologizing of the issue that would efface the specific urgency of an imperative all the more pressing for appearing inevitably too late.

It would in this light be tempting but scarcely sufficient to conclude here, as Adorno winds up *Minima Moralia*, with the observation that "beside the demand thus placed on thought, the question of the reality or unreality of redemption itself hardly matters" (MM sec. 153).

Notes

Unless otherwise indicated, all references to the German edition of Benjamin's works refer to *Gesammelte Schriften*, ed. Rolf Tiedemann and Hermann Schweppenhäuser, 7 volumes (Frankfurt: Suhrkamp, 1980–1991), and will be indicated in the text simply by volume, part, and page number. The following abbreviations will also be used:

Br = German edition of Benjamin's correspondence, *Briefe*, ed. Gershom Scholem and Theodor W. Adorno (Frankfurt: Suhrkamp, 1978).

BW = Theodor W. Adorno and Walter Benjamin, *Briefwechsel 1928–1940*, ed. Henri Lonitz (Frankfurt: Suhrkamp, 1995).

Existing English translations will be cited (modified where appropriate) according to the following abbreviations:

C = *The Correspondence of Walter Benjamin, 1910–1940*, trans. Manfred R. Jacobson and Evelyn M. Jacobson (Chicago: University of Chicago Press, 1994).

CB = *Charles Baudelaire: A Lyric Poet in the Era of High Capitalism*, trans. Harry Zohn (London: Verso, 1983).

ILL = *Illuminations*, trans. Harry Zohn (New York: Schocken, 1969).

OGT = *The Origin of German Tragic Drama*, trans. John Osborne (London: Verso, 1977).

OWS = *One-Way Street*, trans. Edmund Jephcott (London: Verso, 1985).

R = *Reflections*, trans. Edmund Jephcott (New York: Harcourt Brace Jovanovich, 1978).

Works of Adorno will be cited as follows:

AT = *Ästhetische Theorie* (Suhrkamp: Frankfurt, 1972)/*Aesthetic Theory*, trans. Christian Lenhardt (London: Routledge and Kegan Paul, 1984).

DA = (with Max Horkheimer), *Dialektik der Aufklärung* (Frankfurt: Suhrkamp, 1984).

DE = *Dialectic of Enlightenment*, trans. John Cumming (New York: Continuum, 1972).

K = *Kierkegaard: Konstruktion des Ästhetischen* (Frankfurt: Suhrkamp, 1962)/*Kierkegaard: Construction of the Aesthetic*, trans. Robert Hullot-Kentor (Minneapolis: University of Minnesota Press, 1989).

ND = *Negative Dialektik* (Frankfurt: Suhrkamp, 1966)/*Negative Dialectics*, trans. E. B. Ashton (New York: Continuum, 1973).

P = *Prismen* (Frankfurt: Suhrkamp, 1955)/*Prisms*, trans. Sam Weber and Shierry Weber (Cambridge: MIT, 1981).

NL = *Noten zur Literatur* (Frankfurt: Suhrkamp, 1974)/*Notes to Literature*, trans. Shierry Weber Nicholson, vol. 2 (New York: Columbia University Press, 1972).

QF = *Quasi una fantasia*, trans. Rodney Livingstone (London: Verso, 1992).

1. On some of the medieval controversies concerning the role of the body in the *visio Dei*, see Carolyn Walker Bynum, *The Resurrection of the Body 200–1336* (New York: Columbia University Press, 1995), pp. 279–317.

2. See Jaroslav Pelikan, *Christianity and Classical Culture: The Metamorphosis of Natural Theology in the Christian Encounter with Hellenism* (New Haven: Yale University Press, 1993), pp. 120–135, 280–295, 311–326. On the "economy" of resurrection, see pp. 153, 289 f. For the metaphor of the wax seal or stamp in Patristic theology (sometimes related to the parable of the lost coin in Luke 15:10), see pp. 126–128, and Pelikan, *The Christian Tradition: A History of the Development of Doctrine* (Chicago: University of Chicago Press, 1971–1989), 2:96.

3. *Babylonian Talmud*, Sanhedrin 91a–91b, trans. I. Epstein (London: Soncino Press, 1935). On the various senses of resurrection in rabbinic Judaism, see George W. E. Nickelsburg, *Resurrection, Immortality, and Eternal Life in Intertestamental Judaism* (Cambridge: Harvard University Press, 1972); George F. Moore, *Judaism in the First Centuries of the Christian Era: The Age of Tannaim* (Cambridge: Harvard University Press, 1927); Shaye J. D. Cohen, *From the Maccabees to the Mishnah* (Philadelphia: Westminster, 1987).

4. See my "Mourning Work and Play," in *Research in Phenomenology* 23 (1993).

5. "The absolute experience is not disclosure [*dévoilement*] but revelation [*révélation*]." Emmanuel Levinas, *Totality and Infinity: An Essay on Exteriority*, trans. Alphonso Lingis (Pittsburgh: Duquesne University Press, 1969), p. 65 ff.

6. Thus the inevitable link between the prohibition against graven images and the prohibition against incest. See, for example, Jean-Joseph Goux's influential reading of the Mosaic injunction as directed in the first place against fusion with the mother. *Les Iconoclastes* (Paris: Seuil, 1978).

Materialist Mutations of the *Bilderverbot*

7. "Perhaps there is no sublimer passage in the Jewish law than the command, 'Thou shalt not make to thyself any graven image.'" Kant, *Critique of Judgment*, trans. J. H. Bernard (New York: Hafner, 1951), § 29, "General Remark on the Exposition of the Aesthetic Reflective Judgment."

8. Maurice Blanchot, "Interruptions," in Eric Gould, ed., *The Sin of the Book: Edmond Jabès* (Lincoln: University of Nebraska Press, 1985), p. 49.

9. G. W. F. Hegel, *Phenomenology of Spirit*, trans. A. V. Miller (New York: Oxford University Press, 1977), p. 344.

10. Ibid., p. 332.

11. See letters of Scholem to Benjamin of July 9, 17, 1934, in Gershom Scholem, ed., *The Correspondence of Walter Benjamin and Gershom Scholem*, trans. Gary Smith and André Lefevere (New York: Schocken, 1989), pp. xxx, 123, 127. Contrast Adorno, "Notes on Kafka," *Prisms*, esp. pp. 259 f., 268.

12. Friedrich Nietzsche, *Will to Power*, § 603.

13. Gershom Scholem, *Walter Benjamin: The Story of a Friendship* (London: Faber and Faber, 1981).

14. Werner Fuld, *Walter Benjamin: Zwischen den Stühlen* (Munich: Hanser Verlag, 1979).

15. Cf. Jürgen Habermas, "Walter Benjamin: Consciousness-Raising or Rescuing Critique," in Gary Smith, ed., *On Walter Benjamin: Critical Essays and Reflections* (Cambridge: MIT Press, 1988), p. 114.

16. See Rabbi Hiyya b. Abba's representation of Rabbi Johanan's proscription of any prophetic vision of the world "to come" (by way of an idiosyncratic rendering of Isaiah 64:5–"the eye hath not seen, oh Lord, beside thee, what he hath prepared for him that waiteth for him") in Sanhedrin 99a, *Babylonian Talmud*, together with Maimonides' related critique of eudaimonism in *Mishnah Torah*, "Laws of Repentance," and Hermann Cohen's denunciation of the "utopia of mythic belief" in *Religion der Vernunft aus den Quellen des Judentums* (Wiesbaden: Fourier Verlag, 1928), pp. 361–363. The scope of prophesy is here rigorously limited to the messianic (in contrast to the afterlife "to come"). See also Emmanuel Levinas's commentary on the rabbinic subtext: *Difficult Freedom: Essays on Judaism*, trans. Sean Hand (Chicago: University of Chicago Press, 1994), pp. 59–68.

17. Marx, Afterword to the second German edition of *Capital* (Moscow: Progress Publishers, 1959), 1:26.

18. G. W. F. Hegel, *Grundlinien der Philosophie des Rechts* (Frankfurt: Suhrkamp, 1970), p. 27.

19. Letter of October 19, 1877, to Sorge, in Karl Marx and Friedrich Engels, *Selected Correspondence 1846–95*, trans. Dona Torr (New York: International Publishers, 1942).

Rebecca Comay

20. Karl Korsch, *Karl Marx*, p. 53.

21. Immanuel Kant, *Critique of Practical Reason*, trans. Lewis White Beck (Indianapolis: Bobbs-Merrill, 1956), p. 146.

22. "God and eternity in their awful majesty would stand unceasingly before our eyes (for that which we can completely prove is as certain as that which we can ascertain by sight)." Kant, *Critique of Practical Reason*, p. 152.

23. Ibid., p. 153.

24. Benjamin, "Theses on the Philosophy of History," Thesis XII, in *Illuminations*, trans. Harry Zohn (New York: Schocken, 1969).

25. Nietzsche, *Thus Spoke Zarathustra*, "On the New Idol," in Walter Kaufman, trans., *The Portable Nietzsche* (New York: Viking, 1968), p. 162.

26. See Susan Buck-Morss, *The Dialectics of Seeing* (Cambridge: MIT Press, 1989).

27. Cf. Wolfgang Schivelbusch, *Disenchanted Night: The Industrialization of Light in the Nineteenth Century* (Berkeley: University of California Press, 1988).

28. Cf. Lacan, "The Gaze as *objet a*," in *The Four Fundamental Concepts of Psychoanalysis* (New York: Norton, 1978).

29. See "Some Motifs in Baudelaire" (I.2.646; ILL 188). For a discussion of some of the ambiguities of this transaction, see my "Framing Redemption: Aura, Origin, Technology in Heidegger and Benjamin," in Arleen Dallery and Charles Scott, eds., *Ethics and Danger: Essays on Heidegger and Continental Thought* (Albany: State University of New York Press, 1992), and "Facies Hippocratica," in Adriaan Peperzak, ed., *Ethics as First Philosophy: The Thought of Emmanuel Levinas* (New York: Routledge, 1995).

30. See Irving Wohlfarth's comments on this passage, "Resentment Begins at Home: Nietzsche, Benjamin, and the University," in Smith, *On Walter Benjamin*, p. 225 f.

31. "You never look at me from the place from which I see you." Lacan, *Four Fundamental Concepts*, p. 103.

32. Cf. I.1.343; OGT 166. It is perhaps for this reason that Lacan associates Holbein's skull with the melting watches of Salvador Dalí: the anamorphic distortion would correspond to the allegorical disruption of the temporal continuum, exemplified by the revolutionary shooting of the clock-towers, as described in Benjamin's fifteenth thesis on history. See ibid., p. 88.

33. Christine Buci-Glucksmann, *La Folie du voir: de l'esthétique baroque* (Paris: Galilée, 1986). Cf. *La Raison baroque: de Baudelaire à Benjamin* (Paris: Galilée, 1984).

34. Cf. Marcel Proust, *Remembrance of Things Past*, trans. C. K. Scott Moncrieff and Terence Kilmartin (London: Penguin, 1983), 2:35 ff.

35. Louis Aragon, *Paris Peasant,* trans. Simon Watson Taylor (London: Cape, 1971), p. 28.

36. Karl Marx and Frederick Engels, *Werke* (Berlin: Dietz, 1962), 23:15.

37. Br 654; C 482.

38. Cf. Philippe Ivornel, "Paris, Capital of the Popular Front or the Posthumous Life of the 19th Century," *New German Critique* 39 (1986):61–84.

39. Charles Baudelaire, "Salon de 1859," in *Oeuvres complètes* (Paris: Gallimard, 1979), 2:614–619.

40. Cf. Sigmund Freud, *Interpretation of Dreams,* trans. and ed. James Strachey (London: Hogarth Press, 1953), 5:621.

41. Letter of February 23, 1927, to Buber. Also in *Moscow Diary,* trans. Richard Sieburth (Cambridge, Mass.: Harvard University Press), p. 126. Benjamin is here citing Simmel's own citation of Goethe in his *Goethe* (Leipzig: Klinkhardt und Biermann, 1913), p. 57.

42. Compare here Benjamin's comments on Leskov. "The hierarchy of the creaturely world, which has its apex in the righteous man, reaches down into the abyss of the inanimate by many stages. In this connection one particular point has to be noted. This whole creaturely world speaks not so much with the human voice as with what could be called "the voice of nature" in the title of one of Leskov's most significant stories" (II.2.460; ILL 104).

43. Benjamin's interest in Goethe's morphological writings, evidenced as early as in a fragment of 1918 on "Symbolism" (VI.38 f.), is expressed further in the dissertation on romanticism (I.110–119), in *Goethes Wahlverwandtschaften* (I.147), and in a discarded passage of the *Trauerspielbuch* (I.953), and appears finally in the *Passagenwerk* (V.577), where Simmel's presentation in his 1913 *Goethe* plays a decisive role.

44. Simmel, *Goethe,* p. 56, quoted by Buck-Morss, *Dialectics of Seeing,* p. 72.

45. I.2.495 f.; ILL 233 f.

46. " 'To study this period, at once so close and so remote, I compare myself to a surgeon operating with a local anaesthetic; I work in places which are numb, dead; the patient, however, is alive and can still talk.' Paul Morand: 1900 Paris 1931 p 6/7" (V.577).

47. See Irving Wohlfarth's astute comments on this passage in "Et Cetera? The Historian as Chiffonier," *New German Critique* 39 (1985):163.

48. Roland Barthes, *Camera Lucida: Reflections on Photography* (New York: Hill and Wang, 1981).

49. Jean-François Lyotard, "Adorno as the Devil," *Telos* 19 (1974), pp. 127–38; Agamben, "Le prince et le crapaud," in *Enfance et histoire: Déperissement de l'expérience et origine de l'histoire* (Paris: Payot, 1978); Peter Bürger, *The Decline of*

Modernism, trans. Nicholas Walker (University Park: Pennsylvania State University Press, 1992).

50. This point is argued forcefully by Agamben, "Le prince."

51. See the neo-Leninist avowals in the letter of March 18, 1936. I.3.1003 and I.3.1005; Ronald Taylor, trans., *Aesthetics and Politics* (London: Verso, 1977), pp. 122, 125.

52. Cf. H. D. Kittsteiner, "Walter Benjamin's Historicism," *New German Critique* 39 (1986):179–215.

53. Franz Rosenzweig, "The True and the False Messiah: A Note to a Poem by Judah ha-Levi," in Nahum N. Glatzer, *Franz Rosenzweig: His Life and Thought* (New York: Schocken, 1961), p. 350.

12

Hannah Arendt: The Activity of the Spectator

Peg Birmingham

In *Life of the Mind, Thinking*, Hannah Arendt points out that "since Bergson, the use of the sight metaphor in philosophy has kept dwindling, not unsurprisingly, as emphasis and interest have shifted entirely from contemplation to speech, from *nous* to *logos*."[1] Yet Arendt's analysis of vision in the history of philosophy suggests that things are not so simple. In other words, her analysis shows that because emphasis shifts from *nous* to *logos*, the construction of vision in the history of philosophy cannot be so simply characterized as the rise and fall of vision. This is the case for two reasons. First, Arendt argues that in the history of philosophy, *nous* is never found without an accompanying *logos*, making philosophical vision discursive from its beginnings; second, her analysis even suggests that from the earliest Greek beginnings, there is a parallel, albeit implicit, history of the construction of vision, a history that from the beginning does not understand the vision of *nous* as contemplative, but instead, because of the connection between *nous* and *logos*, comes to understand vision differently, as a "theoretical," judgmental *activity* (*theorein*). Here I take up these two parallel histories, arguing that ultimately Arendt's analysis shows that contemporary philosophy is characterized by a construction of vision that makes explicit this implicit history of judgmental vision (*theoria*), although in ways that radically depart from its Greek beginnings.

Peg Birmingham

The Discursive Tension between *Nous* and *Logos*

In her analysis of the construction of vision in the philosophical interpretation of *nous*, Arendt begins by looking at the pre-philosophical assumptions that underlie this construction. Chief among these is the Greek preoccupation with immortality:

Imbedded in a cosmos where everything was immortal, mortality becomes the hallmark of human existence. Men are "the mortals," the only mortal things in existence, because unlike animals they do not exist only as members of a species whose immortal life is guaranteed through procreation. The mortality of men lies in the fact that individual life, with a recognizable life-story from birth to death, rises out of biological life. This is mortality: to move along a rectilinear line in a universe where everything, if it moves at all, moves in a cyclical order.[2]

The concern for immortality is a concern to be at home in a cosmos where everything except humans moves in a cyclical, immortal fashion. Thus, the only way that humans can find a place in such a cosmos is to achieve immortality. This is done "by their capacity for the immortal deed, by their ability to leave nonperishable traces behind."[3] To achieve immortality through greatness of deed is therefore to be of a "divine nature." Such a concern with divine immortality requires that the deed be seen and remembered. In other words, the actor needs a community of spectators who will, watching the event, preserve its memory in their storytelling.

Arendt's argument is that the immortality achievable through *nous* replaces this prephilosophical notion of immortality as achieved through the communal visibility of great deeds. This had to do, she argues, with a decisive flaw in the divine nature of the gods. Although the gods were immortal, they were not eternal; they were deathless but not birthless. Certainly this is evidenced in Hesiod's genealogy wherein the Olympian gods could trace their lineage back to their pre-Olympian ancestors. The gods are temporal, although immortal. Being, on the other hand, is eternal, outside of time altogether. The belief that a contemplation of Being is the way to achieve immortality means that one no longer needs the community of spectators to immortalize the memory of the deed in storytelling. Instead, "the way to the new immortality was to take up one's abode with things that are forever, and the new faculty making this possible was called *nous* or mind."[4] What confers immortality on human beings is now the object of thought, "that which is invariably the everlasting, what was and is and will be, and therefore cannot be otherwise than it is, and cannot not be."[5] The irony is that the philosopher, initially concerned with the immortal, chooses instead the eternal and the necessary: that which is outside time altogether and cannot not be. Thus, *nous* does not bestow immortality. Arendt points out that this has a long tradition, such that even Hegel, when he turned to history, "could do it only on the assumption that not only the revolutions of the skies and sheer thought-things such as numbers and the like followed the iron laws of necessity, but that the course of human affairs on earth followed such laws, the laws of the incarnation of the Absolute Mind."[6]

The grasping of the eternal and necessary by way of *nous* is accomplished through a vision that is speechless, "which to Plato was *arrheton* ('unspeakable') and Aristotle calls *aneu logou* ('without word'), and which later was conceptualized in the paradoxical *nunc stans* ('the standing now')."[7] Moreover, this vision no longer involves an actor and an event; rather it requires contemplation, the cessation of all activity (*a-skhole*). Thus, according to this account offered by Arendt, the earliest construction of vision in the history of philosophy is one that substitutes contemplation for action, solitariness for plurality, the necessary for the contingent, silence for speech, and a vision of the eternal for an immortality awarded by the community in recognition of visibly great deeds. The paradigm for vision is *nous*: eternal, necessary, contemplative, solitary, silent. *Nous* makes humans divine: *theoria*, the vision enjoyed by *nous*, is derived from *theos*, the look of the god who has an immediate access to the eternal object.

And yet Arendt's own account suggests that things are not so simple in this initial construction of the paradigm of *nous* as a contemplative vision. For from the beginning *nous* needs *logos*. Indeed, having argued in *The Human Condition* that Aristotle follows Plato in positing the speechlessness of *nous*, Arendt goes on to argue in the *Life of the Mind* that Aristotle actually showed that the vision of *nous* needs to be translated into words: "This was called *aletheuein* by Aristotle and does not just mean to tell things as they really are without concealing anything, but also applies only to propositions about things that always and necessarily are and cannot be otherwise."[8] The problem with *nous* needing *logos* is that the latter is strictly human and moves vision from the realm of the divine into the realm of human affairs. To overcome this problem, she argues, "the criterion for philosophical speech becomes *homoiosis* (in opposition to *doxa* or opinion), 'to make a likeness,' or assimilate in words as faithfully as possible the vision by *nous*, which itself is without discourse."[9] *Logos* must be mimetic, uncritically and faithfully mimicking what is given to it by this speechless, divine sight—*theorein*. Hence, in the philosophies of *nous*, the paradigm of vision leads to the understanding of truth as *adequatio rei et intellectus*. Certainly the emphasis here is on *nous*. Yet Arendt's analysis reveals that from the outset, the paradigm for vision in the history of philosophy is inherently discursive. From the outset *nous* is bound up with *logos*. In still other words, the self-evidence of noetic insight fails; it is always in need of the *logos*. Here I quote the text at length:

The difficulties to which the "awesome science" of metaphysics has given rise since its inception could possibly all be summed up in the natural tension between *theoria* and *logos*, between seeing and reasoning with words—whether in the form of "dialectics" (*dia-legesthai*) or, on the contrary, of the "syllogism" (*syl-logizesthai*), ie., whether it takes things, especially opinions, apart by means of words or brings them together in a discourse depending for its truth content on a primary premise perceived by intuition, by the *nous*, which is not subject to error because it is not *meta logou*, sequential to words.[10]

This tension between a paradigm in which vision is inherently silent, eternal, and "divine" and one in which vision is intrinsically discursive, active, and finite seems to lead Arendt in *Life of the Mind* (first given as Gifford Lectures in 1973, sixteen years after *The Human Condition*) to rethink the construction of vision in the history of philosophy. It is my suggestion, however, that it is not so much that Arendt rethinks her account of the paradigm of vision in the philosophies of *nous* (having first told this history in *The Human Condition*, she basically retells it in the beginning of *Life of the Mind, Thinking*), as that she discovers in the history of philosophy a parallel although implicit construction of vision. In still other words, it is not that Arendt understands the philosophical discourse of the present as in transition to the affirmation of a different, historically new paradigm of knowledge based on the importance of the *logos*; rather, she discovers that all along in the history of philosophy there is another paradigm of vision: vision, *theorein*, understood as the theoretically guided *activity* of judgment (*theorein*).[11] Thus, while Arendt is quite explicit in her account of how the history of philosophy can be read as a move from *nous* understood as contemplative vision to *logos* understood as speech, she is not so explicit in showing how all along there has been in the history of philosophy an interpretation of *theorein* involving an implicit and ignored notion of *discursive* vision; rather than rejecting the vision paradigm in favor of a hearing paradigm, she tries to bring out and reformulate, through an immanent critique, a very different conception of vision implicit in the notion of critical judgment. To be more precise, it is my argument that the move Arendt describes from *nous* to *logos* can be understood only if *logos* is understood in terms of the discursive vision of the judging spectator and is accordingly interpreted in terms of such a vision.

The Discursive Judgment of the Spectator

At the end of *The Human Condition* Hannah Arendt reveals that not all has gone as expected in her analysis of the distinction between the *vita contemplativa* and the *vita activa*, a distinction that at the beginning of the text is sharp: the *vita contemplativa* is characterized by the quiet and silent gaze of *nous*, while the *vita activa* is characterized by its restless activity within the world of appearances. Yet at the conclusion to the text, she quotes a curious sentence that Cicero ascribed to Cato: "Never is a man more active than when he does nothing, never is he less alone than when he is by himself."[12] The sentence is curious insofar as it is about thinking. The end of *The Human Condition*, then, apparently unravels its beginning—a beginning that made a firm distinction between the life of action and the life of contemplation: thinking is now recognized as an activity and one, moreoever, that is not essentially solitary.

Arendt returns to this sentence attributed to Cato in the Introduction to *Life of the Mind, Thinking*, asking, "What are we doing when we do nothing but think? Where are we when we, normally always surrounded by our fellow-men, are together with no one but ourselves?"[13] Arendt's answer to these questions in *Life of the Mind, Thinking* not only calls into question the inevitability of the rift between thinking and acting, theory and practice, but furthermore shows that all along in the history of philosophy, there is another paradigm of vision, a paradigm that challenges the notion of *theorein* as a contemplative *nous*.

That there is another paradigm of vision in the history of philosophy is apparent by the "curious context in which the word 'philosophize' makes its first appearance."[14] Arendt relates Herodotus's story of Solon, who sets out on a ten-year journey, "partly for political reasons, but also for sight-seeing—*theorein*."[15] Solon meets Croesus of Sardis who addresses him: "Stranger, great word has come to us about you, your wisdom and your wandering about, namely, that you have gone visiting many lands of the earth *philosophizing* with respect to the spectacles you saw."[16] The *theoroi* were philosophers who traveled abroad to study the institutions and laws of other cultures. These were "philosophical" journeys for the sake of *theoria*, a knowledge of what was seen. Solon's theoretical journey was not a turn away from specific regions and local events; rather, in the conversations with people abroad, he could determine which of his laws and institutions were good and which needed improvement.

Here I suggest that Arendt's understanding of the term *theory* must be taken seriously. In *Life of the Mind, Thinking*, Arendt points out that the philosophical term *theory* emerged from the Greek word for spectators, *theatai*. She quotes Diogenes Laertius on this earliest sense of theory: "Life is like a festival; just as some come to the festival to compete, some to ply their trade, but the best people come as spectators (*theatai*), so in life the slavish men go hunting for fame (*doxa*) or gain, the philosophers for truth."[17] Arendt writes: "What is stressed here as more noble than the competition for fame or gain is by no means a truth invisible and inaccessible to ordinary men; nor does the place the spectators withdraw to belong to any "higher" realm."[18] Instead, the spectators are located at the festival, watching the actual event before them. The nobility of the spectators lies in their "active nonparticipation," allowing them to judge the actors involved in the competition.

Indeed, the concern for fame or opinion makes the actor in the event dependent on the spectator's judgment. "For it is through the opinion of the audience and the judge that fame comes about." The actor is not autonomous, since the final verdict concerning the event lies with the spectators. The judgment on the event reflects the plurality of spectators, all contributing their views. Therefore, if theory is that produced by these spectators, then the initial sense of theory (*theatai*) has to do with judgments on events rather than the articulation of eternal and necessary truths.

In the emergence of *theoria* from *theatai*, the term *theoria* continues to retain the significance of a judging spectator. Plato takes up this sense of theory in the *Laws*. He ascribes an important role in the state to the *theoroi* who go abroad to contemplate other systems of laws and other types of institutions. After seeing the institutions of others, the delegation must return and report to the supreme council, whose domain is legislation and education and whose task is the improvement of both. Plato is quite specific that the judgments of the *theoroi* concern actual laws and events and, moreover, are subject to debate and criticism by other members of the council before transforming any of the state's practices. Moreover, the judgments of the *theoroi* are within the context of shared social practices: the justifications of the judgments acquire their rationale only in the dynamic, political discourse.

Finally, Arendt points out that it is Thucydides who best exemplifies this earliest understanding of theory in his attempts,

as a historian, to take up an objective attitude toward the events
of the Peloponnesian War, which is perhaps why Arendt argues
that in thinking the events of history, Thucydides must be looked
to as a guide. Thucydides suggests that the search for the truth
(*theoria*) of the event is possible only by placing in a relation of
contiguity several eyewitness accounts: "In this history I have
made use of set speeches some of which were delivered just
before and others during the war. I have found it difficult to
remember the precise words used in the speeches which I lis-
tened to myself ... so my method has been, while keeping as
closely as possible to the *general sense* of the words that were
actually used, to make the speakers say what, in my opinion was
called for by each situation."[19]

For Thucydides, the position of nobility, that of watching the
conflict from above, is in no sense a position that escapes the
historical event. Moreover, the "general sense" is not obtained
by subsuming the particular situation under an a priori concept
or universal principle gained through the intuitive insight of
nous. The profound sadness of Thucydides' final verdict lies in
the recognition that such a principle could not be given in
advance. In his search for truth (*theoria*), he recognizes that the
truth of the event emerges only in the realm of the political,
where the opinions of the spectators, the plurality of speakers,
give to the situation what is demanded of it.

Thucydides (and this is what interests Arendt) understands
theoria as historical and political. Indeed, only by transfering *theoria* to the sphere of politics is he able to grasp the "demand" of
the situation. The "demand," or, more generally, the truth of
this enormous event, the Pelopponesian War, is determined in
the realm of the political, where each spectator is viewing and
judging the event from a unique perspective and in this sense is
alone—although each view is always only one of a plurality of
views. In this reading, Arendt sheds light on Cato's statement:
"Never is a man more active than when he does nothing, never is
he less alone than when he is by himself."

In her essay "Truth and Politics," Arendt examines a statement by Pericles, an examination that further illuminates a dif-

ferent paradigm of vision in the history of philosophy. Arendt translates the statement by Pericles as, "We love beauty within the limits of political judgment and we philosophize (*theorein*) without the barbarian vice of effeminacy."[20] Several aspects of Arendt's reading must be noted. First, it is the realm of politics that sets limits to the love of wisdom and of beauty. If "limit" is understood as definition, then what gives definition or intelligibility to beauty and wisdom is not the eternal, necessary gaze of *nous* but, instead, the vision of *critical* judgment that remains within and is informed by the political arena. Arendt, understanding the gaze of the philosopher in terms of critical judgment, stresses an experience of vision as a mode of critical reflection. It is an understanding of vision that is much more than a simple, uncritical perception of the given. She recovers from the Greeks the notion of *taste* as precisely that which is capable of such reflection. The love of the philosopher is not the love of eternal forms but the love of beauty, that is, the love of appearances. In other words, the activity of philosophy (*theorein*) is not the contemplative gaze of *nous*, but an activity capable of taking "aim in judgment, discernment, discrimination, in brief, by that curious and ill-defined capacity we commonly call taste."[21]

Taste, according to Arendt, judges the world in its appearance and in its worldliness, but its interest in the world, in the beauty of appearances, which is a public concern, is purely "disinterested" and that means that neither the life interests of the individual nor the moral interests of the self are involved. As Arendt writes, "For judgments of taste, the world is the primary thing, not man, neither man's life nor his self."[22] In her reading of Pericles, Arendt thinks of seeing and looking in terms of the critical judgment of taste because in the realm of politics what is required is independent, discriminating sight (*theoria*) capable of reflecting on the given and distancing itself from it.

Finally, I turn to Arendt's more well-known remarks concerning thinking and judgment—those given in her consideration of Kant. Certainly the discussion of Pericles already betrays a certain debt to Kant, specifically Kant's reflective judgment. And while it is the case that many passages can be found wherein Arendt insists that for Kant thinking has to do with the thinker's relation to itself (certainly all those remarks having to do with the categorical imperative), nonetheless, Arendt argues that the Kant of the *Critique of Judgment* "insisted upon a different way of thinking, for which it would not be enough to be in agreement with one's own self, but which consisted of being able to "think in the place of everybody else" and which he therefore called an "enlarged mentality (*eine erweiterte Denkungsart*)."[23] It is in Arendt's discussion of Kant's reflective judgment that we see her continuing to reformulate this other, implicit paradigm of vision operative in the history of philosophy: one that shows that theoretical vision must be understood as reflective judgment capable of arriving at its own norms and principles rather than acquiescing in what is given by the prevailing historical reality.

For Kant, reason is a "general human need," and there is no distinction between the few and the many. Thus, the philosopher does not occupy any special position outside the realm of human affairs. Moreover, according to Arendt's reading of Kant, thinking is antiauthoritative. It stands the test of open and free communication, which means that the more people who participate in it, the better. Indeed, this is what Kant meant by the "public use of one's reason": thinking requires the company of others. This does not mean that one does not think in solitude, only that one's thoughts must be capable of being communicated either orally or written: company is indispensable for the thinker. In other words, thinking itself can be done only in solitude, but it cannot be done effectively without that freedom to communicate and to exchange one's thoughts in public that enables one to enlarge one's mind by incorporating the insights of others. Furthermore, Arendt argues, thinking not only depends on the public use of one's reason but, at the same time, it "feeds back into public life in its turn by questioning authorities and accepted assumptions." In her reading of Kant, therefore, Arendt is thinking a modern version of the spectator: the thinker who is actively engaged in critically judging and discussing the public affairs of the day. Thinking (*theorein*), as she understands it, is a reflection on others and their taste, and therefore is always the exercising of judgment. Hence the emphasis on taste: "Taste is this 'community sense' and 'sense' means here 'the effect of a reflection upon the mind.' This reflection affects me like a sensation—the sensation of pleasure."[24]

In this process of judgment, the role of the imagination is fundamental. The task, according to Arendt, is to train one's imagination in *theoria*, train it to "go visiting." This is the modern version of Solon's sightseer, the spectator with a philosophical, theoretically critical eye. Arendt cautions that this vision (*theoria*) is not empathy—as if one could visit and read the mind of another. It is the result of first abstracting from the limitations that contingently attach to one's own judgment, of disregarding its subjective private conditions for a more general standpoint. This generality, however, is not the generality of grasping some ahistorical, necessary concept. The concern is with the viewpoint—and the viewpoint is the world. Hence, Arendt finds in Kant's thinking a paradigm of vision (*theorein*) understood in terms of the theoretical spectator—the judge. It is a paradigm in which the vision (*theoria*) of the spectator is truly discursive, needing the company and discourse of others.

The Contemporary Crisis of Discursive Vision: Kafka's Parable "He"

In *Life of the Mind, Thinking*, Arendt performs a type of *epoche* on the framework of metaphysics. She writes: "I have clearly joined the ranks of those who for some time now have been attempting to dismantle metaphysics, and philosophy with all its categories, as we have known them from their beginning in Greece until today. Such dismantling is possible only on the assumption that the thread of tradition is broken and that we shall not be able to renew it."[25] Arendt's dismantling technique certainly draws its inspiration from Husserl and Heidegger but more immediately from Walter Benjamin and Franz Kafka: "What you are then left with is still the past, but a *fragmented* past, which has lost its certainty of evaluation.... It is with such fragments from the past, with their sea-change, that I have dealt.''[26]

If the Greek answer to the question, "What makes us think?" lies in the prephilosophical concern with immortality, a concern that leads the Greeks to substitute the eternal vision of *nous* for the immortal deed, Arendt's own answer lies in closer proximity to the Roman answer to this same question. For both the Romans and Arendt, what makes us think lies in the experience of disunity, of a world torn apart: "Thinking then arises out of the disintegration of reality and the resulting disunity of man and world, from which springs the need for another world, more harmonious and more meaningful.''[27] For both the Romans and Arendt, philosophy arises out of a disintegration of reality: the public world lies in ruins. The Roman answer, however, is in closer proximity to the Greek answer insofar as both posit a model of vision that gazes at another, supersensual world. Arendt's answer resists such an escape impulse. Moreover, for Arendt, the ruins seem more radical insofar as the Romans are able to continue to look to tradition as a source of authority and meaning. As seen in the reference to Benjamin, the past is fragmented and in pieces: "It lies in a veritable rubble heap around us.''[28]

Thus, Arendt's argument is two-pronged. First, she argues that the model for philosophical thinking today is characterized by the notion of the "discursive vision" of the spectator; but second, she argues that the "rubble heap" out of which contemporary culture thinks calls on us to rethink significantly the vision of the spectator. Arendt, reflecting on this rubble heap, attempts to think the *topos* of thinking for contemporary culture. Significantly, she turns to Kafka's parable "He" as a way to answer the question, "Where are we when we think?"

The importance of Kafka's parable "He" for Arendt's reconstruction of discursive vision cannot be underestimated. In both the *Life of the Mind, Thinking* as well as the Preface to *Between Past and Future*, Arendt turns to this parable to designate the *topos* of the contemporary thinker. And in *Essays in Understanding* Arendt devotes an entire essay to thinking, "The No Longer and the Not Yet," the temporality that is at the heart of Kafka's parable.

The contemporary thinker, "He," stands in the fragment, in the gap between the past and the future. Here Arendt pits Kafka against Plato. In Plato's story, the thinker leaves the deceptive and transient appearances of this world, only to return to it with the vision of the world of Being fixed in the eye of *nous*. In Arendt's reading, Kafka's parable begins just at the point where action and the experiences arising from it call for a kind of thinking that will preserve them for the present and allow them to exercise themselves on the future. In the parable, a "he" is engaged in battle with two forces: one coming from the infinite past and the other from the infinite future. The past is driving him into the future, and the future is driving him back to the past. For Arendt this describes the condition of thought that has always existed; however, in other times, this gap was paved over by tradition. It is only with the loss of tradition that the gap has revealed itself in its true character, engaging the thinker in the wearisome struggle Kafka describes.

"He" would like to leap beyond this struggle and assume the role of umpire. For Arendt this is the metaphysical dream of *nous*: to transcend the finitude of existence and to enter a silent realm of the eternal. At this point, Arendt alters the parable. She allows for a deflection produced by the battle. This deflection enables the embattled thinker to move back and forth between past and future along a parallelogram of forces whereby, it is hoped, he can gain enough distance to achieve the impartiality of an umpire without leaving time altogether. She declares that the essays that follow in *Between Past and Future* are exercises, intended to teach not what to think but only how to move in the gap.

Here Arendt departs from the way the spectator is understood in the history of philosophy. The rubble heap includes the dismantled rows of the stadium in which the spectators gained their "noble distance." Thus, Arendt's reformulation of the contemporary vision of the spectator disallows for noble distance.

Nevertheless, the deflection of forces does allow the spectator some distance from the events. Moreover, the description of thinking as "movement" links thinking to acting, for it is precisely the characteristic of movement, of the "being able to," that in *The Human Condition* marked the domain of action. This link completely severs thinking from a model of contemplative vision. Moreover, insofar as movement requires a space of movement, Arendt's analysis suggests that the vision of the spectator is inherently spatial. Thus, her reformulation of *theoria* as the vision of the spectator must include the notion of a "spatial vision" concerned with how things become visible, that is, how spaces are designed such that things are visible. This accounts for Arendt's continuous preoccupation with the very real constitution of political spaces in which power would become visible and public.

At this point in her reading of Kafka, Arendt gives the first clue that the thinker's place is the position of the judge. The temporal duration of this gap between the past and future is the "untimely." Here Arendt is in the tradition of Nietzsche and Heidegger, for whom the "untimely" also plays such an important role: to be untimely in time. This sense of the "untimely" is not the *nunc stans*, the eternal in time. Rather, in *Life of the Mind, Thinking*, Arendt invokes Heidegger's notion of the "*Augenblick*" (moment of vision) and Nietzsche's notion of the "eternal return" to illuminate the temporal duration of this gap. The notion of the "untimely" is understood as "crisis." The untimely is the time of the crisis. The notion of the untimely calls into question the form of history that reintroduces and always assumes a suprahistorical perspective.

To think the untimely is to think *krinein*: critical history as Nietzsche understood it in the second *Untimely Meditations*. And it is suggestive that Arendt at this point thinks together Nietzsche's notion of the eternal return with Heidegger's notion of the *Augenblick* insofar it is Heidegger who argues that one must think together will to power and eternal return, and think them, moreover, as perspective. This perspective is the perspective of the crisis, the *krinein*.[29] *Krinein*, Heidegger argues, is the root of

Entscheidung: a cutting. Thinking is understood here as perspective, located in a particular time and place. *Krinein* is the perspective that distinguishes, separates, and disperses. Thus "He" who moves in the crisis, the gap between the past and the future, is engaged in *krinein*, judgment.

Moreover, in the *Augenblick* (moment of vision), the spectator grasps the specificity of the event. The *Augenblick* is the historical conjunction of traditions, discourses, and practices. Furthermore, as Kafka's parable suggests, the thinker cannot escape the time of the *Augenblick*. This is not the time of the before (tradition) or the after (the future), but the time of the now of historical happening. It is the time that demands a critical response to the specific and the unique. In the moment of vision (*Augenblick*), the critical reply lacks a classical mimetic model on which to base its response. Instead, the spectator, whose vision is neither contemplative nor introspective, looks at the singular and contingent. This vision does not gaze up to the eternal or necessary forms; rather, it looks out to those events through which thinking is given something to think and, moreover, critically to change its ways of seeing.

Here we begin to understand what Arendt means when she argues that "thinking is always out of order." The "out of order" is not such that thinking posits a transcendent object. It is always out of order compared with the ordinary course of events, but it is never unworldly. Thought is inherently bound to the world of appearances. Here we can begin to see why for Arendt the banality of evil is linked to thoughtlessness. If thinking has to do with a crisis of judgment, a fundamental "out of order" with the ordinary course of events, then thoughtlessness is precisely lack of judgment, going along with the course of events in which one is immersed. Certainly Arendt saw that this was the case with Adolf Eichmann.

Discussing G. E. Lessing's notion of *Selbtsdenken*, Arendt gives a further clue as to how she understands the activity of the spectator. *Selbtsdenken* is independent thinking, which does not mean an isolated individual who looks around the world in order "to bring himself into harmony with the world by the detour of thought.''[30] Thought, she argues, does not arise out of the individual and is not the manifestation of a self. This is still another way to understand the deflection of the movement of the ''He'' between past and future: ''Rather, the individual—whom Lessing would say was created for action, not ratiocination—elects such thought because he discovers in thinking another mode of moving in the world of freedom.''[31] Again, Arendt thinks the activity of the judging spectator. But the activity of the judging spectator is not engaged in a means-end relation; it has nothing to do with conclusions or results. Here Arendt reveals how much she removes judging from prescribed categories or standards, arguing that judging is concerned with events, and ''what the illuminating event reveals is a beginning in the past which had hitherto been hidden.''[32] Thus, there is no need to fear that our categories of thought and our standards of judgment lie around us as in a veritable rubble heap. I quote the text at length:

Even though we have lost yardsticks by which to measure, and rules under which to subsume the particular, a being whose essence is beginning may have enough of origin within himself to understand without preconceived categories and to judge without the set of customary rules which is morality. If the essence of all, and in particular of political, action is to make a new beginning, then understanding becomes the other side of action, namely, that form of cognition, distinct from many others, by which acting men ... eventually can come to terms with what irrevocably happened and be reconciled with what unavoidably exists.[33]

At this point we can begin to see how Arendt reconstructs the paradigm of vision in the history of philosophy. Contrary to what it might seem with her emphasis on appearance and her claim that the spectator is essential for the generation of meaning, Arendt dismantles, through her continuous reflection on the active gaze of critical judgment, the conception of vision that makes the passive contemplation of eternal objects paradigmatic. Arendt's reconstruction of vision in contemporary philosophy takes up the earliest notion of *theorein* as the sight of the spectator-judge, insisting on its public and plural characteristics. She insists on a paradigm of vision that is not only discursive but spatial, and therefore active; it is a paradigm of vision that moves critically through the public world making visible not only what has happened and what unavoidably exists but what can be thought and what can be done.

Notes

1. Hannah Arendt, *Life of the Mind: Thinking* (New York: Harcourt Brace Jovanovich, 1971), p. 122.

2. Hannah Arendt, *The Human Condition* (Chicago: University of Chicago Press, 1957), pp. 18–19.

3. Ibid., p. 19.

4. Arendt, *Life of the Mind*, p. 136.

5. Ibid.

6. Ibid., p. 139.

7. Arendt, *Human Condition*, p. 20.

8. Arendt, *Life of the Mind*, p. 137.

9. Ibid., pp. 137–138.

10. Ibid., p. 120.

11. For a discussion of this point see, David Michael Levin, *Modernity and the Hegemony of Vision* (California: University of California Press, 1993), p. 3.

12. Arendt, *Human Condition*, p. 325.

13. Arendt, *Life of the Mind*, p. 8.

14. Ibid., p. 165.

15. Ibid.

16. Ibid.

17. Ibid., p. 93.

18. Ibid.

19. Thucydides, *The Peloponnesian War*, trans. Rex Warner (New York: Penguin, 1954), p. 45.

20. Hannah Arendt, *Between Past and Future* (New York: Penguin, 1967), p. 214.

21. Ibid., pp. 214–215.

22. Ibid., p. 222.

23. Ibid., pp. 220.

24. Hannah Arendt, *Lectures on Kant's Political Philosophy* (Chicago: University of Chicago Press, 1982), p. 71–72.

25. Arendt, *Life of the Mind*, p. 212.

26. Ibid.

27. Ibid., p. 153.

28. Arendt, *Between Past and Future*, p. 123.

29. Martin Heidegger, *Eternal Recurrence of the Same*, trans. D. F. Krell (New York: Harper & Row, 1984), p. 57.

30. Hannah Arendt, *Men in Dark Times* (New York: Harcourt Brace Jovanovich, 1955), p. 8.

31. Ibid., p. 9.

32. Hannah Arendt, "Understanding and Politics," in *Essays in Understanding* (New York: Harcourt Brace Jovanovich, 1994), p. 319.

33. Ibid., p. 322.

13

Keeping Foucault and Derrida in Sight: Panopticism and the Politics of Subversion

David Michael Levin

What is at stake, first of all, is an adventure of vision.
—Jacques Derrida, "Force and Signification"

There are times in life when the question of knowing if one can think differently than one thinks, and perceive differently than one sees, is absolutely necessary if one is to go on looking and reflecting at all.

—Michel Foucault, *The Use of Pleasure*

Is Western culture ocularcentric? Is our culture—for example, the cultural paradigm of knowledge, truth, and reality that has prevailed since Plato—essentially vision generated, vision based, and vision centered? And has it always been so? If our answers are affirmative, what is to be said about modernity—taking this term to refer to the world that began with the Rinascimento? Is modernity ocularcentric, as Martin Heidegger suggests in his essay "Die Zeit des Weltbildes," in any historically distinctive way? What, then, is to be said of the discourse of metaphysics? Is it, and has it, too, always been, ocularcentric? Or has metaphysics functioned, rather, as a cultural counterdiscourse? If we hold that Western culture has indeed always been ocularcentric, do we not have to examine how this visualism has figured in our ethical and political life? Is there a crucial assumption implicit in all these questions, that a grand narrative of epochs is possible? And if so, should we regard such an assumption regarding the telling of history as at all intelligible and legitimate?

David Michael Levin

I am inclined to think that a compelling case can be made for the view that the history of Western culture is a history of ocularcentrism and that, in the modern age, this ocularcentrism has taken on a quite distinctive character—and equally distinctive sociocultural functions. But since I have argued for this interpretation elsewhere, I am not going to argue for it here.[1] Suffice it to say that I would like these questions to problematize epistemic and ontological assumptions that have been, and still are, at work, not only in our philosophical discourse but also in the social and cultural life-world that sustains it. And perhaps these questions will provide a useful framework for our present reading of Michel Foucault and Jacques Derrida.

The reading I wish to propose in this chapter is intended to show that both of these philosophers are convinced that the world of modernity is indeed ocularcentric, and that in the philosophical discourse of this age, in its paradigm of knowledge, truth, reason, and reality, vision—or rather, a particular type of vision, namely, vision with a character that Nietzsche would recognize, through its nihilism, as the will to power—is hegemonic. And since, for them, both this type of character and its hegemony are to be resisted, altered if possible, they engaged their writing, as our reading will show, in an immanent critique of this ocularcentrism. Thus, the philosophical discourses in which they undertook this work are strategically structured, their rhetorical forms, styles, and tropes dictated by the subversive operations of what we might call a postmetaphysical vision. In the texts we shall be considering, they deploy vision strategically—each one exemplifying his own very different way(s) of looking and seeing—in a practice of critique, resistance, and subversion: a politics of subversion.

The hegemony in question here is instituted by, and in turn reproduces, a will to power, a drive to dominate and master, which is the character-potential in vision that prevails in modern times over other, more enlightened potentials. The historical domination of this type of vision in, and as, our cultural paradigm is part of a cultural ideology that the discourse of metaphysics has not only reflected, but also, in effect, assumed it could justify. In the discourse of metaphysics, what is reflected and taken for granted is the domination of a vision of domination, the domination of a vision in which the will to power, not as the affirmation of life but as the will to dominate and master, prevails. This way of looking and seeing, and the optical vocabulary in which it figures, makes metaphysics a metaphysics of presence: a discourse that subjects the presencing of beings, and even the presencing of the being—the inherently open ground, context, and field—of these beings, to reification, reduction, and totalization.

The writings with which we are concerned are on the threshold, the borderline, of another *episteme*, one in which the assumptions of metaphysics—its imperative re-presentation of presencing, its enframing, its totalization and reification of the ground—are no longer compelling, and different possibilities can be explored. This, we might say, is their postmodernism: not at all an absolute or complete break with the past but rather a certain freedom, a freedom achieved through the continuation and persistence of the same self-critical reflectivity that has been from the very beginning constitutive of the spirit of modernity.

In this chapter, we will reflect on certain strategic movements beyond metaphysics as they figure in the philosophical discourses of Derrida and Foucault. More specifically, we will begin to give thought to the experiences with vision—experiences with gazes and glances, moments of insight and blindness, lightness and darkness, visibility and invisibility, grounds, horizons, centers, margins, and frames—that figure in their writings.

Perhaps the entire history of philosophical thinking in the Western world, and indeed, more generally, the entire history of Western culture, has been dominated by vision and a discourse of vision. Although I appreciate the current reluctance to formulate grand narratives of history, I am inclined to believe this narrative interpretation to be true—or say, at the very least, a useful construction. And, according to my reading, Foucault and Derrida, perhaps influenced by Heidegger, would concur. But in any case, I think it would be difficult to deny that the culture of modernity, and the philosophical discourse that has taken place

David Michael Levin

within it, are not only ocularcentric—not only dominated by vision and a paradigm of knowledge, truth, and reality that is vision generated, vision based, and vision centered—but also, in contrast to preceding periods in history, ocularcentric in a distinctively modern way (in accordance with the possibilities and imperatives of late capitalism and its advanced technology) and in terms of a vision with a distinctively modern character (as enframing or, say, reifying and totalizing).

Although I am not going to press the point here, since I have argued for it elsewhere, I do want to suggest that because of the technology-driven economy which prevails in the modern world, ocularcentrism became much more pervasive and much more powerful than it was in earlier times, and that, in keeping with the egocentric, possessive individualism of modernity, the will to power, the will, that is, to dominate, that had always been a latent but very strong predisposition already operative in the very nature of vision, took possession of vision and suppressed other potentialities (e.g., the capacity to be touched and moved by what is seen, what is given to our beholding), so that the character of the vision that became hegemonic turned increasingly willful, and therefore, too, increasingly totalizing and reifying. In the modern period, this ocularcentrism, centering, grounding, and enframing us in a vision of power that alternates between the sovereign position of an outside spectator and the engaged position of a strictly instrumental optics, contributed to the hegemony of a sociocultural paradigm that until very recently subordinated epistemology and ontology to the will to power as the will to dominate and master. The philosophical gaze has always taken pride in its theoretical detachment, its abstractness, its ability to remain untouched and unmoved by what it sees, what it is given to behold. In modern times, it also takes pride in its empiricism, its extensions of the empire of science and technology.

The domination of a vision with this character—the circulation and reproduction of such a vision within our culture—has also made a difference, and continues to make a difference, in the relations of power that structure the public and private spaces of our social interactions. In every social interaction, relations of power, and consequently relations structured by the politics of vision, are involved. All too often, our way of looking at others subjects them to a gaze bent on domination; similarly the numerous administrative extensions of this vision subject people to the visibility of a dominating visual regime. If we are willing to look at our world with care and thought, we will see it as we have made it. We will see that, and also how, the distinctive character of our modern vision has made a world that manifests and reflects this very same character. In other words, if the world that we see around us, when we look at it with a critical gaze, manifests and reflects aspects that appear wrathful, we should take the opportunity to look into the ways in which the character of our vision may be responsible for this condition. In the first instance, responsibility is the exercising of an ability to be responsive. It is a question of our response-ability. When the objects of our gaze look back at us, it is possible to see how our way of looking at them has affected them, making them how we see them, making them what they eventually become. Moreover, as Nietzsche pointed out in *Beyond Good and Evil,* "Whoever fights monsters should see to it that in the process he does not himself become a monster. When you look long into an abyss, the abyss also looks back into you."[2]

Having understood the necessity of a critique of the metaphysics of presence, Foucault and Derrida inscribe and trace the effects, if not also the activity, of a postmetaphysical vision, a way of seeing in which there is a different, historically novel Gestalt formation: the deconstruction of the structural moment, constituted by the simultaneous coemergence of a sovereign subject and its other, takes place in the sites of sight, to the extent that the visionary subject—an individual, a group, or an institution of the state—accepts a different relationship to presence and absence, the visible and the invisible, and the framing of the ground, within the fields of its exercise.

In the realm of perception, the hegemony of a vision of willful character, a vision driven by the will to dominate and master, enframes the field of its exercise in an essentially futile effort to reify and totalize the contextual situation. Instead of letting the ground or field be what and as it is, a dynamically opening openness, this vision is driven by the impossible desire—for the most part unconscious—to end the withdrawal of the horizon and reduce the ground or field to a controllable figure or object presenting itself with clarity and distinctness at the center of focus.

Among other things, what is at stake in this movement beyond metaphysics—beyond the metaphysical appropriation of vision— is the possibility that the subject can enter into a different visual structure, a different visual Gestalt. This freedom would involve a different relationship to the figure that forms at the center of focus; but it would also require, at the same time, since this figure and its (back)ground are interdependent, a different engagement with the (back)ground, the context, the field: a different way of acknowledging the presence-absence of the ground, a different relationship, therefore, to the delimiting horizon, and also a different way of framing.

If, in the philosophical discourse of our time, the movement beyond metaphysics is a movement that simultaneously contests the absolute sovereignty of the center, the absolute authority of the frame, and the absolute grounding originality of the ground, this movement, effecting subversions within the spacing of the text, must also take place outside the boundaries that have separated this discourse from its sociocultural context—in all the different sites, say, where our sight takes place, and in fact is bound to take place. It is accordingly not surprising, then, that in the writing of their texts, Foucault and Derrida demonstrate visions in which center, ground, and frame—and thus, also, the interaction between the subject and its other—are differently articulated, differently structured, differently functioning.

I shall argue, however, that in the texts of Foucault and Derrida, the poststructuralist revisions of metaphysics, revisions that in each case attempt to structure in a process of end-less deconstruction, are interestingly different from one another: two quite different ways of differing from, and deferring, the reifications and totalizations that metaphysical visions always impose.

The discourse of metaphysics is a discourse of grounds, a discourse that has always been determined, in one way or another, by a grounding principle or a principle that calls for grounds. Therefore, one way to challenge this metaphysics is to effect a certain displacement of the principle, citing/siting it within the context of visual experience, interpreting the "ground" in question as the ground that figures in the formation of the visual Gestalt. Shifting the context, the ground for this "ground," by translating it outside the discourse of metaphysics, makes it easier to break the spell of reification and totalization, the spelling of total presence. The translation of this problematic from the discourse of metaphysics into a discourse of vision permits the articulation of a certain *mise-en-abime* that subverts the historical authority of metaphysical representations of the ground; furthermore, this translation cites/sites vision in frame-breaching positions, thus deploying vision—or rather a certain kind of vision—precisely to deconstruct a history of ocularcentrism, the historical hegemony of vision.

Dictated by masterful visions, the discourse of metaphysics is an archive of representations. Now, representation is re-presentation: the subject's deferral of what presences in order to present it again, but this time on the subject's terms, according to the subject's sovereign will. Representation is therefore a strategy for achieving the mastery and domination of a presence, or say a presencing, the contextual openness of which cannot ultimately in fact be mastered and controlled. Both Foucault and Derrida write against the hegemony of representation, seeing in this paradigm an attempt to take control of the ground: to dictate the frame, and all the other terms of the encounter, that make domination of the ground possible. However, they suggest very different—though complementary—ways to breach representational enframing and problematize the reified, totalized presence that representation imposes on the openness, the abyssal originality and end-lessness of the ground. If structuralism is defined as the metaphysical reification and totalization of structure, then they may be read as proposing different but closely related ways of looking beyond the metaphysics of structuralism.

As critics of structuralism, a school of thought with a long history of complicity in the hegemony of representation, both

David Michael Levin

philosophers exhibit ways of exercising, or practicing, their capacity for vision that make major contributions not only to the current critical discourse on modernity, but also to current efforts to think ourselves beyond the metaphysical culture, the metaphysical politics of modernity.

The hegemony of a vision driven by the will to power as the will to dominate and master is not at all restricted to the discourse of philosophy, where it installed a metaphysics of presence; the historical domination of vision is also manifest in, and as, a politics of domination, a politics of presence. To be mastered, all beings, and the very being of beings, must be made constantly visible, constantly present, ready to hand. Thus the politics that is allied with the metaphysics of presence is a politics of invisible surveillance, disciplinary regimes of supervision, the totalitarian administration and authoritarian control of vision and visibility. Panopticism.

I have suggested that both Derrida and Foucault make use of vision in a critique of vision. Thus, we must see that there is a potential in our vision that is opposed to the potential that our modern age has tended for the most part to realize. Our vision also has an emancipatory, or utopian, potential: a potential as a way of contributing to processes of enlightenment. In the reading I am proposing here, Derrida and Foucault each put into writing, in the spirit of the Enlightenment, their own versions of a Kantian critique of (the philosophical vision of) reason and a Kantian critique of (the) reason (in vision). In effect, they not only practice a politics of subversion, using vision itself to resist the willful character of vision, its dreams and images of domination, its ethics, its politics of violence, its metaphysics of presence; they also use their vision to examine the limits and antinomies of vision—and the rationality of vision with this type of character.

Derrida: Ocularcentrism in the Discourse of Metaphysics

After declaring, in words positioned at the beginning of "Force and Signification," a text first published in 1963, that "what is at stake, first of all, is an adventure of vision," Derrida proceeds to articulate a powerful critique of structuralism, targeting "the privilege given to vision" and challenging the "metaphysical eye."[3]

Writing still in the shadows of the Holocaust—the text is haunted by its ghosts, touched and illumined by its flames, disfigured and blinded by its traces—Derrida casts this critique against the historical background of the Enlightenment, the great project of Reason as a natural light. The fateful error consists in the forgetting of force. Seduced by the visualism of thought, we have become obsessed with form, signification, and have ignored events of force, the force of events.

Behind structuralism there is a seemingly harmless desire to impose order and overcome the forces of anarchy that are destroying regularity and conformity of meaning. However, for Derrida, this program is not at all innocent. For structuralism is the project of an unmovable "gaze" that not only totalizes and reifies all that it sees but avoids responsibility for its work of domination. Calling the metaphysics that has given rise to this program "heliocentric," a "photology," and observing that "in this heliocentric metaphysics, force, ceding its place to *eidos* (i.e., the form which is visible for the metaphorical eye), has already been separated from itself in acoustics," Derrida asks: "How can force or weakness be understood in terms of light and dark?"[4]

There is no question, however, about the importance of resisting the language of light. It is difficult, he concedes, "to maintain a discourse against light."[5] But we must nevertheless attempt our "emancipation," our release from its domination. For Derrida, although it is possible to resist the metaphysics of light, we cannot escape its force field.[6] In order to understand "force"— understand, that is, its form or structure—without falling into reductionism, "we would have to attempt a return to the metaphor of darkness and light (of self-revelation and self-concealment), the founding metaphor of Western philosophy as metaphysics.... [For] the entire history of our philosophy is a photology, the name given to a history of, or a treatise on, light."[7]

David Michael Levin

All that one can do, it seems, is problematize the discourse, contesting wherever possible the hegemony of its metaphors— metaphors that have dominated our culture and made of it, despite the Enlightenment, a culture of domination.

The history of this century cannot be overlooked. Forces of hellish violence were unleashed, and they compel our attention. "Force and Signification" is a response to the events we have seen and witnessed. Thus Derrida points out, near the beginning of his essay, that "structuralism is perceived ... at the moment when immanent danger concentrates our vision on the keystone of an institution, the stone which encapsulates both the possibility and the fragility of its existence."[8] Aimed not only at structuralism but also at the discursive field that authorizes it— the field constituted by the vision of metaphysics and the metaphysics of vision—these words suggest the sense in which Derrida's critique boldly stakes out a position with important political implications.

In 1964, a year later, Derrida's "Violence and Metaphysics" appeared in print, a complex meditation on the work of Emmanuel Levinas. In this essay, Derrida undertook a close reading of his friend's thought, a reading that enabled him to continue his own critical reflections on the violence at work in a metaphysics "unable to escape its ancestry in light."[9] (One of the sections of his text bears as its title "The Violence of Light." In 1963, Foucault's *The Birth of the Clinic* appeared, examining in detail what he calls the "majestic violence of light." Coincidence? Synchronicity? Whatever the truth, I note that, for Foucault, this "violence" apparently can be beneficent and progressive, as well as malevolent, for it "brings to an end the bounded, dark kingdom of privileged knowledge" and establishes the more democratic authority of the empirical sciences. In *Discipline and Punish*, a much later work, it is, however, the malevolence of light, used for social control, which finally prevails.)[10]

Derrida examines Levinas's critique of "theoretism," the "imperialism of *theoria*," which he thinks has dominated our cultural world from the very beginning.[11] I would say that Levinas's analysis is similar to, and probably indebted to, the analysis of visualism and theory proposed by Heidegger in "Science and Reflection" (1954) and "The Question Concerning Technology" (also 1954), although Levinas, unlike Heidegger, concentrated his thought on the ethical dimension of the problematic. According to Derrida, Levinas sees "a Greco-Platonic tradition under the surveillance of the agency of the glance and the metaphor of light."[12] In question, for Levinas, is (in Derrida's words) a "heliopolitics," "the ancient, clandestine friendship between light and power, the ancient complicity between theoretical objectivity and technicopolitical possession."[13]

For Levinas, Husserl's phenomenology, under the spell of visualism, unwittingly practices a "transcendental violence," a violence that is most apparent in his descriptions of my experience of others. To make the other an "alter ego" is, according to Levinas, to reduce the other to the same—a violation of the absolute alterity of the other. The problem, as Levinas sees it, is that for a metaphysics that depends on the luminous self-evidence of intuition to resolve the questions generated by purely theoretical reflection, it is inevitable that "everything given to me within the light appears as given to myself by myself."[14] What this means when translated onto the terrain of politics is, as Levinas sees it, all too clear: fascism—authoritarian and totalitarian rule, subjects lost in a "collective representation," a world where "the social ideal will be sought in an ideal of fusion."[15]

Derrida is not unmoved by the dangers Levinas sees, nor does he entirely disagree with Levinas's arguments regarding the historical violence of light and the ocularcentrism of Western metaphysics. However, he wants to insist that "it is difficult to maintain a discourse against light."[16] "How," he asks, "will the metaphysics of the face as the epiphany of the other free itself of light? ... Light perhaps has no opposite."[17] More specifically, he disputes Levinas's claim that as a theoretical intuition under the domination of visualism, Husserlian intentionality can only impose the principle of adequation onto our encounters with one another. Thus, Derrida here defends Husserl against the charge that the requirement of self-evidence "would exhaust and interiorize all distance and all true alterity."[18] While conceding that Husserl's position is, at many points, virtually undecidable, and that it sometimes seems to come very close to an unacceptable idealism—what Foucault, in *The Order of Things,* called "transcendental narcissism"—Derrida nevertheless comes to Husserl's defense: "Who was more obstinately determined than Husserl to show that vision is originally and essentially the inadequation of interiority and exteriority? And that the perception of the transcendent and extended thing is essentially and forever incomplete?"[19] He might also have pointed out here that it is actually, after all, to Husserl that the critical analysis of visualism, theoretism, and objectivism that Heidegger and Levinas elaborate, each in his own way, and in part against Husserl, is principally indebted.

In the final analysis, one cannot definitively position Derrida in relation to the problematic Levinas formulates. In my interpretation of the text, it may at least be said that Derrida is convinced of the need to submit the ocularcentric paradigm that figures in the discourse of metaphysics to the interruptions, the strategic pressures and solicitations, of deconstructive readings. There can be no doubt that Derrida sees this discourse to be vision generated, vision based, and vision centered and that he recognized certain dangers in this paradigm-dominance. The omnipotence of the author, the origin of his authority, is related to the omnipresence of the eye. And this is the eye that desires an ontology reduced to a totalized, reified presence.

In *Speech and Phenomena: Introduction to the Problem of Signs in Husserl's Phenomenology* (1967), Derrida's position seems more determinate. Here he displays Husserl's ocularcentrism and submits the phenomenology in Husserl's texts to the disintegrating operations of deconstruction. In the course of formulating a critique of Husserl's phenomenology of language—of, in particular, his theory of meaning—Derrida demonstrates how Husserl's visualism commits him to a metaphysics of presence that is at odds with the intentionality and temporality he himself was the first to disclose.

In concluding this work, Derrida declares that "the thing itself always escapes." Thus, "contrary to the assurance that Husserl gives us . . . , 'the look' cannot 'abide.' "[20] This summarizes Derrida's critique of Husserl, a critical reading in which he displays Husserl's ocularcentrism and subjects the phenomenology in Husserl's texts to the disintegrating operations of deconstruction.

Derrida notes that, in his *Cartesian Meditations*, Husserl stated his intention to "exclude all 'metaphysical adventure', all speculative excesses" (sec. 60). But Derrida's critical reading of the text is a solicitation that brings out Husserl's ocularcentrism, his own speculative excesses—or, rather, reading him, as Derrida does, from a different point of view, a different slant, that this critical reading brings excesses to the light that Husserl never suspected: excesses that ironically were set in motion by the very metaphorics of vision on which Husserl thought he could depend in order precisely to exclude them.

According to Derrida, the texts of Husserl's transcendental phenomenology are constituted, saturated, by the metaphorical vocabulary of an ocularcentrism that continues the historical hegemony, here in the West, of an ancient metaphysics of presence—a metaphysics for which mastery of sense, control over meaning, and domination of the totality are of the essence.

Thus, in *Speech and Phenomena*, Derrida argues against the primacy of "perception" in Husserl's sense of the term, contending that the embeddedness of the act of perception in its situation, its context, its circumstantial field, will always deny perception its metaphysical claims—not only to absolute finality but also to absolute originality. The advent of perception is always dependent on the "convenience" of a preceding interpretation, a sense of the field, a clearing or opening, later called "différance," that is always already laid down for it, and that this perception, never simultaneous with the opening up of the field, always too late (*nachträglich*) for that, can never retrieve and master. "There never was any 'perception,'" he says, "and 'presentation' is a representation of the representation that yearns for itself therein as for its own birth or death."[21] What is called "an act of perception" is merely an artifact, a conceptual construction. No matter how early one attends to such an "act," a phenomenology free of metaphysical agendas compels one to admit that the event has always already taken place in a time that eludes meta-physical mastery.

This position is elaborated in a footnote, where we read: "In affirming that perception does not exist, or that what is called perception is not primordial, that somehow everything 'begins' by 're-presentation' (a proposition which can only be maintained by the elimination of these last two concepts: it means that there is no 'beginning' and that the 'representation' we were talking about is not the modification of a 're-' that has *befallen* a primordial presentation) and by reintroducing the difference involved in 'signs' at the core of what is 'primordial', we do not retreat from the level of transcendental phenomenology toward either an 'empiricism' or a 'kantian' critique of the claim to enjoy primordial intuition."[22] Instead, we move in the direction (*sens*) of a much more radical deconstruction of the metaphysics implicit in perception: a deconstruction set in motion by our acknowledgment of the temporality constitutive of all perceptual experience.

Thus, in a chapter bearing the title "Signs and the Blink of an Eye," Derrida maintains that "as soon as we admit the continuity of the now and the not-now, perception and nonperception, in the zone of primordiality common to primordial impression and primordial retention, we admit the other into the self-identity of the *Augenblick*; nonpresence and nonevidence are admitted into the *blink of an instant*. There is a duration to the blink, and it closes the eye. This alterity is in fact the condition for presence, presentation, and thus for *Vorstellung* in general."[23] The domination, the mastery of the field that Husserl claims for his ocularcentric phenomenology, is thus subverted by something he failed to see: the blink of an instant, a closure that denies constant surveillance, abolishes continuous possession, and opens the field that the eye had vainly tried to delimit to all that is its other. This blink, for Husserl as for Descartes, functions, in the production of their texts, as a sort of "blind spot." What Derrida enables us to see is that, and also how, in each case, there is, as he says of Rousseau, a text, a "system" of writing and reading, "which we know is ordered around its own blind spot."[24]

Continuing his reflections on Husserl in "Form and Meaning: A Note on the Phenomenology of Language" (also published in 1967), Derrida examines Husserl's concepts of intuition, self-evidence, and apodeicticity and notes that "the metaphysical domination of the concept of form [*morphe, eidos*] is bound to occasion some submission to sight. This submission always would be a submission of sense to sight, of sense to the sense-of-vision.... One could elaborate the implications of such a placing-on-view."[25] Here he explicitly connects the domination of a metaphysics of presence to the hegemony of vision in our paradigm of knowledge, truth, and reality, problematizing this metaphysics by challenging the authority of a vision-generated, vision-centered theory of meaning.

Of Grammatology, first published, like all the other texts we have considered so far, in 1967, also gives some attention to the problem of visual hegemony. For example, in a section entitled "Writing before the Letter," Derrida calls our attention to "the field of vision" that "a certain concept of the sign" and "a certain concept of the relationship between speech and writing" have "controlled for a few millennia."[26] And he declares it his project, there, to effect what he terms a "dislocation" in, and also of, the discourse of vision that has determined philosophical thinking since Plato.

What disturbs him is the privilege given to speech: a privilege that we might consider to be peculiarly ironic, if not indeed paradoxical—since it is only writing, and not speech, that must address, and submit to, the desire of the gaze for presence—but that we would have expected him to explain, not only by noting our questionable assumptions about the immediacy and presence of face-to-face speech, but also by pointing out that it is precisely because our thinking is dominated by vision, bedazzled by a vision of absolute presence, that we have persisted in these assumptions, and therefore in this privileging of speech. A strong case can be made, as I think Heidegger has shown,[27] to support the argument that the dominance of vision has seduced us into the delusions of power, the narcissistic delusions of omnipotence and omniscience, that are enshrined in our metaphysics—an ancient "metaphysics," as Derrida calls it, "of presence."

According to Heidegger's reading of the history of metaphysics, it is vision, with its power to survey, to encompass and
comprehend, as a totality, a field of simultaneously co-present
objects, that seduces us into the fatal delusions of this metaphysics, convincing us that totalization—total visibility, total
clarity, total presence, total determinacy, total control over
meaning—is not only desirable but actually possible. Thus one
would have expected Derrida to argue that it is precisely this
vision-generated metaphysics that compels us to privilege speech,
for we have somehow become convinced—as Derrida points out,
Plato is perhaps the first to have formulated the argument—that
in the face-to-face immediacy of speech a full presence of meaning is actually possible, whereas in the case of writing, a use of
language from which the author is always eventually, and therefore essentially absent, this presence cannot, of course, be
assumed.

It could thus be argued that even the metaphysical prioritizing
of *phone* (sound, voice, speech) is actually motivated by an attachment to vision: that it is precisely a certain way of seeing, a
seeing the character of which is dominated by ocularcentrism,
which has led philosophers to favor speech over writing, despite
the fact that it is writing which addresses, which appeals to, the
eyes. What this argument suggests is that, strange as it may seem,
to prioritize writing and show its disseminative operations would
be, in effect, to subvert the metaphysics of presence, using the
eyes as witnesses for the prosecution, getting them to betray their
own power—and also their "blind spots," "the not-seen that
[simultaneously] opens and limits visibility."[28]

It is vision, with its power to survey, to encompass and comprehend, as a totality, a field of simultaneously co-present objects,
that seduces us into the fatal delusions of metaphysics, convincing us that totalization—total visibility, total clarity, total presence, total determinacy, total control over meaning—is not only
desirable but actually possible. And we become convinced that
in the face-to-face immediacy of speech, but not in writing, the
ideal projected by our visual metaphysics—the ideal of a full
presence of meaning—is actually possible. Given this history, the

priority that Derrida has accorded to writing makes good sense. Showing the disseminative operations of writing does work to subvert the metaphysics of presence, requiring eyes bent on domination to read texts that have been deliberately constructed to catch the eyes with their optical properties—an opticality that resists and betrays their will to power.

In fact, however, Derrida's analysis, worded in a way that leaves his meaning exceedingly confusing, seems on one reading to subordinate ocularcentrism to phonocentrism, ascribing primacy to the latter in accounting for the interpretation of being as presence; but on another reading, to think the two together, as factors both responsible for, and yet also accorded "legitimation" by, the historical determination of being as presence. He says:

Phonocentrism merges with the historical determination of the meaning of being in general as *presence*, with all the subdeterminations which depend on this general form and which organize within it their system and their historical sequence (presence of the thing to the sight as *eidos*, presence as substance/essence/existence (*ousia*), temporal presence as point (*stigme*) of the now or of the moment (*nun*), the self-presence of the cogito, consciousness, subjectivity, the co-presence of the other and the self, intersubjectivity as the intentional phenomenon of the ego, and so forth). Logocentrism would thus support the determination of the being of this entity as presence.[29]

The problem with both these interpretations, however, is that they do not propose any account of what we might call, after Nietzsche and Foucault, the "genealogy" of the discourse of presence. All Derrida seems willing to say, in the passage quoted above, is that somehow phonocentrism, logocentrism, and ocularcentrism are all crucially implicated in the historical determination of being as presence: "implicated," that is, in a sense that leaves mysteriously unanswered the historical question that Heidegger's work was the first to formulate and the first, also, to attempt to answer: How (why) did the meaning of being eventually receive its historical determination as presence in the discourse of metaphysics? What, in other words, accounts for the imposition of this determination?

David Michael Levin

Since Heidegger himself attempted to answer this question, Derrida's reticence and vagueness are all the more surprising. To be sure, this was, for Heidegger, an extremely difficult question; but as early as 1929, in a lecture entitled "Was ist Metaphysik?" he was already using the vocabulary of his phenomenological hermeneutics to elaborate the ocularcentric genealogy of Western metaphysics.[30] And in 1935, in an important series of lectures that were published in 1953 under the title *An Introduction to Metaphysics*, this analysis was continued and amplified. In fact, Heidegger carried forward this narrative account in many other subsequent texts, among which some of the texts published in *The End of Philosophy* ("Metaphysics as History of Being" and "Sketches for a History of Being as Metaphysics") are perhaps of special significance.

I think it can be argued that Derrida's critique of the philosophical privileging of *phone*, the immediacy of voice and the presence of speech, is based on his seeing the paradoxical fact that this prioritizing is actually ocularcentric: vision generated and vision motivated. For it is a certain way of seeing, a vision hegemonized by an ocularcentric paradigm of knowledge, truth, and reality, a vision of completeness and permanence, that has (mis)led philosophers to value speech over writing, despite the fact that writing is *for the eyes*. Once the vision of these eyes has been internalized, withdrawn into the inner light of the mind, where it is transformed into the "I see" of understanding, it is readily confused with the sound of inner speech—and with the truthful voice of reason.[31] Derrida's insistence on writing, and on the necessity for philosophy to acknowledge its being-written, its being-as-writing—an insistence on the visual appeal of philosophical thought—is actually a strategically effective way for him to deconstruct the ocularcentrism of philosophy. In a double bind, he always deploys a paradoxical, ironic, double gesture. He uses (his) writing to appeal (in both senses of this term) to our vision, only to seduce it into acknowledging dissemination, invisibility, absence, alterity—vision's failure to achieve metaphysical totalization and plenitude.

A crucial text we shall be considering to determine Derrida's position with regard to ocularcentrism and metaphysics is "White Mythology: Metaphor in the Text of Philosophy," first published in 1971. The English translation of this text has been included in *Margins of Philosophy* (1982), which begins with a short text bearing the title "Tympan." In beginning this text, Derrida promises that "we will analyze the metaphysical exchange, the circular complicity of the metaphors of the eye and the ear."[32] And indeed he does, particularly in "White Mythology," which is, as the subtitle indicates, an examination—a deconstructive reading—of philosophical texts, focusing attention on how philosophical discourse has made use of metaphorical language—how metaphors function, how they work, or rather play, within the architecture of this discourse.

Here is how, at the beginning of his essay, Derrida's formulates his concern. He wants to reflect, he says, on "the white mythology which reassembles and reflects the culture of the West: the white man takes his own mythology, Indo-European mythology, his own *logos*, that is, the *mythos* of his idiom, for the universal form of that he must still wish to call Reason."[33] Derrida's deconstruction of this mythology, this discourse, may thus be read as a political act, a gesture of defiance aimed at locating and remarking the continuing traces of our ethnocentrism, our racism, our colonialism insofar as they still figure in the metaphorics that carries our philosophical thought.

As we shall see, however, this "white mythology" also refers to all the "heliotropes," all the metaphorics of sun and light, vision and visibility, around which our metaphysics has been constituted: "The very opposition of appearing and disappearing, the entire lexicon of the *phainesthai*, of *aletheia*, of day and night, of the visible and the invisible, of the present and the absent—all this is possible only under the sun."[34]

Following Heidegger's example, Derrida proposes, then, to examine some of the "founding" concepts. Naming *theoria*, *eidos*, and *logos*, all of them concepts that Heidegger had studied before him and had connected to the historical privilege of sight,

Derrida adds this comment, with his characteristically dry humor: "And let us not insist upon the optic metaphor that opens up every theoretical point of view under the sun."[35]

Returning, like Heidegger, to the work of Plato, Derrida notes that "in *The Republic* (VI–VII), before and after the Line which presents ontology according to the analogies of proportionality, the Sun appears. In order to disappear. It is there, but as the invisible source of light, in a kind of insistent eclipse, more than essential, producing the essence—Being and appearing—of what is. One looks at it directly on pain of blindness and death. Keeping itself beyond all that which is, it figures the Good of which the sensory sun is the son: the source of life and visibility, of seed and light."[36]

"This metaphorics," he says, "is of course articulated in a specific syntax; but as a metaphorics, it belongs to a more general syntax, to a more extended system that equally constrains platonism; everything is illuminated by this system's sun, the sun of absence and presence, blinding and luminous, dazzling."[37] Here he articulates what looks like, and what one might easily take to be, a "real connection" between the heliotropes around which the discourse of metaphysics (unquestionably) turns and the obsession of this discourse with the goodness, the truth, and the beauty of presence—the light of presence and the presence of light. (But of course "real connections" are as problematic as their opposite, and Derrida's vision ceaselessly slips back and forth between "literal" and "figurative" senses of "vision," problematizing the textual boundaries with which metaphysics has always protected and consoled itself.)

Without disputing the heliocentrism and ocularcentrism of metaphysics, Derrida will argue, however, that, contrary to first appearances, the logic of this sun-and-light-centered discourse does not in fact entail, or necessitate, a metaphysics of presence—on the contrary, the more one thinks about the matter, the more one will be compelled to acknowledge that the logic of this metaphorics actually resists, and even subverts, the possibility of presence.[38] Thus he asks us to reflect on the phenomenology actually implicit in the logic of this metaphorics: "Presence disappearing in its own radiance, the hidden source of light, of truth, and of meaning, the erasure of the visage of Being—such must be the insistent return of that which subjects metaphysics to metaphor."[39] Here we can see Derrida's deconstructive strategy at work—that is, at play: he uses the metaphorics of light to deconstruct the metaphysics of presence, that very presence that the visual generation of metaphyics has been thought to support. If this is a Hegelian *Aufhebung*, it is a sublation with a mischievous, chiasmic twist: "la métaphysique—relève de la métaphore."[40]

According to Derrida, it must of course be recognized that

the tenor of the dominant metaphor will return always to the major signified of ontotheology: the circle of the heliotrope. Certainly the metaphors of light and the circle, which are so important in Descartes, are not organized as they are in Plato or Aristotle, in Hegel or Husserl. But if we put ourselves at the most critical and properly Cartesian point of the critical procedure, at the point of hyperbolic doubt and the hypothesis of the Evil Genius, at the point when doubt strikes not only ideas of sensory origin but also 'clear and distinct' ideas and what is mathematically self-evident, we know that what permits the discourse to be picked up and pursued, its ultimate resource, is designated as *lumen naturale*. Natural light, and all the axioms it brings into our field of vision, is never subjected to the most radical doubt. The latter unfolds *in* light.[41]

(One is reminded here of Heidegger's contention that we tend not to notice the circumambient lighting, the being of the light itself and as such, a light that is the lighting of being, but see only the beings that this lighting makes visible.)

Derrida attempts to establish that "the determination of the truth of Being in presence passes through the detour of this tropic system. The presence of *ousia* as *eidos* (to be placed before the metaphorical eye) or as *hypokeimenon* (to underlie visible phenomena or accidents) faces the theoretical organ; which, as Hegel's *Aesthetics* reminds us, has the power not to consume what it perceives and to let be the object of desire. Philosophy, as a theory of metaphor, first will have been a metaphor of theory.

David Michael Levin

This circulation has not excluded but, on the contrary, has permitted and provoked, the transformation of presence into self-presence, into the proximity or properness of subjectivity to and for itself."[42]

Derrida is not the first philosopher to remind us that metaphysics uses and depends on metaphors, but he is perhaps the first one to call attention to the subversive implications, using one of the favorite tropes to make his point: just as the sun, the source of light, hides itself, can become invisible and elude our efforts at mastering the power of its light, so all metaphors are ultimately going to be disruptive of and resistant to the impulse behind metaphysics—its drive to "dominate" presence through intuition ("vision or contact"), concept (the mental eye's "grasping" of the signified), and consciousness ("proximity or self-presence").[43] And if all metaphors transgress the "proper meaning" of words, establishing affinities that are never more than partially "appropriate," and, in general, introduce uncontrollable semantic play into the discursive field, then metaphors of light and vision will be doubly disruptive and resistant: "this supplement of a code [is one] which traverses its own field, endlessly displaces its closure, breaks its line, opens its circle, and no ontology will have been able to [master or] reduce it."[44]

For Derrida, then, metaphysics is indeed ocularcentric. And he contests this encoding of the discourse, just as he will contest all forms of domination—hence, all frames and margins, all centers and totalities. He also believes that metaphysics has been, and still is, written under the authoritarian spell of presence, and that this too must be questioned and contested. But what he shows is that the metaphorical code cannot be reduced—not even by metaphysics—to any essentially fixated ontology. Thus, the use of a vocabulary generated by light and vision, far from supporting a metaphysics of presence, will actually negate its very possibility. He suggests, moreover, that our metaphysics, though proud of its generation by light and vision, conveniently forgets and conceals its production through writing, a technology specifically constituted by and for light and vision. Consequently, Derrida's strategy is to use his own writing—the visibility of a writing, a medium expressly ordered and encoded for the eyes to see and read—in order to force metaphysics out into the open, so that we can see, exemplified in his own writing, just how *écriture* inevitably problematizes the (authoritarian) presence of meaning, making visible its disseminations, disruptions, decenterings, and slippages—and therefore just why the very fact that metaphysics is written spells out the impossibility of such presence. In this way, deploying the metaphorics of light in a "double gesture," he forces the eyes to see—or rather, "see," with scare-quotes, since it is precisely a question, here, of a certain "blind spot," the "not-seen"—that to which, in their insolent assumption of an ocularcentric ontology and epistemology, they have for too long been blind: neither the encoding of metaphysics in writing, nor the privileging of the eyes in the discourse written for them, can give support to this presence—and to the authoritarian, totalitarian politics that accompanies its rule. Although it is a vision—a vision, let us say, of the open— that opens the discourse of metaphysics, this opening is always also a closure, a self-limiting of the visibility of the visibile. This closure is its blind spot: and precisely this is repeated in the foreshadowing of a dark political state, a place that is a nonplace: an Attica, for example, or a gulag, or even worse, an Auschwitz.

It is to call attention, then, to this blind spot that Derrida introduces the concept of 'supplementarity,' signifying that which, when acknowledged, thoroughly alters the visual field in which its recognition places it: "The concept of the supplement is a sort of blind spot ..., the not-seen that opens and limits visibility."[45] But if "blindness to the supplement is the law,"[46] then it is on the exclusionary essence of the law that our attention should be critically focused. Laws can be changed. And the principle for reflecting on them and altering them is a principle of reason: a principle of practical reason that opens the eyes to that which lies beyond its present horizons.

In 1983, in a lecture at Cornell University, "The Principle of Reason: The University in the Eyes of the Pupil," Derrida continued his ruminations. "Metaphysics," he said, "associates sight with knowledge.... We give preference to sensing 'through the eyes' not only for taking action, but even when we have no praxis in view. This one sense, naturally theoretical and contemplative, goes beyond practical usefulness and provides us with more to know than any other; indeed, it unveils countless differences. We give preference to sight just as we give preference to the uncovering of difference."[47] But then he asked, thinking about "knowing how to learn and learning how to know," "Is sight enough?" Answering his own question, he joined in a debate comparing the virtues of seeing with those of listening, a quarrel much older, as Hans Blumenberg has documented it, than that between the Ancients and the Moderns,[48] and declared that "we must also know how to hear, and to listen. I might suggest somewhat playfully that we have to know how to shut our eyes in order to be better listeners."[49]

Derrida then proceeds to argue, agreeing with Heidegger, that "the modern dominance of the principle of reason had to go hand in hand with the interpretation of the essence of beings as objects, an object present as representation (*Vorstellung*), an object placed and positioned *before* a subject. This latter, a man who says 'I', an ego certain of itself, thus ensures his own technical mastery over the totality of what is.... But this dominance of the 'being-before' does not *reduce* to that of sight or of *theoria*, nor even to that of a metaphor of the optical ... dimension. It is in *Der Satz vom Grund* that Heidegger states all his reservations on the very presuppositions of such rhetoricizing interpretations. It is not a matter of distinguishing here between sight and non-sight, but rather between two ways of *thinking* of sight and of light."[50]

This textual passage calls for comment. It must be observed that Derrida does not deny here the dominance of visualism, nor does he deny that visualism has played a role in the formation of metaphysics. Rather, all that he denies is that this formation can be reduced to visualism, or totally explained by it. Like Heidegger, he rejects oversimplifications. The final sentence supports this reading, refusing both the reduction to visualism and the total denial of visualism.

But this leaves us with a question: what are the two ways of thinking of sight and light? What are these ways? Derrida's answer is deeply encrypted, but we do get some hints: (1) when he adds, in his next sentence, that "it is true that a caricature of representational man, in the heideggerian sense, would readily endow him with hard eyes permanently open to a nature that he is to dominate, to rape if necessary, by fixing it in front of himself, or by swooping down on it like a bird of prey";[51] (2) when, in the sentence following, he asserts that the principle of reason "installs its empire only to the extent that the abyssal question of the being that is hiding within it remains hidden, and with it the question of the grounding of the ground itself";[52] (3) when, nearing the end of the lecture, he briefly indicates his vision of the university, seeing it not only as a place that gives time for reflection but as a place that gives time for a reflection willing to turn back, "in all the senses of that word," on the very conditions of reflection, thereby looking at itself, at its way of looking at things; and (4) when, finally, he speaks in favor of the *Augenblick*, Heidegger's "moment of vision," which he prefers to describe in a more Nietzschean way, as a "wink" or a "blink," "the twinkling of an eye."[53]

It may thus be conjectured that, for Derrida, what is at stake is the possibility of thinking vision and light, not in the familiar terms of "representational man," but rather in terms of a very different character—in sum, a character open to difference and other perspectives.

Derrida's 1983 lecture, "The Principle of Reason," marks, perhaps, a transitional phase in his thinking about vision and light in the discourse of philosophy, for it shifts several times— one might say, in an *Augenblick*, "in the twinkling of an eye," but also, perhaps, "with the shutting of an eye"—between reflections that concern metaphysics (*theoria*) and reflections that concern ethics and politics (*praxis*). But in "The Laws of Reflection: Nelson Mandela, in Admiration," a text published in 1987, Derrida is not concerned with the logic of visualism in metaphysics—a problematic about which he first started to write in the early sixties. Instead, continuing his thinking about "heliopolitics" ("Violence and Metaphysics"), his concern is entirely given over to the ethics and politics of vision and light. The questioning of metaphysics, of the logic of ocularcentrism in metaphysics, withdraws into the background, giving way to questioning that is, in a very important sense, more practical than theoretical.

In fact, this text signifies much more than a shift from reflections on metaphysics to reflections on ethics and politics. It also represents a shift from a deconstructive critique of vision to a deconstructive use of vision in social and political critique. In "The Laws of Reflection," Derrida explains his admiration for Mandela. Mandela, he says, is "a man of reflection." But that accounts only in part for his admiration. Derrida also admires Mandela's admiration for the law—the character of Mandela's admiration for the law, or, say, Mandela's way of demonstrating his admiration for the law. No blind fascination, no bedazzled devotion, no fanaticism, but rather "a force of reflection" that knows how to admire the law: how to admire it in a way that enables others, enables us, to see what he sees.

There are, according to Derrida, "specular paradoxes in the experience of the law."[54] And perhaps nowhere else have these paradoxes been more acute than in South Africa. But "there is no law," he says, "without a mirror."[55] Thus, an admiring mirror of law, and an admirably critical reflection of the law, is precisely what Mandela becomes. "This inflexible logic of reflection was Mandela's practice."[56]

Let us look into this critical practice. Mandela, of course, was summoned many times to appear before the law—before the law of a state founded not on principles of justice and equality but on the principles of apartheid. And always, when he appeared before this law, he would attempt, as Derrida puts it, to ask "the question of the subject responsible before the law."[57] This question, reflecting his critical reflections before this law, deflects the accusations against him and accuses those who have accused him, setting up "an optic of reflection" that forces his accusers to look at themselves, to recognize the racism in their blind spot. He attempts to make them see what and how he sees, how he sees what and how they see. He gets them to look at both their admiration for a law his gaze of contempt reflects and also at their contempt for the law his admiring gaze reflects. Mandela comes "before a law he rejects, beyond any doubt, but which he rejects in the name of a superior law, the very one he declares to admire and before which he agrees to appear."[58]

Mandela rests his case on "the tradition inaugurated by the Magna Carta, the Universal Declaration of the Rights of Man under their diverse forms (he frequently calls upon 'human dignity', upon what is 'human' and 'worthy of that name')."[59] Is he then "a simple inheritor" of this tradition? Derrida replies: "Yes and no, depending on what is meant here by inheritance. You can recognize an authentic inheritor in the one who conserves and reproduces, but also in the one who respects the logic of the legacy enough to turn it upon occasion against those who claim to be its guardians, enough to reveal, despite and against the usurpers, what has never yet been seen in the inheritance."[60]

Mandela's eyes, the gaze he directs, the glances he casts in the direction of his accusers, make visible—beautifully, admirably visible—the truth of the moral law they have scorned. In his eyes, there is a deeply rooted respect for this law. Thus: "His reflection ... shows what phenomenality kept in hiding. It does not reproduce; it produces the visible."[61] Moreover: "This production of light is justice—moral or political.... It translates here the political violence of the whites."[62] By a "specular inversion," the truth of justice is brought to the light.

But as he stands before the pure white laws of apartheid, Mandela's eyes also look beyond the visible, reflecting a vision of what does not yet exist. He looks forward to a time of mutual respect, when the exchanging of glances and gazes between whites and blacks will be the practical ground of reciprocity. And he projects—or say, foresees—another time, a time in which the potential for a truly just and egalitarian society, and for a state founded on the principle of democratic pluralism, has finally been achieved.

This essay on Mandela represents an important new phase in Derrida's thinking about light and vision. We may call it, perhaps, "heliopolitics," but what matters is the fact that although he is still thinking theoretically—that is, with a theoretical eye, he is looking away from the texts of metaphysics, where he documented the operations and effects of ocularcentrism, in order to see, inscribed in the very prose of the world, the ethics and politics of light and vision, and read, there, the "writing" of light and the "logic" of the gaze.

In reflecting on Mandela, Derrida brings to the light not only a gaze of deep respect but also a gaze of defiance, a deconstructive gaze effectively resisting conditions of oppression: a fearless gaze, rooted in the truth, rooted in a vision of justice.

However, considering Nietzsche's influence on Derrida's thinking, it is surprising that Derrida has not given more thought to the embodiment of deconstructive strategies in the mobility (*écriture*) of the gaze and that he has not made visible, in the doctrine of perspectivism, the existence of a multiplicity of gazes, gazes that have the power to decenter authoritarian institutions, subvert totalitarian regimes, and cast the principles of democratic pluralism in a new and different light.

Such limitations must themselves be put in proper perspective. Derrida's texts are constructed to engage the reader's eyes in deconstructive practices, readings that repeatedly displace and decenter them, force them out of line, subject them to the play of uncertainty, and draw them into the undecidability of double binds. What readers may learn to see, and learn, reflectively, about the character of their seeing, in the course of reading such texts, could subvert the authority of metaphysics, turning its ocularcentric claim of presence into an absurdity.

This breaching of our metaphysics is not without ethical and political significance. But so far Derrida has not reflected on, or made visible, how deconstructive readings of his texts can set processes in motion that will transform the metaphysically disposed gaze. When the texts one is reading are Derridean texts, the process of reading will have its effects—effects, I mean, on the reading gaze. How is this gaze affected by its readings of such texts? Derrida has left it to us, his readers, to see how these deconstructive readings, into the play of which his writing seductively draws us, can constitute, and in the process also transform, both the reader's habitual way(s) of looking and seeing and the reader's reflectively formed understanding of the experience of looking and seeing.

In "Structure, Sign and Play in the Discourses of the Human Sciences," Derrida tells us that it has become "necessary to think both the law which somehow governed the desire for a center in the constitution of structure, and the process of signification which orders the displacements and substitutions for this law of central presence—but a central presence which has never been itself, has always already been exiled from itself into its own substitute.... Henceforth, it was necessary to begin thinking that there was no center, that the center could not be thought in the form of a present being, that the center had no natural site, that it was not a fixed locus but a function, a sort of nonlocus in which an infinite number of sign-substitutions came into play."[63]

The experience with reading that Derrida gives to his readers shows—teaches—the eyes the truth in this analysis. This it accomplishes by making the eyes—eyes that have been governed by a desire for the center and disciplined to obey the order of the straight line—actually pass through precisely those movements about which Derrida is writing in this passage. For Derrida, processes of enlightenment, the difficult work of learning that ethics and politics demand, can take hold anywhere—even there, for example, where our reading eyes are solicited by a provocative text.

If the gaze of the philosophical tradition is the gaze that produced the metaphysics of presence, then the gaze that Derrida's writing seduces us into pursuing is a gaze that will have no center, no permanence, no stability, no determinacy, no predictability. It is an aleatory, nomadic, outlaw gaze that he inscribes in his texts, inducing the reader's eyes to abandon their tyrannical discipline. The experience with reading that Derrida gives to his readers is one that continually frustrates the eyes' linearity, their claims to hold a privileged position, their desire for a fixed center, and their assumptions regarding closure, totality, visibility, and transparency. Reading Derrida multiplies points of view, calls for an acknowledgment of perspectives from the margins, and opens "the text" to the interminable play of the visible and the invisible. No metaphysics of presence is possible for a gaze that has allowed itself to become inscribed, or say implicated, in the construction of Derridean texts. Thus, for example, Derrida frequently writes in a way that deliberately risks confusing what the eyes can see with what the ears will hear. This in itself, of course, contests the hegemony of vision, using vision against itself by using the sounds proposed to vision to deconstruct this hegemony. Moreover, what reading his texts makes visible to the eyes— what reading them brings to the light in the most sensible way— takes the gaze through gestures that trace out, before them, the practical possibility of an enlightened ethics and politics. (But the texts always also trace out warnings, for at the center of all the enlightened texts within which such ethics and politics emerge as possible, there will be at work an unavowed, unavowable blind spot, visible only belatedly as a limit on visibility and a danger for processes of enlightenment.)

In his essay on Kant, "Of an Apocalyptic Tone Recently Adopted in Philosophy," Derrida declares that "we cannot and we must not—this is a law and a destiny—forgo the *Aufklärung*. In other words, we cannot and we must not forgo what compels recognition as the enigmatic desire for vigilance, for the lucid vigil [*veille*], for clarification, for critique and truth."[64] However, he also expresses strong reservations about the Enlightenment project: concerns, in particular, regarding the extent to which, despite, and in audible contradiction to its own most noble intentions, it has succeeeded in avoiding, or even *can* avoid, the assumption of an "apocalyptic tone"—a tone of voice, of address, that betrays a certain impatience with *différance*, and communicates the intolerance of a vision already convinced of its universality.

I suggest that Derrida's years of thinking about ocularcentrism in metaphysics, as well as his more recent thinking about the ethics and politics of light and vision, represent a strong commitment to continuing the Enlightenment project. He continues this project by thinking critically about the light its discourse sheds on social and political questions. And yet I think it must in the end be noted that, in his passion to combat the ocular support for the metaphysics and politics of presence, he gives little recognition to the way vision and its discourse have figured in the histories of rationalism and empiricism, both of them implicitly—or potentially—democratic movements of liberation and enlightenment. In the rationalisms of Descartes, Spinoza, Kant, and Hegel, one can discern, despite all their differences, an unwavering commitment to promoting the capacities of all people for reflective self-direction: the empowerment in and of ideas and ideals, and the rational liberty in assenting only to what our own intellects can see with clarity and demonstrate to and for themselves. Similarly, in the empiricisms of Hobbes, Locke, and Hume, one can discern, despite their differences, an equally strong passion for submitting the words and displays of authority to the power of factual evidence, the power in observation and the testimony of experience—what we can see and verify with our own eyes. The text on Mandela's powers of reflection could serve as a beginning for an account in which the politics of vision, a major subtext of signifiers operative in these histories of rationalism and empiricism, would be brought out, rendered visible, and subjected to critical analysis.

Whereas Heidegger made vision hermeneutical, in keeping with the unconcealment (presence/absence) of the truth of being, Derrida makes vision textual. Addressing the same problematic—the reification and totalization of being in a metaphysics of presence—but from a different angle, Derrida demonstrates a postmetaphysical vision by inscribing and encrypting his glances and gazes within the movement of *écriture*, subverting the metaphysical eye in the articulations of his texts. In effect, he articulates a "*vision écriture*": in a style of writing that insists on being strictly optical, he inscribes a vision, a gaze, that has no identity apart from the operations and effects of the text. If, for Heidegger, what was crucial is the figure-ground formation, what is crucial for Derrida is the deconstruction of the absolute frame, the metaphysical delimitation of inside and outside, center and periphery, and the corresponding assignment of epistemic (or say power/knowledge) privileges (i.e., an apodeictic gaze at what is present) to the position at the center.

Derrida's strategy throughout his texts is to use his own writing—the visibility of a writing, a medium expressly ordered and encoded for the eyes to see and read—in order to force metaphysics out into the open, so that we may *see* the undoing of a metaphysics of presence taking place in the very writing of the discourse assumed to affirm it.

Derrida textualizes the gaze in an optical writing, a writing that is intelligible to the gaze alone. This *vision écriture* becomes a vehicle not only for the deconstruction and decentering of the absolute gaze proclaimed by metaphysics, but also, at the same time, for the display of the possibilities open to vision in a post-metaphysical context. *Vision écriture* is Derrida's strategy for dis-spelling the spell-binding power of the center and its frame and releasing the anarchic play of possibilities inherent in the ground. This strategy works, of course, by enacting sudden, unforeseeable shifts in point of view, in angle, in proximity and distance, in centrality and marginality, in sharpness (or specificity) and diffuseness (or generality) of focus. If at first Derrida calls our attention to something commonly assumed to be central, something we have mastered by putting it right in front of our eyes, he soon gets us to notice something that would be considered marginal or even irrelevant. If at one moment he has us attending to something very closely, the next moment he gets us to look at it from afar, or with a squint and a sideways glance. If there is something we have always viewed with admiration, then at that he may get us, with a turn of phrase that turns our eyes, suddenly to look askance. If at one moment we are looking at a problem from a position that seems to be inside, then in the next moment, in a leap without any warning, any transition, we find ourselves looking at this "same" problem from a position we had only been able to think outside. If he wants us to think about a problem to which we are accustomed to give only passing notice, he gets us to stay with the problem and look at it with a steady gaze, only to position us so that he can catch us by surprise and reveal the existence of a blind spot, a failure to see something crucial that all along has been right before our eyes. Wherever we are accustomed to assume a frame; wherever we are accustomed to seeing only with clarity and distinctness; wherever we are used to a direct frontal view; wherever we can see only an object-like ground, Derrida's writing compels us to see otherwise.[65] Weaving his sight into his texts, he is able, simply by a turn of phrase or a grammatical construction, to disarm the sovereign gaze of metaphysical thought, casting it into the end-less play textual configurations. Reading Derrida's writing, our vision is shifted to the margins, the footnotes, the signature, the title, the white spaces surrounding the words. Inscribed in the text, in the very writing of the text, Derrida's point of view is likely to erupt anywhere, interrupting logical sequences of thought and catching the philosopher whom he is critically reading in a momentary blink, a moment of inattention. Using words to articulate spaces of play and indeterminacy, Derrida challenges the sovereign gaze of the philosopher, rational, immobile, fully open, exactly centered and strictly frontal, with a texture that admits not only looking and seeing, insight and intuition, speculation and reflection, but also blindness, distance, indistinctness, confusion, ambiguity, and opacity; a texture traversed by glimpses and glances, winks and blinks, squints and saccades. *Vision écriture*, vision textualized in a Derridean style of writing, is decentered and de-essentialized, its origins and ends disseminated among the shadows of ink that play on the surface of the paper; and it loses not only its prized self-possession but also its power to possess what it perceives.

Just as the Principle of Sufficient Reason has depended on a framework of assumptions to ensure the closure of the metaphysical ground, so our vision has depended on the enframing and confronting of its ground to ensure its metaphysical power. Derrida denies vision the security of this frontality and enframing, but in releasing the ground from a metaphysical structure, he actually gives to vision a different freedom, a freedom quite inconceivable within the philosophical discourse of modernity. Looking beyond enframing and frontality with a vision no longer settled into structuralism, a vision no longer hostage to epistemology,

David Michael Levin

Derrida seems to suggest a new possibility: that we could finally draw on the invisible to see with truly aesthetic eyes.

Derrida's "adventure" with vision continues. His latest is the writing of *Mémoires d'aveugle: L'autoportrait et autres ruines*.[66] In this text, written for an exhibition at the Louvre that Derrida himself organized (October 1990–January 1991), Derrida gives us his meditations on vision and blindness, memories and musings that he relates to works of art in the Louvre collection. Although, to be sure, the text is all "about" blindness, "what one learns here," as Françoise Viatte and Régis Michel, curators at the Louvre, have noted in their Preface, "are the ways of *opening eyes*." In this regard, the final pages are of singular importance. Derrida reflects on the significance of the fact that our eyes can weep as well as see—and that only human eyes are capable of tears.[67] Thus, at the closing of this text, he broaches very directly the ethical character—or the ethical destination—of our capacity for vision. And he seems to recognize, at least implicitly, that there is a potential in this capacity not only for aggression, but also for sympathy and compassion: the eyes can be touched and moved, moved even to tears, by what they see, what they are given to see. There is, then, a blindness that is moral—a trait of character—and an indebtedness that vision incurs: a beholdenness for what we are given to behold. But the text ends with Derrida's insistence on a certain irremediable tension between skepticism and faith, a tension in which our vision is drawn toward the illumination of a transcendental ground, but also, and precisely because of this attraction, it is drawn, or rather finds itself drawn, into the passion of a fateful sacrifice, a sacrifice, in the end, of sight to sight. What is at stake here is indeed the "adventure of vision" to which Derrida alluded some time ago in "Force and Signification." In these *Mémoires*, however, Derrida has come out of the text to reflect on, and directly intervene in, the force fields within which the spectacles of vision and blindness are inscribed. These interventions continue to question, problematize, and subvert the vision that dominates our culture, multiplying and encrypting points of view while resisting the ontotheology of apocalyptic visions and indefinitely deferring the equally dan-

gerous temptation to invoke the powers of vision with a prophetic discourse.

Foucault in the Empire of the Gaze

In "What Is Enlightenment?" Foucault ponders the question,
"How can the growth of capabilities be disconnected from the
intensification of power relations?"[68] Much of the thinking
behind this question draws us into a questioning of the role of
vision in our culture. Already, as early, for example, as his work
on *Madness and Civilization* (1961), Foucault took a critical interest
in ocularcentric questions. And, like Derrida, he used vision to
undermine vision—or, more precisely, he strategically deployed
his own way of seeing things, and the images this way of seeing
can produce, to problematize the mode of vision that has been
and still is hegemonic, and to challenge the complicity of this
mode of vision in our disciplinary practices and institutions of
power. Researching the treatment of madness during the classical period (1650–1800 more or less), he found that "madness
had become a thing to look at" and that in fact it "no longer
exists except as *seen*."[69] Thus, in this book, he gave thought to
the history of images of madness, a history inseparable from the
legitimation of Reason through its use in the classification of
madness. Looking into the archives, what caught Foucault's historical eyes were the spectacles that were made of the mad, and
the spectacles through which physicians looked at their patients.
What do people see? To what are they blind—in effect, shutting
their eyes? How can some people not see the same suffering
and cruelty that others see? What is necessary for suffering and
cruelty to be seen as such? What accounts for our cultural
perceptions?

In *Madness and Civilization*, Foucault takes notice of the asym-
metry, the nonreciprocity, that defines the optics of the normative space of the asylum and comments on the ocularcentric
refusal of dialogue: "The science of mental disease, as it would
develop in the asylum, would always be only of the order of
observation and classification. It would not be a dialogue."[70]

Dialogue requires proximity and participation; the gaze can be distant and detached, a useful instrument of Reason, occupying the position of spectator the better to observe and classify.

Foucault's next major work, *The Birth of the Clinic* (1963), bears the subtitle *An Archaeology of Medical Perception.* It thus brings these questions—"the themes," as he puts it, "of light and liberty"—to the fore and attempts, for the first time, to lay bare and make visible the historical correlations that connect the perceptual practices, technologies, and institutions of medicine to the formation of medicine as a scientific discourse and a discourse about man.[71] Sharpening his focus and exemplifying the "glance," which, unlike the "gaze," always "strikes at one point, which is central or decisive,"[72] Foucault quotes from a scientific treatise published in France in 1797: "One must, as far as possible, make science ocular."[73] Contesting "the great [Enlightenment] myth of the free gaze," which, "freed from darkness, dissipates all darkness,"[74] Foucault tells us that, for him, "the most important moral problem raised by the idea of the clinic was the following: by what right can one transform into an object of clinical observation a patient whose poverty had compelled him to seek assistance at the hospital?"[75]

Foucault communicates his concern for the ethical and political dimensions of our culture of vision in the form of questions that focus our sight on our practices and institutions and make them visible in a critical light: "But to look in order to know, to show in order to teach, is not this a tacit form of violence, all the more abusive for its silence, upon a sick body that demands to be comforted, not displayed? Can pain be a spectacle?"[76]

His book is thus a careful historical analysis of the "sovereignty of the gaze," above all, "the eye that knows and decides, the eye that governs."[77] Foucault accordingly documents the moment in European history—a moment we may associate with Descartes and the seventeenth century—when "the eye becomes the depository and source of clarity."[78] This is also the moment when light, "anterior to every gaze," an "element of ideality" and "the unassignable place of origin where things were adequate to their essence," becomes instead a purely subjective light, an interior "light of reason," which the eye obeys and reproduces.[79] This eye "has the power," he says, "to bring a truth to light that it receives only to the extent that it has brought it to light; as it opens, the eye first opens the truth: a flexion that marks the transition from the world of classical clarity—from the 'enlightenment'—to the nineteenth century."[80]

According to Foucault, "the cosmological values implicit in the *Aufklärung* are still at work."[81] The later, modern gaze enjoys a certain privilege, and even a certain preeminence, among the five senses. In this regard, it is not different from the gaze of earlier ages. But it differs from its ancestors in that its tendency to serve the desire for mastery and domination—what Nietzsche called the will to power—has joined forces with modern technology and technocracy: "the gaze that sees is a gaze that dominates; and although it also knows how to subject itself, it dominates its masters."[82] Even in the clinics of the late seventeenth century, the "loquacious," discursively constituted gaze was becoming a gaze that "atomizes the most individual flesh and enumerates its secret bits, [and] is that fixed, attentive, rather dilated gaze which, from the height of death, has already condemned life."[83] Increasingly, its attention to qualities will give way to analytic and quantitative reductions of the visible. Where is there "the gaze of compassion"?[84] What happened when the "Dialectic of the Lumières [was] transported into the doctor's eye"?[85]

Before continuing our chronological reading of Foucault's "ocularcentric" works, I want to call attention to a sentence that Foucault undoubtedly meant to convey something of the spirit of the Enlightenment (at least, as Kant understood it in his essay "Was ist Aufklärung?"), but that one might also ponder in the light of Derrida's critique of an ocularcentric metaphysics of presence. Foucault's asseveration reads: "The eye, which is akin to light, supports only the present."[86] As we shall see, however, Foucault's way of working with "the present" decisively problematizes its metaphysical reduction to a state of pure presence. The Foucauldian gaze *is* cast on the present, but this present is thoroughly historical.

David Michael Levin

Vision and the light of the Enlightenment also figure prominently in *The Order of Things* (1966), Foucault's next work on the human sciences. In the Preface he states what is perhaps the primary methodological assumption behind this work: "The fundamental codes of a culture—those governing its language, its schemas of perception, its exchanges, its techniques, its values, the hierarchy of its practices—establish for every man, from the very first, the empirical orders with which he will be dealing and within which he will be at home."[87]

Thus, in his interpretation of *Las Meninas*, a painting by Velázquez that he discusses in the first chapter of his book, Foucault calls our attention to its peculiar optics: the mirror and its reflection, the position of the spectator, the making of a spectacle, the role of observation, the sovereignty of the gaze, the subjection of the subject under observation, questions of power and the total clarification of knowledge in the lines of sight and the crisscrossing of gazes, and finally, questions of centrality and marginality, foreground and background, presence and absence, visibility and invisibility:

Man appears in his ambiguous position as an object of knowledge and as a subject that knows: enslaved sovereign, observed spectator, he appears in the place belonging to the king, which was assigned to him in advance by *Las Meninas*, but from which his real presence has for so long been excluded. As if, in that vacant space towards which Velázquez's whole painting was directed, but which it was nevertheless reflecting only in the chance presence of a mirror, and as though by stealth, all the figures whose alternation, reciprocal exclusion, interweaving and fluttering one imagined (the model, the painter, the king, the spectator) suddenly stopped their imperceptible dance, immobilized into one substantial figure, and demanded that the entire space of the representation should at last be related to *one* corporeal gaze.[88]

Here, at the end of this textual passage, where Foucault sees, in the field of forces constructed by the articulation of different perspectives, the operations of a structural logic calling for the imposition of unity, stability and totality, and relating this order to a sovereign gaze, strong and authoritative, we find what I believe to be the first traces, the first textual foreshadowings, of his later critical analysis of panopticism.

In fact, near the beginning of this book, in an attempt to formulate the difference between an imposed order and a freely created order, Foucault is already giving us a glimpse into the significance of the relationship between sight (*le voir*), power (*pouvoir*), and knowledge (*savoir*), for he wrote: "Order is, at one and the same time, that which is given in things as their inner law, the hidden network that determines the way they confront one another, and also that which has no existence except in the grid created by a glance, an examination, a language."[89]

According to Foucault, each historical age has inaugurated a different *episteme*, a different paradigm of rationality, and "a new field of visibility."[90] Thus, in *The Order of Things*, he studies the transition from the *episteme* dominant during the classical period—the period spanning the seventeenth and eighteenth centuries—to the *episteme* the emergence of which, late in the eighteenth century, constituted the beginning of the "Age of Man." Documenting the classificatory rationality of the "table" and the later, more empirical rationality of the observable specimen, he differentiates classical order from modern order by showing their different ways of encoding the hegemony of vision—the "almost exclusive privilege of sight."[91]

For Foucault, much of the significance of *Las Meninas* lies in the way it relates to questions of representation. Observing that there is a window to the left through which light comes and floods the room, he comments: "This extreme, partial, scarcely indicated window frees a whole flow of daylight which serves as the common locus of the representation.... [It is] a light which renders all representation visible."[92] We *see* this light, but not its source, which is outside the room. This he takes to be emblematic of the classical period and its Enlightenment.

It was in this period, according to Foucault, that rationality first began to adopt the functions of representation ("representation" in both senses of this term), assuming the possibility of forming a complete and accurate picture of the true order of the world and ordering signs and representations into tables and systems able to mirror, or reflect, the corresponding order of the world.

David Michael Levin

It eventually became apparent that total illumination, total clarity, total visibility, and therefore total knowledge are not possible. Even the possibility of a total knowledge of oneself— a knowledge such as Descartes once claimed—was eventually regarded with suspicion. Moreover, it gradually became apparent that in the representations of the classical period, the sovereign could not be represented, even though his sovereign gaze was powerfully organizing the spectacle it surveyed. In fact, there was no place for Man as both a subject who sees and an object who is visible and seen. The double nature of Man, as both the source of representation and also the object of his representation, could not itself be represented. And this was not the only blindness of that time, for the classical period did not see, did not notice, this absence, this missing constitutive subject. Modernity inherited a wealth of encyclopedias—nomenclatures, taxonomies, tables. But nowhere in these documents does the subject's activity of representation itself appear, recognized for what it is.

For Foucault, what makes *Las Meninas* historically significant is the fact that its subject matter, what it represents for us, is representation. The painting, as he sees it from our contemporary vantage point, is a representation of representation, a narrative *tableau*, laying out, as if in the clarity of a classical table, the various "functions" of representation: the model (the object of the representation), the painter (the one whose activity has produced this representation), and of course the spectator (the one who views this representation), to each of which there correspond distinctive representational gazes, both subjective and objectivating. But the one position that the picture leaves out, and indicates only obliquely, is the position occupied by the subject whose activity is responsible for this representation.

In the narrative Foucault tells, the constitutive gaze of this sovereign subject, the singular absence of which Velázquez secretly contributed to making visible, only began to emerge, with Kant, in the "Age of Man." As we shall see, Foucault's subsequent work enables us to understand the emergence of this gaze—and, above all, to understand the political significance of its coming to light and its increasing visibility.

The Archaeology of Knowledge (1969), Foucault's next major work, marginalizes the problematic of light and vision that was so central to his earlier thinking. The subject matter in this work is, rather, discourse. Here Foucault undertakes an archaeological excavation of the "rules of formation" that are involved in the constitution of the discourses contributing to the human sciences. We shall therefore turn our attention to "Nietzsche, Genealogy, History," a text published in 1971 in a volume paying homage to Jean Hyppolite.

The text is an argument against "traditional history" and a defense of what Nietzsche called "effective history." In a striking passage, and perhaps under the influence of Derrida as well as Nietzsche, Foucault at last brings together his old problematic of light and vision with critical reflections on the discourse of metaphysics and attempts to go beyond critique to bring into being the freedom and empowerment of a new way of seeing: "Once the historical sense is mastered by a suprahistorical per-spective, metaphysics can bend it to its own purpose.... On the other hand, the historical sense can evade metaphysics and become a privileged instrument of genealogy if it refuses the certainty of absolutes. Given this, it corresponds to the acuity of a glance that distinguishes, separates, and disperses; that is capable of liberating divergence and marginal elements—the kind of dissociative view that is capable of composing itself, capable of shattering the unity of man's being."[93] Here, in a text that announces his shift from archaeology to genealogy, Foucault formulates a contrast between the "suprahistorical perspective," which he associates with metaphysics and traditional historio-graphy, and the critical "glance," which he associates with "effective history."

Like Nietzsche, Foucault scoffs at the possibility of any abso-lutely "comprehensive view of history." Such a view can only fabricate a historical narrative "whose function is to compose the finally reduced diversity of time into a totality fully closed upon itself."[94] Opposed to this is a way of looking at history that "will uproot its traditional foundations and relentlessly disrupt its pre-tended [natural or teleological] continuity."[95] "Effective history" requires a different optics. In order to document singularities, contingencies, and discontinuities, it "shortens its vision to those things nearest to it."[96] And although it "has no fear of looking down" from the heights, it always also "descends to seize the various perspectives, to disclose dispersions and differences."[97] He says:

The final trait of effective history is its affirmation of knowledge as perspective. Historians take unusual pains to erase the elements in their work which reveal their grounding in a particular time and place.... [By contrast,] Nietzsche's version of historical sense is explicit in its perspective.... Its perception is slanted, being a deliberate appraisal, affirmation, or negation.... It is not given to a discreet effacement before the objects it observes and does not submit itself to their processes; nor does it seek laws, since it gives equal weight to its own sight and to its objects. Through this historical sense, knowledge is allowed to create its own genealogy in the act of cognition; and *wirkliche Historie* composes a genealogy of history as the vertical projection of its position.[98]

One cannot overestimate the significance of this text for understanding the evolution of Foucault's way of working with, and working through, the problematic of light and vision. What Foucault discovered in reading Nietzsche was an accurate articulation of the very technique, the very style of looking and seeing, that he had already been practicing, but only unconsciously and gropingly. Reading Nietzsche, then, he learned more about how and what to look for, how and what to notice and observe, and how to clarify, mirror, and reflect what he saw in a way that is critical, subversive, and effective. And he learned something about the importance of recognizing and multiplying perspectives, thereby decentering the "sovereign gaze," the gaze that figures not only in traditional historiography but also in the discourse of metaphysics and in the politics of all monarchies and hierarchies.

Positioned in the margins and on the borderlines, positioned, always, where one would least expect it, the Foucauldian gaze exposes the secret workings of power. Moved only by the light of truth, it turns our attention to the cruelty and violence we do not want to see. It insists on looking at what others have kept invisible. It questions both the visible and the invisible, requiring that we justify the institutions that determine them. Henceforth, the sovereign gaze of an ocularcentric metaphysics, a gaze whose will to power pressures this discourse to require absolute presence in a center of focus, and whose character readily collaborates with social processes to install authoritarian and totalitarian regimes of power, will be challenged and resisted by a positioning of the gaze, and a way of looking and seeing, that put into effect a continual process of decentering and dispersion. The anarchic gaze that organizes Foucault's discourse and speaks from its marginal and invisible positions: this gaze, with its strange angles and optics, subverts the hegemonic vision. To understand how it works, we must adopt its positions, its angles, its optics; and we must follow its radically democratic proliferation of perspectives and viewpoints, its demonstration of a gaze that enjoys exceptional mobility and freedom, and its vigilance as a theoretically informed vision capable of subjecting regimes of power to continuous public scrutiny.[99] What Foucault learned from Nietzsche continued the evolution of his thinking about light and vision, and it encouraged him to put into practice a sight singularly well adapted to what I would call his "politics of positions."

In closing "What Is Enlightenment?" an essay that represents his homage to Kant, Foucault asks: "How can the growth of capabilities be disconnected from the intensification of power relations?"[100] Foucault's answer, I suggest, would be that there cannot be any disconnection, but capabilities—our willingness, for example, and our capacity to look and see things fearlessly and honestly, as they actually are—can nevertheless grow and develop in ways that make them powerful and disciplined challenges to oppressive forms of power. Sight is not only a natural endowment; it is also the gift of a capacity that can be developed. And since it is a "power" in its own right, sight can learn and mature in its discipline, its vigilance, its fearlessness, its ability to exercise its open freedom, its skillfulness and resourcefulness as a critical witness to power. It is precisely because the growth of our capabilities—our sight, for example—cannot be disconnected from relations of power that these capabilities can function critically and as a source of resistance. This function is made possible precisely when, and precisely where, the growth of our capacities encounters oppressive orders of power and suffers as a result.

Thus it was that with increasing consciousness and understanding, Foucault turned his gaze, his seeing, into a finely disciplined practice—and not only an exercise of the freedom to contest and resist but also an exercise in the ethics and politics of respect, caring for the marginalized and occluded, the positions and perspectives of our invisible others. In "Body/Power" (a 1975 interview), Foucault articulates this moment of vision: "What's effectively needed is a ramified, penetrative *perception* of the present, one that makes it possible to locate lines of weakness, strong points, positions where the instances of power have secured and implanted themselves."[101] A year later, in an interview with the title "The Politics of Health in the Eighteenth Century," he expressed his position thus: "One of the tasks that seems immediate and urgent to me, over and above anything else, is this: that we should indicate and show up, even where they are hidden, all the relationships of political power which actually control the social body and oppress and repress it."[102] In part, this task is a project of and for our vision.

In an important sense, *Discipline and Punish: The Birth of the Prison* (published in France in 1975) represents the capstone of Foucault's work on the problematic of light and vision, as well as an exemplary practice of this project. Although he spoke about this problematic in at least one major interview—"The Eye of Power" took place in 1977—*Discipline and Punish* is, I believe, the last text he wrote on light and vision. It is concerned, he says, with "the subjection of those who are perceived as objects and the objectification of those who are thus subjected."[103]

Looking closely, then, at modernity, the "Age of Man," what Foucault saw—what his eyes witnessed and attested—was a new organization of power: a regime of power no longer founded, as he argued in a 1976 lecture, in the physical existence of the sovereign but rather in "continuous and permanent systems of surveillance."[104] Reminding us that "the 'Enlightenment', which discovered the liberties, also invented the disciplines,"[105] he called this new ordering of power, spectacularly different from all preceding orderings of power, "disciplinary power." But what makes this particularly interesting is that he also saw the connection between this form of "governmentality"—disciplinary, administrative technologies and apparatuses of power—and the hegemony of the gaze.

It may be true that even in ancient times, the power of sight played a major role in the formation of Western culture. It may also be true that both the Renaissance and the classical period were governed—albeit in very different ways—by the sovereign gaze. But according to Foucault, the "Age of Man" inaugurated an extremely different relationship between power/knowledge and the light of the gaze.

Focusing this new relationship in a word, Foucault began speaking about Jeremy Bentham's blueprint for a Panopticon, a model prison, and about "panopticism," the institutional forms that disciplinary power assumes when hegemonized by ocularcentrism. Panopticism is the political equivalent of the metaphysics of presence: social control—the order in stability and integration—by means of the new technologies of oversight and supervision, and a network of disciplinary practices and institutions penetrating and circulating through all spheres of the social world, ensuring the constant and permanent regulation of daily life.

In "Types of Lighting," Walter Benjamin called attention to the fact that soon after the invention of electricity, there were projects for city lighting based on the eighteenth-century Enlightenment "idea of universal illumination," and recalled how, as early as 1836, Jacques Fabien warned against the effects of an overabundance of light.[106] Foucault saw what Benjamin saw: the dangerous connection between the Enlightenment and administrative panopticism, which modern technologies and technocracies have finally made possible. Only in modernity does the ocularcentrism of our culture appear as panopticism: the system of administrative institutions and disciplinary practices organized by the conjunction of a universalized but instrumental rationality and advanced technologies of visibility.

In the early years of his career, it happened that Foucault found employment in psychiatric hospitals, where he positioned himself primarily in the roles of spectator, observer, and witness. His experiences working in these institutions made a deep and lasting impression on him. Thus, it is not surprising that as his early work on psychiatric institutions and the practices and institutions of medicine abundantly document, Foucault began to see, in the world around him, signs and symptoms of what he later would describe as an ever-increasing panopticism. This perception was confirmed and strengthened by his reading of Bentham's design for a "Panopticon." Here he found the frightening prospect of a "transparent society," "power through transparency," "a visibility organized around a dominating, overseeing gaze," and a totalitarian politicization of space in the form of "a project of universal visibility."[107] Consequently he saw the need for studies that would make the apparatuses and workings of "the eye of power" visible—visible, that is, *as* the disciplinary power of surveillance, a "new type of gaze," keeping individuals and populations as much in sight as possible.[108] And he saw the need to reflect on the historical relationship between this increasing panopticism and the ideals and illusions of the Enlightenment. For whereas the Enlightenment thought of illumination only as a rational liberation of the subject, one of the legacies of this *episteme* is a light of violence, a light that involves the subject not only in social relations organized for increasing subjection but also in the normalization of self-regulatory processes—the forever vigilant inner eye of "conscience."

Foucault has shown how it is possible to trace the connection between conditions of our lives—the economy of capitalism, the imperatives of a patriarchal culture, the persistence of racism—and the gaze of power—even the more enlightened gaze achieved by the Enlightenment. He has shown, moreover, that even after the historical changes of the Enlightenment, this gaze, produced in and by a patriarchal white culture, has continued to function under the spell of the will to power, reproducing this culture and its violence, reproducing through the very structure of perception—through the very structure of intentionality—an economy based on possessive and aggressive ambitions and a social world in which subjects encounter one another in cruel and destructive ways.

This is the "dark side" of the Enlightenment, that "terror" of a Reason turned exclusively instrumental, technological, against which Max Weber first warned us, and which Horkheimer and Adorno, as survivors of the Holocaust, felt compelled to confirm in their *Dialectic of Enlightenment*. Foucault elaborates on their analysis:

Historically, the process by which the bourgeoisie became in the course of the eighteenth century the politically dominant class was masked by the establishment of an explicit, coded and formally egalitarian jurid-ical framework, made possible by the organization of a parliamentary, representative regime. But the development and generalization of dis-ciplinary mechanisms constituted the other, dark side of these pro-cesses. The general juridical form that guaranteed a system of rights that were egalitarian in principle was supported by these tiny, everyday, physical mechanisms, by all those systems of micro-power that are essentially non-egalitarian and asymmetrical, and that we call the dis-ciplines.... The real, corporal disciplines constituted the foundation of the formal, juridical liberties. The contract may have been regarded as the ideal foundation of law and political power; panopticism con-stituted the technique, universally widespread, of coercion. It continued to work in depth on the juridical structures of society, in order to make the effective mechanisms of power function in opposition to the formal framework that it had acquired. The "Enlightenment" which dis-covered the liberties also invented the disciplines.[109]

Instead of extending liberation, the Enlightenment's light of Reason has, according to the Foucauldian narrative, turned into external and internal (public and private) surveillance, processes of "rationalization" that only increase and strengthen the forces of domination. It is necessary to ask ourselves, however, whether this normalization is the work of Enlightenment Reason, or whether it is instead the work of a counter-Enlightenment irra-tionalism the unleashed forces of which the Enlightenment has not yet succeeded in transforming. Foucault's own vision, here, is not sufficiently clear.

In any event, despite the momentum of these historical pro-cesses, Foucault did not get caught in Weber's "iron cage," nor did he fall into Adorno's bleak despair. Although, for Foucault, panoptical power is everywhere, this does not mean that there is no place for liberty—that freedom is not possible. On the contrary, the omnipresence of power (power relations) means that wherever one is, there is always something one can do, always a position one can take, in relation to an oppressive form of power: "In relations of power, there is necessarily the possibility of resistance.... If there are relations of power throughout every social field, it is because there is freedom everywhere."[110] Freedom, in fact, is "all the more real and effective" when it is formed right at the point where relations of power are operative: "It exists all the more by being in the same place as [the oppressive] power; hence, like [this] power, resistance is multiple and can be integrated in global strategies."[111] Thus, no matter how oppressive conditions may be, "we can never be ensnared by power; we can always modify its grip in determinate conditions and according to a precise strategy."[112]

Since power as a matter of sovereignty has all but vanished, displaced by power as a matter of panoptical disciplines, Foucault substitutes a strategic model of power for the model based on law. According to this strategic model, the abolition of the sovereign juridical subject opens the political field to acts of subversion and resistance—a multiplicity of deconstructive strategies that "operate a decentering that leaves no privilege to any center."[113] Power for Foucault "is everywhere; not because it embraces everything, but because it can come from everywhere."[114] Foucault rejects theories that can see power only in terms of an oppositional duality: the position of domination and the position of subordination. This picture is disempowering. Foucault shows us that power can come "from below" and that it "is exercised from innumerable points."[115] In fact, since power can exist only in a relationship, it follows that wherever there is power, there is resistance: not a resistance to power that is itself outside of power, but rather a multiplicity of "points of resistance" that are "present everywhere within the power network": local articulations of power, some significantly visual, locally confronting other articulations of power.[116]

Now that governmental power has changed, no longer classi-
cally centralized; now that it circulates in the form of disciplinary
regimes, colonizes the life-world, and increasingly organizes and
regulates the institutions and practices of civil society, new forms
of critical social analysis and new strategies of resistance and
reform are needed. What, for Foucault, corresponds to this new
situation is a politics of strategic positions: a theory, or analysis,
of power, and a multiplicity of practices, which are capable of
confronting and challenging oppressive disciplinary regimes,
oppressive technologies of power, according to a logic of differentiation. Since the power of the state is now decentralized,
divided, multiplied, dispersed, mobile, and heteromorphous,
capable of reaching into the farthest extremities and the inner-
most recesses, resistance and reform must abandon the classical
logic of identity and begin working with a logic of difference.
Instead of attacking a central authority, the origin of power that
Foucault has exposed as myth, enlightened politics must henceforth work by multiplying points of difference, proliferating sites
for democratic struggle, and organizing discursive relays between
these points, these sites.[117]

Whether, even today, our lives are to some extent still oppressed by a "sovereign gaze" or whether the "sovereign gaze"
of the state has been transformed, along with the dissemination
of state power in general, into multiple points of oppressive disciplinary surveillance, the politics of liberation must be a politics
that multiplies and proliferates a subversive gaze at all points of
contact. It is my contention that in working out an appropriate
model for political analysis and action, Foucault arrived at what I
shall call a "politics of strategic positions" and that the formulation of this politics enabled him to conceptualize and practice a way of seeing that could function critically, subversively,
and deconstructively, resisting the power of panopticism. To the
hidden eye of disciplinary power that creates practices and institutions to see and control everything while itself keeping out of
sight, Foucault opposes a gaze that can pop up anywhere and
always where it is least expected; a gaze that adopts odd angles
and lens; a gaze that keeps out of sight in order to be free of

surveillance, free to see the workings of power and subject them to a critical scrutiny capable of deconstructing their intricate webs of authority. Thus, just as Derrida evolved strategic textual positions and strategies for textual deconstruction in order to oppose the domination of an ocularcentric metaphysics of presence, so Foucault evolved strategic political positions and strategies for political deconstruction in order to oppose the domination of ocularcentric disciplinary practices and institutions. And since, for Foucault, these regimes of disciplinary power are "panoptical," he evolved an appropriately "optical" politics of resistance and reform: a deconstructive way of seeing that finely matched his deconstructive politics of strategic positions. And it is precisely this way of seeing things that is his most lasting contribution to the human sciences.

Instead of encouraging the shutting of eyes, moral blindness, the gaze of cruelty, the predatory, aggressive stare, the fixed, impassive, sovereign gaze, the abstract theoretical gaze, the god's-eye vantage point, the comprehensive, transhistorical gaze, the timeless gaze of contemplation, the private eye of introspection, and the pure, self-evident transcendental intuition, Foucault encouraged acts of watching, examining, scrutinizing, penetrating, and observing; he multiplied his perspectives; he praised eyes that are open to the truth; he invoked a gaze of compassion; he held himself open to different points of view; he kept the operations of power in sight; and he surveyed the field of political struggles, not from the air but from the ground of the action.[118]

Admirable though this is, however, we must not overlook the fact that Foucault had a serious deficiency: in truth, a debilitating blind spot. There is no recognition in his writings of the different contemporary gazes, multiplied and strengthened by our visual technologies, in which the actions of public officials, and the practices and institutions of civic life, are subject to public scrutiny. Much can be said about how investigative reporting, making visible the concealed operations of government, and the televising of courtroom proceedings, debates in the halls of Congress, and special congressional hearings serve the visibility conditions essential to a participatory democracy. Just as women are now "taking back the night," so there are citizen groups taking back the light, deflecting the panoptical spotlight of disciplinary regimes of power and turning it on the agents of public trust. Foucault seems not to have seen the various ways in which our contemporary democracy encourages the proliferation of citizen interest groups and popular organizations with the power to make government visible, keeping public officials in sight and overseeing their actions. Foucault did not see that critical eyes like his can actually be incorporated and institutionalized, operating through an array of public instruments and a multitude of citizen associations and organizations.

Like Derrida, Foucault was committed to a liberal politics of individualism. Although they both eschewed the traditional discourse of sovereign rights, there is no question of their support for struggles to secure new freedoms. But this focus on liberty tends to marginalize questions of equality and social justice and to reduce our field of action to a choice between resistance or acquiescence. Understood in the context of their strong individualism, the politics of resistance tends to marginalize collective will-formation—the processes of social interaction and coalition building constitutive of participatory democracy. Correspondingly, their understanding of vision tends to be limited to seeing it in its critical roles, blind to the roles of the gaze in mutual recognition and reciprocity, blind to the roles of the gaze in building a sense of community. One has reason to fear repressive unities, the totalist collective, the "we" of fascism; but in the politics of Foucault and Derrida, I see this fear condensed into a tragic blind spot.

Nearing the abrupt end of his life, it seems that Foucault began to realize that it is not enough to think and practice a vision of resistance, a vision of subversion. Very slowly, tentatively, and awkwardly, he even began to acknowledge, not only in his practice but also in his thought, a vision of mutual recognition, a vision of reciprocity. In "The Concern for Truth" (May 1984), Foucault argued, with words that echo Habermas, that the intellectual must renounce the god's-eye vantage point in order to "participate in the formation of a political will," bringing the workings of power to the light, making them visible, and problematizing practices and institutions that have been naturalized, or falsely assumed to be based on consensus.[119] In effect, Foucault was thus suggesting that resistance and reform must learn to adapt the skirmishing strategies of guerrilla warfare to the rationality-conditions of discursive will-formations. Presumably, there would be a corresponding change in the micropractices of a vision committed to such formations.

An interview with the title "How Much Does It Cost for Reason to Tell the Truth?" adds a crucial dimension to this suggestion. After telling us that "reason is a long narrative, which ends today and makes room for another," Foucault assures us that the historical contingency of forms of rationality "doesn't mean that these forms of rationality are irrational. They rest," he says, perhaps reminded of Levinas, "upon a foundation of human practices and human faces."[120]

Surprising language! Near the end of his life, as the certainty of death gradually inhabited him, it seems that he began to shift his position, putting away his topological maps of the political terrain, maps drawn as if from an imperial height, and began moving closer to people, closer to the positions of the practical subject. What concerned him, he said, is "politics as an ethics."[121] What exactly this means he has left to us. However, there was an interview conducted by Paul Rabinow in May 1984, just before his death, on the basis of which one might infer that what he meant was a politics of dialogue, a "discourse ethics," with the subjects opposing one another positioned face to face—procedurally, if not necessarily literally.

Instead of warfare, polemics, confrontation, subjects are now peacefully engaged in rational discussions, arguing and debating, questioning both others and themselves, examining their motives, their perceptions, their viewpoints, and the reasons claimed to justify their respective positions, and cooperating in the attempt to work through their differences and conflicts. Resistance and subversion, the moment of transgression, are still important to him, but he now gives more attention to actions that are symmetrical and constructive. There are, perhaps, some faint echoes here of Habermas. There is a surprising reliance here on the concepts of "rights," "reciprocity," "responsibility," and "obligations," although the way in which he speaks of rights implicitly breaks with the "sovereign natural rights" of the classical juridical discourse, moving, rather, in the direction of a conception of dialogically constituted rights—rights recognized and established as constitutive of the conditions necessary for a discursively legitimated social formation:

In the serious play of questions and answers, in the work of reciprocal elucidation, the rights of each person are in some sense immanent in the discussion. They depend only on the dialogue situation. The person asking the questions is merely exercising the right that has been given him: to remain unconvinced, to perceive a contradiction, to require more information, to emphasize different postulates, to point out faulty reasoning, etc. As for the person answering the questions, he too exercises a right that does not go beyond the discussion itself; by the logic of his own discourse he is tied to what he has said earlier, and by the acceptance of dialogue he is tied to the questioning of the other. Questions and answers depend on a game ... in which each of the two partners takes pains to use only the rights given him by the other and by the accepted form of the dialogue.[122]

Here, at last, going beyond the politics of opposition and resistance, Foucault explicitly recognizes a politics that positions subjects face to face (literally or figuratively) in the ethical space of public discourse. However, nothing is said explicitly in this text about a democratic, egalitarian reciprocity of gazes, even though the dialogical situation certainly implies the recognition of a gaze that one cannot see in any of his earlier work. Admittedly, between a gaze of resistance and a gaze of reciprocity, there is, in a sense, an abyss. But I cannot resist the temptation to venture a certain speculative hypothesis. In my hermeneutical reading of his words, I am convinced—whereas Martin Jay is not—that Foucault was on the verge of recognizing a reciprocity of gazes.[123] Thus, if his recognition of politics in, and as, a discourse ethics represents, as it seems, an important step—and, as fate would make it, the last step—in his thinking about a politics of strategic positions, then his final recognition of the gaze in reflective reciprocity would represent, correspondingly, a decisive last step in his thinking about light and vision—and indeed an equally decisive last moment in his reception of the legacy of the Enlightenment.

Until this final phase in his thinking, Foucault concentrated on the orders imposed by the eye of power—the sovereign gaze of the classical period, followed by the disciplinary gaze of the modern—and on their correspondingly evolving opposites, the enlightened vision of Reason, followed by the look of defiance— and ultimately by the transgressive, critical, metaphorical, and deconstructive gaze that he celebrated and described in great phenomenological detail but never explicitly acknowledged to be his own.

There is a surprising irony here. By not acknowledging as his own this critical gaze, the gaze from the standpoint of which he in fact thought and wrote and acted, Foucault thereby reenacted the very spectacle he analyzed in the painting by Velázquez. For Foucault's own gaze, the gaze that saw what he wrote about, the gaze that is the source of his critique of power, is not signified and acknowledged as such. The critical activity of representation and deconstruction, the work of his eyes, is not itself rendered visible. And yet it is precisely his strategic praxis—his positions, his sites, his angles, his focus, his lenses—that is ultimately most important—even more important than the different things that Foucault's eyes have showed us. What we need most to see is not what it is that he makes visible, but rather how it is that he can bring to the light what we others have not seen, not been able to see. Foucault's subversive gaze instantiates, exemplifies, his political engagement. But precisely this gaze is kept invisible. Withdrawn from visibility, of course, in order to avoid drawing our attention away from the objects of his concern—but also, perhaps, in order to avoid being caught within the scope of the scopic regimes he is attempting to subvert.

A similar observation may be made about Derrida. The vision that figures in his texts is operated through sudden glances, surprising angles, occasional interruptions in the form of squints, winks, and blinks, odd choices of focus, that reverse our sense of what is important and what is not, sentencing what we consider important to the background and the margins of visibility. Sometimes he plays on our curiosity and vanity, drawing us on with mere peeks and glimpses. Sometimes he uses words, letters, the visible marks that appear on the page, to hide what he means from vision; and sometimes he uses them precisely in order to heighten the disclosure of what he means by communicating it in a way that speaks only to the eyes. Important though these inscriptions of vision are, Derrida does not thematize, does not acknowledge the deconstructive acts of seeing that are responsible for the processes of writing and reading into the play of which his texts seductively draw our sight. To be sure, the sight involved in such processes—a multiplicity of quick, extremely mobile glances, darting unpredictably to and fro, rather than a monadic, stationary and unmovable gaze—cannot be made fully present. But it is never even acknowledged, as such, in his texts. Like Foucault's own way of seeing, the presence of his gaze has remained concealed, for the most part showing itself rather in its critical operations and deconstructive effects, and of course, but more obliquely, in descriptions of the panoptical gaze of metaphysics, an always "other" way of seeing.

It is not, then, until—under the influence, certainly, of Habermas—Foucault began to think in earnest about discourses as dialogical situations, and not only as objects of study in the human sciences, and began, in consequence, to formulate an ethics of politics, a practice of politics as ethics, that he moved into the proximity of gazes reciprocating mutual recognition and reflecting mutual respect in the harmony of collaboration.[124] Had Foucault actually reached this political terrain and explicitly articulated his vision of its problems and its promise, he would have brought to the light, for our vision, the distinctive opportunities of the present, a radically new moment in the dialectical history of light and vision: the visionary moment of pluralistic democracy.

In a recently published book, *The Descent of Icarus: Science and the Transformation of Contemporary Democracy*, Yaron Ezrahi has attempted a genealogy of the gaze that complements and (in

Derrida's sense) supplements Foucault's: a genealogy concerned not with the gaze of the sovereign, the gaze of the dominant central authority, but rather with the gazes of the subjected, the dispersed multitude.[125] Distinguishing the gaze constitutive of the period that Foucault would call the classical from the enlightened gaze of modernity, Ezrahi argues that the popular gaze of the earlier period was essentially "celebrative" (participating in the spectacle of a sovereign power, a center of power, to which it was subject), whereas, by contrast, the civic gaze of the modern citizen, an essentially republican and liberal gaze, has been, rather, "attestive" (empirical, experimental, analytic, independent, and critical, deeply informed by the spirit of modern science and technology).

If this account is right, then, according to my hermenutical reading of Foucault, the gaze that figured in the production of most of Foucault's discourse, a gaze that was always, in Ezrahi's sense, "attestive," or critical, has finally perhaps undergone a major evolutionary transformation, or rather, given birth to a gaze with a distinctive new vision: a gaze different from the "attestive," or critical, a gaze that not only understands itself as inevitably situated, contextualized, relativized, multiplied, perspectival, and textualized, but now also recognizes itself as participatory, finding its identity in and through the other—a "late modern" gaze (or say, with Ezrahi, who concludes his study by recognizing, with a debt paid to John Dewey, the recent emergence of an intensely reflexive "postmodern" gaze), opening up new public spaces and new prospects for democratic politics. Instead of the governmental panopticon keeping everyone in sight and in line, there can be a reversal of this gaze. Indeed, one can easily find today, in many democratic states, a multitude of sites where spontaneously organized associations of citizens are policing, or keeping watch over, the operations of their government. Moreover, one can also find many sites opening up for the peaceful and cooperative exchange of different points of view: enlightened spaces where gazes will reciprocate demonstrations of respect and where the discursive interactions of democratic politics can take place. The reflexivity of the "postmodern" way of seeing problematizes the complicity of vision in relations of power, but it also introduces subversive ambiguities into the system of assumptions that have traditionally authorized the gaze of respect and reciprocity—assumptions, for example, regarding the relationship of this gaze to the perception of identity and difference—and ultimately to the perception of the invisible.

According to my reading, a similar evolution appears in the work of Derrida, whose deconstructive gaze—a gaze at once present and absent in the play of *écriture*, a gaze that moves metaphorically, endlessly encoding and decoding the logic of difference—is transported and resited (also resighted and recited) in South Africa, where, in the light of Nelson Mandela's critical and subversive reflections, it is touched for the first time by a vision of reversibilities and reciprocities and begins to see the possibility of justice not only in deconstruction, but also in the projection and construction of a new social order, created out of the recognition and respect that racially heterogeneous gazes accord one another in civil space.

In this regard, I would like to draw on Nietzsche's interpretation of perspectivism to formulate a position that he is commonly thought to oppose. In note 470 of *The Will to Power*, Nietzsche proclaims his "profound aversion to reposing once and for all in any one total view of the world."[126] This aversion, which both Derrida and Foucault share, to totalitarian and identitarian thinking, to all forms of prejudice, intolerance, and dogmatism, lies at the very heart of Nietzsche's perspectivism. Now, most readers interpret Nietzsche to draw an extreme doctrine of relativism from this perspectivism. And there is certainly some justification for this reading, as a hasty and incomplete persual of a note (sec. 374) from *Joyful Wisdom* indicates: "the human intellect," he says, there, "cannot avoid seeing itself in its perspective forms, and only in them. We cannot see around our corner: it is hopeless curiosity to want to know what other modes of intellect and perspective there might be."[127] However, if one continues reading, Nietzsche also says: "But I think that we are today at least far from the ludicrous immodesty of decreeing from our nook that there can be legitimate perspectives only from that nook. The world, on the contrary, has once more become 'infinite' to us; insofar we cannot dismiss the possibility that it contains infinite interpretations.'' It may come as a surprise to readers who can see Nietzsche only within the discourse of postmodernism that, in this passage, his version of perspectivism does not in principle exclude a concept of legitimacy. There may be an infinity of interpretations, but Nietzsche does not in any sense deny the possibility that some interpretations could be better than others.

When this passage is read in conjunction with a note from *The Genealogy of Morals*, the position where I am locating Nietzsche finds further support. Nietzsche says: ''The more affects we allow to speak in a given matter, the more eyes, different eyes, we can use to view a given spectacle, the more complete will be our 'conception' of it, the greater our 'objectivity.' ''[128] This clearly is not the kind of thinking popular in postmodernism. What especially interests me in Nietzsche's position here is that it suggests the possibility of combining a certain doctrine of perspectivism with the ''regulative ideal'' of a vision that is, or attempts to be, universal. In other words, it suggests the possibility of a common, or universal, point of view, a political consensus—a political position—achieved through dialogue and pragmatically constructed out of a multitude of different perspectives. Unfortunately, Nietzsche never pursued this thought, undoubtedly worried about the problem of distinguishing such a vision from the God's-eye vision he rightly rejected. With perhaps less justification, Foucault and Derrida also leave this possibility, which would connect the justice in postmodernism with the justice of the Enlightenment, very much in the dark.

L'Aveu de l'Aveugle: Miroirs, Mémoires, et la Question de Voir

Let us return to Derrida's *Mémoires de l'Aveugle*. Recently, in conjunction with an exhibition at the Louvre showing works of art on the theme of blindness, Derrida focused his attention as never before on the problematic of vision and blindness, writing a major essay for the exhibition. I cannot hope to do justice to this very intricately woven text. But I do not want to leave this remarkable text without remark. The artist's fascination with blindness, a fascination that in many cases can only be called an obsession, is not difficult to understand. Depending so utterly on their gift of vision, would they not practice their art with a certain anxiety, a certain dread of blindness? The loss of their eyesight would, of course, be annihilating. But it would be a mistake to give their portraits of blindness such an interpretation—or at least to assume that this was their only or even their primary motivation, be it conscious or unconscious. For just as many works of art are a celebration of the realm of vision—and by that I mean a celebration not only of the visible, but also, if often by indirection, of the gift of vision itself—so the works in the Louvre exhibit are philosophical reflections on the human significance of this gift.

Some of the portraits are reflections in the sense that they were drawn from images in a mirror, but even those not drawn in this way are reflections in the sense that they *function* as mirrors, as *mémoires*, as reminders. Those of us who enjoy the gift of sight need to be reminded of the gift—and reminded, too, that the presence in our midst of people without sight constitutes a moral claim on our solicitude, our generosity and compassion. The mirrors, then, are memories that refuse to be forgotten: they are drawings that draw us into an ethic of lucidity.

They are also reminders of our finitude, our limitation, our ruin: they show us our proximity to the invisible; they show us touched by the invisible; they show us inhabiting the invisible. It is not only the blind who dwell in the invisible; nor is it that those of us who can see are touched by the invisible only through the presence of the blind. In truth, we are all, in a sense, immersed in blindness, inhabitants of the invisible—and most of all precisely at that moment when we who can "see" are quite sure that we are seeing what is given us to see. Inseparable from the nobility of sight, there is the temptation of pride. Thus it was the questioning of our most comfortable assumptions, conventions, and distinctions that I think drew Derrida's attention to these works. Where are the borderlines that would securely locate us—

David Michael Levin

those of us who can "see"—within the realm of the visible? We who can "see" believe ourselves to be different from those who are blind. We see the blind immersed in darkness; we regard them as denizens of the invisible—all the while forgetting the extent of our own blindness.

Seeing cannot be a metaphysical comprehension of the visible. Total metaphysical presence is not possible: all seeing is unconcealment, and thus also, inevitably, the very ruination of vision. Buried within *l'aveugle*, encoded within the French word for "the blind," I see *l'aveu*, the French word for avowal, acknowledgment, confession. Do we not indeed, we who claim to see, have something to avow, to acknowledge, to confess? The blind in the Louvre portraits are mirrors, and their blindness is a reminder to those of us who can "see," bringing us back to our memories of that invisible without which nothing at all could be visible—and reminding us to confess our limitation, our necessary blindness. This blindness is like the libation, the pouring off of some wine as a gift of gratitude to the deities: it may be thought of as the sacrifice exacted in return for our sight.

Before the blind, we are called to account, compelled to look into ourselves, compelled to acknowledge that all too often we have turned away or shut our eyes to that which we did not want to see. Thus, the art in the exhibition double-crossed the borderlines that separate the sighted from the blind: in the very act of recognizing the other as blind, we are compelled to avow our own blindness. We are already the other. The artifice of the art is a questioning of seeing (*de voir*). It is also, however, the questioning of our response-ability (*devoir*). An ethics of lucidity—and an avowal of its ruination.

The Philosopher's Positions: In and Out of Sight

In closing, I once again invoke the wisdom of Nietzsche, a philosopher from whom both Derrida and Foucault enjoyed learning. Believing, as he says in *Twilight of the Idols*, that "one has to learn to see," he warns us, in *Daybreak: Thoughts on the Prejudices of Morality*, that "even they [the gods] have not acquired this eye [of gay wisdom] at a single stroke: seeing needs practice and preschooling, and he who is fortunate enough will also find at the proper time a teacher of pure seeing."[129] Foucault and Derrida were fortunate and learned well: they learned how to keep out of sight, how to elude disciplinary supervision, how to elude being framed and held captive within any framework, any visual regime, in order to have the freedom to observe as much as possible. It certainly is not easy to keep them in sight.

But the titular words, "keeping in sight," suggest more than one scenario. Let us consider another scenario and generate another narrative to interpret the difficulty of keeping them in sight. Perhaps we cannot keep them in sight because they ceased to think of politics in exclusively ocularcentric terms and began instead to think in terms of a dialogical model. Hannah Arendt reminds us that "since Bergson, the use of the sight metaphor in philosophy has kept dwindling, not unsurprisingly, as emphasis and interest have shifted entirely from contemplation to speech, from *nous* to *logos*."[130] Both Foucault and Derrida immersed themselves in language. First of all, they studied discourses, studied their histories, their rules of formation, their ways of working, their effects; but they also invented new, critical uses of discourse, using the discourses of their artifice to resist, subvert, and deconstruct the authority and legitimacy of other discourses. And as we have seen, both of them eventually reached a point in their thinking where they began to formulate—say, constructively —an ethics and politics of discourse. If this position signifies a paradigm shift, from an ordering of rationality centered in the domination of vision to an ordering of rationality founded on the justice of communicative processes, then perhaps we should rather delight in not keeping them any longer in the empire of sight.

And yet, once politics is thought according to the normative logic of the dialogue situation, with all the different viewpoints facing one another, perhaps we should regard as a welcome advance that moment of enlightenment when finally, at long last, setting the stage for a third scenario, we let these dangerous philosophers emerge from the shadows and come into our sight, with words of reflection that oblige us to open our eyes.[131]

David Michael Levin

Acknowledgments

I thank Martin Jay for reading an earlier draft of this chapter and for making many useful and thought-provoking criticisms. Our only point of difference is that we have somewhat different interpretations of the extent to which Derrida and Foucault can be situated within the Enlightenment project. I read them as moving closer to this project in their later work, although I also want to point out that each one stands in a very complex relationship to this project.

Notes

1. See my "Decline and Fall: Ocularcentrism in Heidegger's Reading of the History of Metaphysics," in D. M. Levin, ed., *Modernity and the Hegemony of Vision* (Los Angeles: University of California Press, 1993).

2. Friedrich Nietzsche, *Beyond Good and Evil* (New York: Random House, 1966), §146, p. 89.

3. See Jacques Derrida, "Force and Signification," in *Writing and Difference* (Chicago: University of Chicago Press, 1978), pp. 3, 28, 27.

4. Ibid., p. 27.

5. Derrida, "Violence and Metaphysics," in *Writing and Difference*, p. 85.

6. Ibid., p. 28.

7. Ibid., p. 27.

8. Ibid., p. 6.

9. Derrida, "Violence and Metaphysics," in *Writing and Difference*, p. 118.

10. Foucault, *The Birth of the Clinic: An Archaeology of Medical Perception* (New York: Random House, Vintage Books, 1975), p. 39.

11. Derrida, "Violence and Metaphysics," pp. 84–85.

12. Ibid., p. 88.

13. Ibid., pp. 90–91.

14. Ibid., p. 92.

15. Ibid., p. 90.

16. Ibid., p. 85.

17. Ibid., p. 92.

18. Ibid., p. 118.

19. Ibid., p. 120.

20. Derrida, *Speech and Phenomena, and Other Essays on Husserl's Theory of Signs* (Evanston: Northwestern University Press, 1973), p. 104.

21. Ibid., p. 103.

22. Ibid., pp. 45–46.

23. Ibid., p. 65.

24. Derrida, *Of Grammatology* (Baltimore: Johns Hopkins University Press, 1976), p. 164.

25. Derrida, *Speech and Phenomena*, pp. 108–109.

26. Derrida, *Of Grammatology*, p. 4.

27. See David Michael Levin, *The Opening of Vision* (London: Routledge, 1988) and "Decline and Fall: Ocularcentrism in Heidegger's Reading of the History of Metaphysics," in Levin, *Modernity and the Hegemony of Vision*.

28. Derrida, *Of Grammatology*, p. 163.

29. Ibid., p. 12.

30. See Martin Heidegger, *Was ist Metaphysik?* (Frankfurt: Vittorio Klostermann, 1949), p. 7. The text opens with the question, "Deeply considered, what is metaphysics?" To which he replies: "It thinks beings [*das Seiende*] as beings. Everywhere, wherever it is asked what a being [*das Seiende*] may be, beings as such stand in sight [*steht in der Sicht*]. The metaphysical representation [*Vorstellung*] owes this sight to the light of being. The light, i.e., that which such thinking experiences as light, does not itself come further into the sight [*Sicht*] of this thinking, for it represents beings always and only in reference [*in der Hinsicht*] to beings."

31. See John McCumber, "Derrida and the Closure of Vision," in Levin, *Modernity and the Hegemony of Vision*. McCumber also proposes a nice analysis of the "blind spot" as it figures in the (de)structuring of textuality.

32. Derrida, "Tympan," *Margins of Philosophy* (Chicago: University of Chicago Press, 1982), p. xiii.

33. Derrida, "White Mythology," *Margins of Philosophy*, p. 213.

34. Ibid., p. 251.

35. Ibid., p. 224.

36. Ibid., p. 242.

37. Ibid., p. 267.

38. Ibid., p. 250.

39. Ibid., p. 268.

40. Ibid.

41. Ibid., p. 266.

42. Ibid., p. 254.

43. Ibid., p. 270.

44. Ibid., p. 271.

45. Derrida, *Of Grammatology*, p. 163.

46. Ibid., p. 149.

47. Derrida, "The Principle of Reason: The University in the Eyes of Its Pupils," *Diacritics* 13, no. 3 (Fall 1983):4.

48. See Hans Blumenberg, "Light as a Metaphor of Truth," in Levin, *Modernity and the Hegemony of Vision*. Also see Hans Jonas, "The Nobility of Sight: A Study in the Phenomenology of the Senses," in S. Spicker, ed., *The Philosophy of the Body: Rejections of Cartesian Dualism* (New York: Quadrangle, 1970), pp. 312–333; Hans Jonas, *The Phenomenon of Life: Toward a Philosophical Biology* (New York: Harper & Row, 1966), pp. 135–156; and Hannah Arendt, who, in *The Life of the Mind* (New York: Harcourt Brace Jovanovich, 1978), pp. 110–112, confesses that she has begun to "wonder why hearing did not develop into the guiding metaphor for thinking." Also see David M. Levin, *The Listening Self: Personal Growth, Social Change, and the Closure of Metaphysics* (London: Routledge, 1989).

49. Derrida, "The Principle of Reason," p. 4.

50. Ibid., pp. 9–10.

51. Ibid., p. 10.

52. Ibid.

53. Ibid., p. 20.

54. Derrida, "The Laws of Reflection: Nelson Mandela, In Admiration," in J. Derrida and Mustapha Tlili, eds., *For Nelson Mandela* (New York: Henry Holt, Seaver Books, 1987), p. 14.

55. Ibid.

56. Ibid., p. 17.

57. Ibid., p. 26.

58. Ibid., p. 27.

59. Ibid., p. 16.

60. Ibid., p. 17.

61. Ibid., p. 34.

62. Ibid.

63. Derrida, "Structure, Sign and Play in the Discourses of the Human Sciences," in *Writing and Difference* (Chicago: University of Chicago Press, 1978), p. 280.

64. Derrida, "Of an Apocalyptic Tone Recently Adopted in Philosophy," *Semeia*, vol. 23 (1982), p. 82.

65. See Derrida, *The Truth in Painting* (Chicago: University of Chicago Press, 1987), for a sustained critical reading of philosophical texts—principally Kant's *Critique of Judgment*—with regard to the problematic of representation, frame, and context. This work, however, is only indirectly concerned with vision—with ocularcentrism and the philosophical discourse on/of vision.

66. Derrida, *Mémoires d'aveugle: L'autoportrait et autres ruines* (Paris: Edition de la Réunion des Musées Nationaux, 1990), translated as *Memoirs of the Blind* (Chicago: University of Chicago Press, 1993).

67. Derrida's discussion of the weeping of the eyes, the water of tears, and the moment of unveiling recalls my own discussion of these themes in *The Opening of Vision* (London: Routledge, 1988), where I argued that vision, as an act of beholding, is correspondingly beholden, that *crying is the root of seeing*, that vision needs to stay in contact with the body of feeling, that crying manifests this need, that the water of tears temporarily sacrifices vision, but is ultimately a purification and clarification that puts it in touch again with our capacity to be touched and moved by what we see, and that tears are a veiling of sight that unveils the deeper nature of vision.

68. Foucault, "What Is Enlightenment?" in Paul Rabinow, ed., *The Foucault Reader* (New York: Pantheon Books, 1984), p. 48.

69. Foucault, *Madness and Civilization: A History of Insanity in the Age of Reason* (New York: Random House, 1965), pp. 70, 250.

70. Ibid., p. 250.

71. Foucault, *Birth of the Clinic*, p. 52.

72. Ibid., p. 121. Also see p. 165, where he distinguishes two kinds of gaze: "a local, circumscribed gaze" and "an absolute, absolutely integrating gaze that dominates and founds all perceptual experience." "It is this gaze," he tells us, "that structures into a sovereign unity that which belongs to a lower level of the eye, the ear, and the sense of touch." In *Vision and Painting: The Logic of the Gaze* (New Haven: Yale University Press, 1983), Norman Bryson suggests a distinction

between the "Gaze" and the "Glance," arguing that the first, synoptic and temporally enduring, enacts a metaphysics of presence, whereas the second, narrowly directed and temporally brief, enacts a perpetual subversion of this ontology and epistemology. See esp. pp. 121–122.

73. Ibid., p. 88.

74. Ibid., p. 51.

75. Ibid., p. 83.

76. Ibid., p. 84.

77. Ibid., p. 89.

78. Ibid., p. xiii.

79. Ibid.

80. Ibid.

81. Ibid., p. 52.

82. Ibid., p. 39.

83. Ibid., p. 166.

84. Ibid., p. 40.

85. Ibid., p. 52.

86. Ibid., p. 65.

87. Foucault, *The Order of Things: An Archaeology of the Human Sciences* (New York: Random House, Vintage Books, 1973), p. xx.

88. Ibid., p. 312. Italics added.

89. Ibid., p. 13.

90. Ibid., p. 132.

91. Ibid., p. 133.

92. Ibid., p. 6.

93. Foucault, "Nietzsche, Genealogy, History," in Rabinow, *The Foucault Reader*, p. 87.

94. Ibid., p. 86.

95. Ibid., p. 89.

96. Ibid.

97. Ibid.

98. Ibid., p. 90.

99. See, in this regard, Bryson, *Vision and Painting*, esp. pp. 121–122. As I noted earlier, Bryson distinguishes the "Gaze" from the "Glance," and argues that the "Gaze" enacts a metaphysics of presence, while the "Glance" enacts a perpetual subversion.

100. Foucault, "What Is Enlightenment?" in Rabinow, *The Foucault Reader*, p. 48.

101. Foucault, "Body/Power," in *Power/Knowledge: Selected Interviews and Other Writings, 1972–1977* (New York: Pantheon, 1980), p. 62. Italics added.

102. Foucault, "The Politics of Health in the Eighteenth Century," pp. 170–171.

103. Foucault, *Discipline and Punish: The Birth of the Prison* (New York: Random House, Vintage Books, 1979), p. 185.

104. Foucault, "Two Lectures," in *Power/Knowledge*, pp. 104–105.

105. Foucault, *Discipline and Punish*, p. 222.

106. See Susan Buck-Morss, *The Dialectics of Seeing: Walter Benjamin and the Arcades Project* (Cambridge: MIT Press), p. 308.

107. Foucault, "The Eye of Power," in *Power/Knowledge*, pp. 152, 154. This interview took place in 1977, after the publication of *Discipline and Punish*.

108. Ibid., p. 146.

109. Foucault, *Discipline and Punish*, p. 222.

110. Foucault, "The Ethic of Care for the Self as a Practice of Freedom," in J. Bernauer and D. Rasmussen, eds., *The Final Foucault* (Cambridge: MIT Press, 1988), pp. 12–13.

111. Foucault, "Power and Strategies," in *Power/Knowledge*, p. 142.

112. Foucault, "Power and Sex," in *Michel Foucault: Politics, Philosophy, Culture* (London: Routledge, 1990), p. 123.

113. Foucault, *The Archaeology of Knowledge*, p. 205. Also see *Power/Knowledge*, pp. 98 and 102.

114. Foucault, *The History of Sexuality* (New York: Random House, 1978), 1:93.

115. Ibid., p. 94.

116. Ibid., pp. 94–95.

117. See Foucault, "Two Lectures," in *Power/Knowledge,* p. 80; "Revolutionary Action: Until Now," in *Language, Countermemory, Practice* (Ithaca: Cornell University Press, 1977), p. 230; and "Power and Sex," in *Michel Foucault: Politics, Philosophy, Culture,* p. 124.

118. See Gilles Deleuze, *Foucault* (Minneapolis: University of Minnesota Press, 1988), esp. pp. 46–49, and an excellent study by John Rajchman, "Foucault's Art of Seeing," *October* 44 (Spring 1988):89–117.

119. Foucault, "The Concern for Truth," in *Michel Foucault: Politics, Philosophy, Culture,* p. 265.

120. Foucault, "How Much Does it Cost for Reason to Tell the Truth?" in *Foucault Live* (New York: Columbia University Semiotext(e), 1989), pp. 242, 252.

121. Foucault, "Politics and Ethics: An Interview," in Rabinow, *The Foucault Reader,* p. 374.

122. Foucault, "Polemics, Politics, and Problematizations," in Rabinow, *The Foucault Reader,* pp. 381–382.

123. See Martin Jay, "In the Empire of the Gaze," in David Hoy, ed., *Foucault: A Critical Reader* (Oxford: Basil Blackwell, 1986), p. 195. Jay contends that, "unlike many non-French commentators on the implications of vision, he [Foucault] resisted exploring its reciprocal, intersubjective, communicative function, that of the mutual glance.... As de Certeau has pointed out, Foucault focused so insistently on the dangers of panopticism that he remained blind to other micro-practices of everyday life that subvert its power." Jay's study is an important one, and I concur with much that he has to say. But this chapter argues that Foucault comes closer to recognizing reciprocity in vision than Jay is willing to grant.

124. Concerning the reversibility of reflective gazes as the embodied, experiential ground of ethical reciprocity and social justice, see David M. Levin, "Justice in the Flesh," in G. Johnson and M. Smith, eds., *Ontology and Alterity in Merleau-Ponty* (Evanston: Northwestern University Press, 1990), pp. 35–44, and "Visions of Narcissism: Intersubjectivity and the Reversals of Reflection," in M. Dillon, ed., *Merleau-Ponty Vivant* (Albany: State University of New York Press, 1991), pp. 47–90.

125. See Ezrahi, *The Descent of Icarus.* I cannot recommend this book too highly. It tells a familiar story from an excitingly new angle, making visible an important but long marginalized field of experience and enriching our public vision. Also see Thomas Flynn, "Foucault and the Eclipse of Vision," in David M. Levin, ed., *Modernity and the Hegemony of Vision* (Los Angeles: University of California Press, 1993).

126. Friedrich Nietzsche, *The Will to Power* (New York: Random House, 1967), p. 262.

127. Nietzsche, *Joyful Wisdom* (New York: Frederick Unger, 1960), p. 340.

128. Nietzsche, *The Genealogy of Morals* (New York: Doubleday, 1956), p. 255.

129. Nietzsche, *Twilight of the Idols* (New York: Penguin Books, 1968), p. 5, and *Daybreak: Thoughts on the Prejudices of Morality* (New York: Cambridge University Press, 1982), p. 203.

130. Hannah Arendt, *The Life of the Mind* (New York: Harcourt Brace Jovanovich, 1978), p. 122.

14

Difference and the Ruin of Representation in Gilles Deleuze

Dorothea Olkowski

Anyone who has followed feminist film theory over the last decade is aware of the extent to which vision and the act of looking have been problematized and politicized by feminist critics of film.[1] While the Lacanian-psychoanalytic approach to conceptualizing vision has drawn attention to the "scopophilia" inherent in both the production and the spectatorship of classic Hollywood film, its weaknesses are those inherent in any attempt to claim that certain characteristics inflexibly and essentially constitute the *telos* of vision.[2] Psychoanalytic film criticism relies on a conception of vision developed by theorists like Jean-Louis Baudry, who claims that cinema is merely the final and most perfected material realization of the return to the scene of the unconscious. This realization began, he proposes, in Plato's cave, a prehistoric cinema that produced the first simulated and displaced dream state wherein the unconscious could represent itself.[3] Thus, he proposes, film's special function is to satisfy narcissism by providing the subject with visual representations that reproduce images from the unconscious, images that represent a world ordered by active male subjects and passive females objectified by a controlling male gaze.[4]

But such claims have not been able to withstand the critique of their teleological aims and visual presuppositions. For example, in the essay "Geometry and Abjection," the British artist and critic Victor Burgin points to the "reductive and simplistic equation of *looking* with *objectification*'' (emphasis added) that underlies our current reception and recognition of images as objectified representations.[5] This particular way of seeing is, Burgin contends, not a necessity but is related to a conception of space that is only one in a long line of spaces that constitute what he takes to be the history of culturally constructed spaces.

Burgin, whose art is well known in the contemporary international art scene for challenging visual norms, has a particular problem with equating vision with objectification insofar as it is an equation drawn from Euclidean physiological optics, which does not, he believes, adequately describe the changed apprehension of space that corresponds to contemporary life. Euclidean geometry, he points out, was based on visual evidence, on what could be seen, rather than on technical or even practical considerations, and it appeals to the Classical Greek cosmological model that reemerged in the Middle Ages as the locus of human action. In Aristotle's version of the Greek cosmos, each body is located in a continuum of actual and potential places that constitute space. For the Middle Ages this meant a sphere with a center and a circumference wherein each being is assigned a place preordained by God.[6] In this, Burgin follows Michel Foucault, who also characterizes the space of the Middle Ages as a hierarchic ensemble of places, though Foucault specifies that it is defined by particular oppositions: sacred and profane, protected and open, urban and rural.[7] And although Newton later conceived of space as absolute, homogeneous, and immovable, that is, as extensive, the Aristotelian-medieval conception remained operative, constituting specific social and/or political localizations within an absolute space. As such, Burgin claims, for humanist-derived political philosophy, space is organized in accordance with this determinate conceptual hierarchy. Thus, it is impossible that objectified visual representations dominate our looking by necessity, as Baudry claims; rather, insofar as such representations dominate vision, they do so merely for political and/or social reasons. That is, they are relatively unmotivated by, and thus unrelated to, the so-called necessities and truths of scientific discovery or invention.

What I will try to show is that the spatial hierarchy that Burgin critiques is neither simply a historical fact—random and unmotivated—nor something absolutely necessary, preordained, and unalterable. As a historical fact, spatial hierarchy would be unmotivated by what is usually taken to be its opposite, that is, any force that philosophy takes to be metaphysically necessary. Thus, while spatial hierarchy constitutes the very *logos* of visual representation, this means only that it is what we mean by visual representation, it is the very definition of visual representation, and that, though such vision and the space in which it takes place are constructed (so they have no inherent teleological necessity), they still are not simply contingent or unmotivated. While Burgin emphasizes the social and political dimensions of visual representation, that is, the degree to which it grants privilege to human beings so as to justify their claims to inherent social and or natural qualities,[8] I will begin by articulating the conceptual schema that constitutes such a vision in order to engage in the "ruin of representation."[9] It should then be possible, by considering actual practices, to suggest alternative modes of vision and how they are constructed.

Burgin's notion of culturally constructed spaces proves to be of great use in carrying out the ruin of representation, for he continues, beyond these preliminary remarks, to document what he takes to be the historical eras that have lent their names to various definitions of space. He claims (again following Foucault) that *premodern space* is organized by location; *modern space* by Euclid's infinite, extensible, boundless geometry; *early modern space* by the humanist subject; *late modern space* by industrial capitalism's imperative to disperse, displace, and disseminate; and *postmodern space* by monetary capitalism's imploding and infolding. However, it strikes me that there is a disjunction between the claim that space has a history and the fact that theories (and in most instances practices) of representation have tended to remain constant, faithful to the Euclidean, geometrical-optical metaphors of the modern period, which themselves fall back on Aristotelian representational schemas.

The Italian Renaissance conceived of the picture plane by combining the medieval notion that space has a center with Euclidean optics, according to which seeing is produced in a "cone of vision" that the picture plane intersects. The Renaissance privileged this cosmological model, and contemporary culture continues to maintain, as its dominant system of space, one in which socially inscribed human beings are deployed in a space that is more or less uniform in itself. The cone of vision model, however, insofar as it is adopted from the Renaissance, operates to deny the key feature of postmodern space: that space is not geographical but governed by the electronic speed of the computer and the video.[10] Having admitted to the fact that representation does not seem to adhere to the space of its history, I wonder how Burgin can possibly maintain that space has a history except in the purest, most positivist scientific sense? Still, Burgin is on to something important if he is right that the Renaissance pictorial model of looking still dominates our seeing. And if this is the case, it says something important about vision: that it is not simply an accident of history, but also not preordained by nature, insofar as the dominant mode of vision, the Renaissance representational model, was constructed by combining several different conceptualizations of space, attached, according to Burgin, to several different phases of history.

If the so-called history of space has not coincided with the dominant mode of vision derived from Greek cosmology and Renaissance science, and consequently has not challenged the hegemony of representation, this incongruity needs to be accounted for. It is likely that some more complex and perhaps more abstract factors are at work, factors that are not clearly inscribed in the general history of scientific inquiry. It may in fact be the case that the enigma of representation is part of some more complex and hidden structure, so that its explanation is less than apparent to the generalized nature of historical inquiry. Gilles Deleuze has put forth the thesis that visual representation has always been linked to the development of the Western metaphysical framework that guarantees a particular kind of order and truth. Above all, visual representation is used to justify certain types of rooted social and political as well as philosophical regimes.

In his early book, *Différence et répétition*, Deleuze is primarily interested in discovering a way to think the notion of difference apart from the Aristotelian metaphysical framework in whose terms it was originally conceived, at least among Western thinkers.[11] In doing so, he seems to have recovered the philosophical underpinnings of representation as the dominant mode of seeing the world regardless of which historical conception of space obtains at any given moment. The discovery that Deleuze makes is that visual representation has been constituted, in Western philosophy and visual practice, in terms of the Aristotelian framework. This discovery may be why, following *Différence et répétition*, Deleuze engages in numerous efforts to analyze visual representation as a particularly restricted form of imaging; thus it may also be the case that this first analysis remains the heart of all his other thinking on the question.[12]

For Deleuze, the bias that has constructed representation as the standard and norm for all visual images, and so for vision, is not merely part of a historical moment. It is grounded in something more profound whose persistence and effects I will take up at the end of this chapter, but whose cause may well lie in philosophy's answer to the question: What is difference? In asking this question, Deleuze is clearly not interested in empirical differences, or in things insofar as they are already distinguished from one another and so remain outside the notion of difference. He wants to ask about difference itself. Deleuze's description of this notion is so evocative and creates such a strong image that it merits quoting at length:

Let us rather imagine something which is distinguished—and yet that from which it is distinguished is not distinguished from it. The flash of lightening for example, is distinguished from the black sky, but must carry the sky along with it.... One would say that the bottom rises to the surface, without ceasing to be the bottom. There is, on both sides, something cruel—and even monstrous—in this struggle against an elusive adversary, where the distinguished is opposed to something which cannot be distinguished from it, and which continues to embrace that which is divorced from it. (p. 43)

A number of considerations can be discerned in this analysis. Consider the norm for all visual representation: single-point perspective. In his treatise, "On Painting," Alberti laid out the rules of representation in painting. The image must appear within the boundaries of a rectangle or framed window that maintains the image at a distance from the viewer who views it as if through a window.[13] The canvas itself is divided geometrically so that the illusion of three dimensions can be produced on the canvas by establishing an infinitely receding horizon, in the center of the flat surface, that constitutes a hierarchy in terms of the proportionate sizes of the objects that appear within the grid. Those objects closest to the viewer appear to be the largest; those farthest removed are the smallest and become smaller as they recede toward the infinite horizon. Within this space, the figures are carefully modeled with light and shadow, furthering the illusion of depth and three dimensions. Drawing is emphasized over color insofar as it meets the demand for planar, symmetrical, and conceptual surfaces conveying more intelligible and less optical images. However, numerous Renaissance scholars attest to the fact that while Renaissance artists battled against the restrictions of the theorists, preferring the living quality of images in movement to the mirrored perfection of nature, nonetheless this more static conception of representation prevailed in the end.[14]

We find it, for example, in the work of Nicolas Poussin (1593–1665), who wrote that the highest aim of painted imagery is to represent noble and serious human actions, shown in a logical and orderly way—not as they actually happen but as they would happen were nature perfect.[15] In Poussin's painting, the impressions of nature are ordered according to laws of visibility that create the topographical exactitude required for idealized landscapes. Figures are frozen in the moment of action in landscapes that are hierarchically ordered spaces. But if we follow Deleuze's prescription, we must think about the bottom of such images rising to the surface, that is, the background rising up onto the surface of the image. The result is distortion of the image, a distortion that decomposes the planar and symmetrically arranged bodies and objects. When, as Deleuze says, the bottom rises to the surface, the grid is effaced, modeling is defeated, and form is destroyed. This is the monstrosity, the cruelty of difference in the image. Such cruel or monstrous distortion of the hierarchically composed representational image, the three-dimensional illusion, and the plastic technique of relief produces irregular and sometimes disturbing images.

Goya's *Executions of May 3, 1808* offers a grisaille of soldiers that form a solid, nearly undifferentiated plane, each one a repetition of the next, while the surface of the canvas becomes a site of murder and carnage. In William Blake's primal scenes of awe, terror, or creation, an emblematic figure blazes in the center of a depthless surface. These paintings and drawings manifest no respect for norms of proportion or sense, the key elements of perspectival visual representation. Such distortion is not limited to the nineteenth century; that is, it is not tied to a particular historical era in the west. Giotto's fourteenth-century Arena Chapel interior also articulates a highly differentiated kind of pictorial space that sharpens the viewer's awareness of the picture surface. In the scene of Hell, in particular, there is a total collapse of hierarchized space: shattered architecture, a completely flat surface, fading and disappearing color and bodies.[16] In none of these cases does what appears on the surface correspond to what we would expect from the so-called history of space.

In each case, form is destroyed, figure-ground relief renounced, and a determination is made (p. 44). Far from being the materialization of irrationality and chaos, what emerges in these images is a profound and difficult kind of vision where, as Deleuze notes, "determination is made by dint of supporting a precise and unilateral relationship with the indeterminate" (p. 44). The bottom rises, the form dissolves, yet a determination is made, perhaps the most important determination of all: one that has been routinely and without thought compromised by the categorical orientation of Western philosophy since Aristotle, who articulated the demand for coherence and hierarchy in the organic representation and who, according to Deleuze, inscribes all difference in a general concept.

While the detour through Aristotle is complex, it is absolutely necessary for insight into how hierarchical representation came to be established as the single and authoritative source of visual intelligibility and political stabilization. According to Deleuze, it is Aristotle who, to a far greater degree than Plato, refused to recognize difference and who is thus responsible for the establishment of the hegemonic reign of representation. On the level of practice, when visual representation is taken to be the only intelligible regime of visibility, then hegemonic and rigid social and political practices embrace representation to justify their existence.

For Aristotle, Deleuze states, terms differ through the mediation of something else, but there are degrees of mediation and thus degrees of difference. True difference, in Aristotle, is located only in the greatest of these, but not so distantly that there is no basis for comparison: "That contrariety is the greatest difference is made clear by induction. For things which differ in *genus* have no way to one another, but are too far distant and not comparable; and for things that differ in *species* the extremes from which generation takes place are the contraries, and the distance between extremes—and therefore that between the contraries—is the greatest."[17]

Merely material contraries would of course be accidental; generic differences are too great and cannot even be considered together; individual differences are too small (p. 46). Only the genus is divided by specific differences; that is, the differences modify the subject in its form such that the genus remains the same for itself (identical), yet becomes other in the differences that divide it (p. 47).

Aristotle is not even considering differences that are merely other and do not differ in a particular respect, that is, do not begin with something in common. This is why the organic unity of the representation of a genus in a concept is what is at stake for him: "For ... that which is different is different from some particular thing in some particular respect, so that there must be something *identical* whereby they differ."[18] Difference is only allowed to exist in terms of identity with regard to a generic concept (p. 48). What gets constituted in Aristotle is thus the very ruin of difference itself. There is and can be no concept proper to difference, for difference is always inscribed within the genus, the concept in general, and difference is no more than difference within identity. The result is that "one confuses the determination of the concept of difference with the inscription of difference in the identity of an indeterminate concept" (p. 48).

While this approach provides coherence and intelligibility through the hierarchy imposed by identical generic concepts and their specific differences, it restricts difference to the role of a predicate of concepts. But the restriction is not absolute, for precisely at this point something happens that amounts to a "crack" in thought through which another notion of difference will emerge. Genera are, in Aristotle's account, "ultimate determinable concepts [categories]," so they are not conditioned by a higher-level concept or meta-genus common to them all. As Aristotle insists: "But it is not possible that either unity or being should be a single genus of things; *for the differentiae of any genus must each of them both have being and be one.*"[19]

Differences have being; differences themselves are. Yet in the same breath, Aristotle also maintains that no genus can be predicated of its differentia. The point to note here is that if differences are, then the genus should be able to be predicated of or attributable to its differences. But as I will make clear, Aristotle's overall framework makes this impossible.

In Aristotle, being subsists as an identical or common concept that functions distributively and hierarchically (p. 49). This means that being is not a genus whose species would be the categories; such a division would make being *univocal* which, for Aristotle, it is not. Rather, the unity of being is that of an analogy. Franz Brentano has clarified this:

Thus *Metaphysics* V. 10 claims that, since being is said in several ways, the same follows for all other concepts which are attributed to it, so that the identical, the different, and the opposite ought to be recognized as something different for each category.... Similarly, *Metaphysics* V.28 states peremptorily that whatever belongs to different categories does not have a common genus and that the categories can be reduced neither to one another nor to a single higher entity.[20]

As for the unity of being lying in *analogy*, Aristotle states that unity comes from number, species (those whose definition is one), genus (those with common attributes), or analogy (those that are relative to one another).[21] Analogy, Brentano points out, operates specifically in relation to "one definite kind of thing." In Aristotle's examples, all that is healthy is relative to health and all that is medical is relative to the medical art.[22] As Aristotle writes: "And that which is medical is relative to the medical art, one thing being called medical because it possesses it, another because it is naturally adapted to it, another because it is a function of the medical art. And we shall find other words used *similarly* to these."[23] In the specific case of being, being refers primarily to substance, and all other categories only have being in reference to substance.[24] Or, as Deleuze notes, being is hierarchically primary and distributively common to all categories; thus insofar as it operates analogically, being is equivocal and will never give us a proper concept of difference (pp. 49, 50).

Specific difference determines difference only in the identity of the concept in general, while generic difference is no more than analogy. Between these two kinds of differences "a bond of complicity is formed in *representation*." Thus, what we are witnessing is the very formation of representation, the *logos* of representation mentioned above, which is always composed of the differences (conceived in terms of analogy) between species subsumed under the identity of a genus that itself stands in relations of analogy with other genera. However, this abstract representation, insofar as it subsumes species, also relies on what constitutes them, namely, resemblances that presume the continuity of the sensible intuition in a concrete representation (p. 51). The effect of this dual system of classification is to erase difference as a concept and as reality. This occurs, of course, in the process of reflection, the judgment according to which these determinations are made and according to which difference is made to submit to representation: "In the concept of reflection, indeed, the mediatory and mediatized difference submits itself fully to the *identity* of the concept, to the *opposition* of predicates, to the *analogy* of judgment, and to the *resemblance* of perception. We find here again the essentially quadripartite character of representation" (p. 52).

Deleuze characterizes representation as "organic" insofar as it is constituted in terms of this four-part judgment, in accordance with which difference is excluded from representation. If difference were to show itself at all as a concept and reality, it could do so in this model only as a crack, a catastrophe, a break in resemblance or as the impossibility of claiming identity, opposition, analogy, or resemblance where reflection demands they should occur.

It is clear to Deleuze that in most political, social, artistic, ethnic, economic, scientific, linguistic, and philosophical practices, the Aristotelian model of organic representation—organized around identity, opposition, analogy, and resemblance—dominates. This development is motivated by the intelligibility and simplicity of organic representation as revealed in political and visual practices. As Poussin discovered, organic representation perfects vision and idealizes the real; and as the Italian Renaissance proves, organic representation offers visible intelligibility and coherence.

Two key questions emerge out of this problematic. First, under what, if any, conditions is difference a concept and real? Second, what accounts for the domination of the occurrence according to which difference is made to submit to organic representation? Is it, as Burgin implies, a choice made in favor of certain historical constructions, or is representation part of some other more determined and less contingent structure? Beginning with the first question, I would argue that to conceptualize real difference, the model of judgments must be abandoned, for it is by means of judgment or "good sense" that difference is lost. Foucault has remarked on this specifically: "But *what* recognizes these similarities, the exactly alike and the least similar—the greatest and the smallest, the brightest and the darkest—if not good sense? ... And it is good sense that reigns in the philosophy of representation."[25]

Deleuze suggests that an appropriate though contingent replacement for judgment is the proposition. This is not to insist that the conceptualization of difference as real can only emerge in linguistics. Difference is not principally linguistic either in scope or origin, for as I shall make clear below, the linguistic formalization is only one expression of the science of multiplicities.[26] However, the propositional model explains multiplicities in a rather simple manner, which can serve as an introduction to other kinds of material multiplicities that themselves implicate language. Deleuze offers the well-known example of "evening star–morning star." He writes: "The distinction between these meanings is certainly a real distinction, but there is nothing numerical about it, and much less anything ontological: it is rather a formal, qualitative, or semiological distinction.... The important thing is that we are able to conceive of several formally distinct meanings, which nonetheless are related to being as to a single, ontologically one referent" (pp. 52–53). Not only is being the ontologically one referent, but it is in no sense equivocal; being is expressed in one and the same sense in each of its (numerically) distinct expressors. Being is (ontologically) one, and the meaning of *being* is ontologically one.

In this crucial shift of expression, being is not said in several ways; being is expressed in one and the same sense of each of its (numerically) distinct designates (*le designé*), yet each difference has its own essence; they do not have the same meaning (p. 53). If being speaks with a single voice in the proposition, and being is "said" of difference itself, then being is not equivocal; it is univocal and being is said of differences, none of which have the same meaning. The effect of this is to conceptualize difference as real, to conceptualize it differentially, and not to submit it to representation, which always searches out the common elements underlying difference.[27] Of course, mere univocity does not guarantee that individual differences are not somehow the same or equal, that they do not have the same meaning. Everything

Difference and the Ruin of Representation in Gilles Deleuze

depends on how distribution is governed. In Aristotle, entities have different degrees of being, as if there were only so much being available for distribution. This occurs because "there is a hierarchy which measures beings according to their limits, and according to their degree of proximity or distance in relation to a principle" (p. 55). For Deleuze, such a measure of being is also a measure of law and the limits of law.

Having found the crack in thought in Aristotle's notion of being, Deleuze proposes to articulate this crack, and he lays out a different kind of law and measure for the "being which is said of difference." The articulation of this kind of "monstrosity" (monstrous in relation to the rigid hierarchies of organic representation) is yet another thought and practice (in addition to the proposition above) of difference, one that is more easily related to vision and visual practices. It would be more comfortable to imply that there is nothing out of the ordinary in what Deleuze is suggesting here; however, insofar as this is not the case, I do not want to domesticate this concept. While Deleuze's logic and semiotics are enormously sophisticated, still there is an element of danger in what he is suggesting. The monstrous nature of difference in the face of the stability and hierarchy of representation is undeniable. It is not a safe way to act or to think, because in the judgments of what Deleuze calls "State power," difference is heretical and must be scapegoated. In the eyes of State power, difference *is* monstrous. Thus, I want to make use of this word that Deleuze introduces in *Différence et répétition* because it reflects what is at stake in Deleuze's work.

The sort of measure Deleuze proposes to account for monstrous difference is the "*nomadic nomos,* without property, enclosure or measure ... an allocation of those who distribute *themselves* ... in a *space without precise limits*" (p. 54; final emphasis added). Such a "wandering distribution" is not the Aristotelian space (adopted by Renaissance perspectivism) that is divided, shared, and hierarchized in accordance with the principle of proximity to being and degree of being. It is easy to see that the "fixed and proportional determinations" of Aristotelian hierarchies correlate very well with the fixed and proportional determinations of objectified and perspectival visual representations, whether those of the Italian Renaissance or those of feminist film theory. It is beyond the scope of this chapter to follow Deleuze through an account of various philosophies that have supported hierarchized accounts of space and those that have taken up the space of univocal being, the space of the surface. However, what does emerge from this analysis is the realization that the space of difference, thought and practiced differentially, is not subject to historical interpretation, even though its absence is certainly a reflection of the prevailing forms of social and political life.

I have noted that the great Renaissance artists opposed the demand for planar, symmetrical, and conceptual images, and that they did so, perhaps surprisingly, for the sake of movement: "As has been said, illusion was partly realized in the simple creation of virtual three-dimensional forms (*rilievo*), in convincing relationship (perspective). But surpassing these ... was the representation of movement."[28] Yet in Aristotle, organic visual representation is distributed hierarchically around "one center, a sole and elusive perspective," analogous to Aristotle's distribution of being. Thus "it mediatizes everything, but mobilizes and moves nothing (p. 78). Movement, however, accords with the nomadic *nomos* insofar as it involves a plurality of centers (of differences, each of which *is*), superimposing and mixing perspectives and points of view and effecting the distortion of representation in the visual field (p. 79). Such an effect is not the product of the multiplication of representations for "the infinite representation comprises precisely an infinity of representations, whether it ensures the convergence of all points of view on an identical object or an identical world, or whether it creates the properties of an identical Self from different moments. But, in this way, it keeps a single center which gathers and represents all the others as a unity of a series that orders and organizes, once and for all, the terms and their relations" (p. 79). In the system of hierarchical distribution, regardless of the number of representations, the conceptual form of the identical, that is, the concept in general, subordinates all differences. In order for there to be movement and mobility, the nomadic *nomos*, distortion must somehow destabilize representation, representation must be torn from its center and from the identity of the concept, as well as from the perfect hierarchy of distribution that Aristotle establishes (p. 79).

For Deleuze, Aristotle's conceptualization does not simply create hierarchies of thought; rather it serves to legitimate or justify certain visual, linguistic, social, and political practices that developed around the demand for intelligibility, rigidity, and hegemony. Therefore, merely reconceptualizing difference is not enough to restore difference as difference; rather, the ruin of representation can be accomplished only on the level of actual practices. This is why Deleuze claims that the modern work of art, more than anything, "tends to realize these conditions," the conditions effecting representation's demise. Painting and sculpture distort visual representation so that we have to combine the view from above and the view from below, or we have to go up and come down in space (p. 79). And as I have tried to show, these distorting tendencies (distorting in relation to the rigid hierarchies of representation) have always been present in selected works of art and, to some extent, even in the work of representational artists, as the crack or the catastrophe that emerges in the midst of representation.

Along these same lines, art historian Svetlana Alpers points out that under the influence of Aristotelian cosmology, Italian artists were normally unwilling or unable to sacrifice either the authority that single-point perspective attributes to the viewer or the unity that it provides to the image. Italian artists, she continues, turned away from individuation for the sake of general human traits and truths and resemblance to an ideal of appearance and action (p. 78). Alpers contrasts this with the work of Dutch artists like Samuel von Hoogstraten, who urges young artists to be humble and to paint the diversity of things in the world where each face is created to be different (p. 77). She cites an illustration of Jean Perlerin's (called Viator) geometry: "One plate, 'Perspective,' shows a multiplication of distance-points leading the eye to a variety of views up and down, in and out of an empty room, *adding* on views of the moving eye."[29] Perlerin's illustration makes possible the construction of a mobile image. Deleuze and Félix Guattari offer their own mobile image. In the visual work of art, difference refers to other differences that never identify but only differentiate it, such that each difference stands in relation to other differences all of which are without a center and without convergence both in relation to themselves and in relation to one another (p. 79). In this way each work of art is "a true *theatre*, made of metamorphoses and permutations [and].... The work of art leaves the domain of representation in order to become 'experience,' transcendental empiricism, and the science of the sensible" (p. 79).

The second question that I posed above remains to be addressed. Why has representation succeeded in dominating difference? The question is difficult to answer directly without falling into a trap that once again submits difference to identity by positing the answer (which has two faces) in terms of contrariety, as Aristotle does. One approach might be to concentrate on the nomadic *nomos* as an anarchic organization of elements.[30] Another approach, one I find preferable and closer in spirit to Deleuze's own writing, might be to explore the nomadic *nomos* as ethical and aesthetic variations without a theme.[31] Given Deleuze's claim that practice is what realizes movement, a practical formulation may serve as the best guide to envisioning the nomadic *nomos* in Deleuze's work, as well as to an explanation of why there is a tendency for representation to dominate both the practical and the conceptual fields.

Deleuze and Guattari recognize the existence of a double articulation that takes into account both Aristotle's hierarchical distribution of being and their own preference for difference. These two articulations, alone and in combination, produce an unlimited number and kinds of organization of elements. *Representations* are produced by a certain organization of elements in the assemblage (any collection of molecular or quasi-molecular elements). The production of representation is a second-level articulation that establishes functional, compact, and stable forms (objects) that simultaneously actualize in molar compounds or substances (Deleuze and Guattari, p. 41). The resultant stable, functional structure is the type that represents differences as different only in relation to identity. Thus, objectification also refers to the second level of articulation. It is both a matter of reification and making or taking something to be an object, that is, static, inherently necessary, the product of a judgment.

The nomadic *nomos*, on the other hand, is constituted in the first articulation, on which the second, that of representation, is based. It begins with substances that are molecular or quasi-molecular elements—assemblages—and imposes on them a form that consists only of connections and successions (p. 41). "Assemblage" sounds chaotic, though clearly this is not the case. In an assemblage, there are two divergent orientations: "There are lines of articulation or segmentarity, strata and territories; but also lines of flight, movements of deterritorialization and destratification. Comparative rates of flow on these lines produce phenomena of relative slowness and viscosity, or on the contrary acceleration and rupture. All this, lines and measurable speeds, constitutes an assemblage. A book is an assemblage of this kind, and as such it is unattributable. It is a multiplicity" (Deleuze and Guattari, pp. 9–10).

An assemblage is a multiplicity. If it is "territorialized" and "stratified," it is organized according to the principles of categorical reflection. Such an assemblage is slow and viscous, that is, stable, and makes possible "a kind of organism, in the sense of an organic whole, a signifying totality, or a determination attributable to a subject" (Deleuze and Guattari, p. 10). As such, it is representational. Turned toward lines of flight that are *movements* of "deterritorialization" and "destratification," that is, of destabilization, the assemblage is dismantled as an organism. This means that it is not an organic representation attributable to a subject; it is the monstrosity.

Complete and total destratification or pure becoming, pure differentiation without limit is not the goal of destratification. This is the life of submolecular unformed matter, chaos, void, and destruction, and as has been the case with so many revolutionary movements in politics and even in the arts, insofar as they are wildly destabilized, they are able to be reclaimed even more easily by organic representation (Deleuze and Guattari, p. 503). Thus, while the assemblage cannot be identified as either a subject or an object (only representation does this), neither is it the indeterminate chaos of unformed matters. Rather, it is a configuration of speeds, intensities, and varying distributions of its elements. Such an image of thought is necessary to the articulation of difference thought differentially and to the realization of mobility.

So while the first articulation of the assemblage does order elements, it does not do so in the same way as the second articulation; for, in the first, the elements remain "supple," while the latter centers, unifies, integrates, hierarchizes, and finalizes its elements (Deleuze and Guattari, p. 41). Substances and forms constitute both articulations, so clearly they form no opposition to one another. As Deleuze and Guattari point out, substances are always already formed matters, and forms always indicate that some coding, some organization of the field is taking place. Any assemblage (whether it be a work of art, a painting, a book, a subject) is subject to double articulation. This means that organic representation is more than a historical phenomenon; it is an effect of the double articulation that operates everywhere. This is not to say that the choice that double articulation opens up to us is not historical. The choice of perfection over movement, stability over nomadism, and viscosity over flows does seem to be historically, that is, politically motivated. Functionally, there is a choice between the stability and immobility of identity in the concept in representation with its hierarchic distribution, and something that is not its opposite, but simply the first level of articulation, the level of multiplicity. The level of the first articulation is what I have referred to at the beginning of this chapter as "monstrosity," making the determination that is difference: the mobility and therefore distortion of the perfected representation.

On the political level, which feminist film theory and Burgin first alerted us to, Deleuze and Guattari connect the second articulation that produces representation to the hierarchical distribution of power that characterizes the state apparatus. By this they do not mean to imply that all state governments are somehow corrupted and anarchy should reign. The state apparatus is merely the name they give to the most static and stratified organization of power, an organization that makes use of representation's intelligibility and rigidity to justify its existence: "Undoubtedly, the great collective bodies of a State are differentiated and hierarchical organisms that on the one hand enjoy a monopoly over a power or function and on the other hand send out local representatives" (Deleuze and Guattari, p. 366). Functioning according to a vision that imposes the order of representation, the state is an organism that appropriates a military war machine to serve its political needs; regulates bands or clans, as conquerors imposing law on the conquered; reduces the scientific model of problems and accidents that condition and resolve them to a model based on the distinction of genus and species or essence and properties; defines thought as either the *imperium*, that is, the "whole" as final ground of being, or as the "republic," that is, a system in which the "sovereign" subject figures as legislative and juridical ground. The hierarchical and static articulation of representation is, according to this analysis, a function of a state apparatus and state power. State power, as Deleuze and Guattari define it, is made visible in the game of chess: "Chess is a game of State, or of the court: the emperor of China played it. Chess pieces are coded; they have an internal nature and intrinsic properties from which their movements, situations, and confrontations derive. They have qualities; a knight remains a knight, a pawn a pawn, a bishop a bishop" (Deleuze and Guattari, p. 352). Chess pieces act only biunivocally with one another so that the war they enact is institutionalized, regulated, and coded. It takes place in an arranged, closed space, the hierarchized space of the Aristotelian cosmos and organic representation.

Deleuze and Guattari compare this representational game of centralized and rigidly hierarchized states to the game of Go. The game pieces in Go are anonymous and collective "its": "It could be a man, a woman, a louse, an elephant" (Deleuze and Guattari, p. 353). Their properties are thus subject to continuous change depending on what sort of configurations appear on the board. Go is thus a game of pure strategy since by itself, a single Go piece can synchronically destroy a whole constellation (p. 353). Alphonso Lingis has characterized the difference between these two types of organization beautifully in his essay, "The Society of Dismembered Body Parts," in which he describes the practices of the Quechua people who live in the Andes and discovers the simultaneous existence of a nomadic *nomos* and a representational power structure: "You can wander the high Andes and, by night, hear the murmurs of the people around the fire, hear their Quechua tongue without understanding it, hear the light, subtle, supple tripping of their sounds, hear their intonations and their murmurs, hear it as the very resonance of their substance, their gentle, unassertive, vibrant, sensitive way of vocalizing together."[32] Here Lingis focuses on the first articulation, the nomadic *nomos* where the voices of the tribesmen distribute themselves in space: voices speak and are heard by others that respond, but unevenly, with murmurs, pauses, silences. But when the second articulation asserts itself, the voices can be represented: "But if you were to drink some magic potion, some cocktail of coca tea and whisky, and suddenly understood their language, and abruptly understood that they are speaking about 'transporting cocaine into the hands of the Colombian agents,' then abruptly you have subjected yourself to the codings of imperial society; you have suddenly related their sounds not to their own throats and substance but to the international code established by the reigning barbarian empire in Washington and Bonn and Tokyo, where cocaine means the same thing—crime."[33] Represented under the category of "crime," the murmurs of the Quechua become subject to the international code: they are criminals, identified as outlaws in accordance with the laws of the hierarchic institutions of capitalist nations.

Thus, for Deleuze and Guattari, what is at stake politically is historical. There are always particular persons acting according to the demands of their era. In the case of the smuggler, a particular assemblage, that of the state apparatus, judges that any element it cannot organize according to its hierarchized demands must be guilty of heresy or treason. From the standpoint of the state apparatus, the nomad is always deterritorialized, always a heretic or a criminal. The nomad, who only ever moves, whose very home is mobile, is thus distributed in a space without borders or enclosure, and so creates what Deleuze and Guattari call a "war machine," not an army or a guerrilla force, but a mode of organization that is exterior to any "state apparatus," outside what I have been referring to as hierarchized representations (Deleuze and Guattari, p. 471).

Double articulation, however, does not limit the types of political or social regimes to two. In fact, for Deleuze and Guattari, double articulation in the organization of assemblages effects a multiplicity of different regimes which, following a semiotic model, they refer to as regimes of signs. While it is not possible to discuss this in depth here, I do want to make clear that these "semiotics" or organizations of assemblages are mixtures— mixtures of presignifying, countersignifying, postsignifying, and signifying elements: "Assemblages determine a given people, period, or language, and even a given style, fashion, pathology, or minuscule event in a limited situation can assure the predominance of one semiotic or another" (Deleuze and Guattari, p. 149).[34] Deleuze and Guattari claim that there is no limit to the number of these social and political assemblages.

My point here is to show how the construction of vision, which I have discussed principally in terms of painting, is an effect of social and political practices whose organization consists of mixtures of signifying regimes. That this is a more abstract level of thinking than the historical is, I hope, clear. Exactly how social and political life (including vision) is constituted cannot be entirely arbitrary, thus simply a matter of contingent historical choice; but neither is it limited by a single dominant *logos*. Rather, the double articulation that operates in all strata makes it necessary for us to reformulate not only our notions regarding the cultural construction of vision but also our ways of thinking about all social and political life. Regimes of signs are not merely chance events, but assemblages organized in accordance with certain practices specific to a culture or way of life. They have neither the status of historical contingency—which may be explicable after the fact but remain contingent—nor that of an unalterable *telos* in nature. They are fluid structures with efficient causes. As Deleuze and Guattari conclude, "We are not, of course, doing history: we are not saying that a people invents this regime of signs, only that at a given moment a people effectuates the assemblage that assures the relative dominance of that regime under certain historical conditions" (Deleuze and Guattari, p. 152).

I have noted that, for Deleuze, only signifying practices effect the ruin of representation. The political representation of the law is just another aspect of the organic representation that dominates vision. So to break with this representation, to find ways to bring about the "ruin of representation," is intrinsic to the practice of artists and nomads. Ultimately, double articulation is a function of the practical and ethical level: it is a question of life itself and the value of life. Feminist film theory is correct in assuming that there is a political and social impetus organizing our modes of seeing, our very vision. And because, for Deleuze, this impetus is neither teleologically preordained nor radically contingent history, but part of a grab for power based on irrefutable conceptual claims for intelligibility, coherence, and hierarchic distribution, it is Deleuze's project to point to other ways to see, to open up the field of our vision to the nomadic *nomos* that creates wandering distributions of assemblages, distributions whose plurality of centers mix perspectives and points of view and open up the structures of power to create truly democratic institutions.

Notes

1. For a critique of the psychoanalytic approach to vision see my "Bodies in the Light, Relaxing the Imaginary in Video," in Juliet Flower MacCannell and Laura Zakarin, eds., *Thinking Bodies* (Stanford: Stanford University Press, 1994), pp. 165–180.

2. For a particularly nuanced Lacanian reading of feminist film theory, see Joan Copjec, "The Orthopsychic Subject: Film Theory and the Reception of Lacan," *October* 49 (Spring 1989).

3. Jean-Louis Baudry, "The Apparatus," *Camera Obscura* 1 (1976):113.

4. This is, of course, the famous thesis of Laura Mulvey in "Visual Pleasure and Narrative Cinema," in Gerald Mast and Marshall Cohen, eds., *Film Theory and Criticism* (New York: Oxford University Press, 1985).

5. Victor Burgin, "Geometry and Abjection," in James Donald ed., *Psychoanalysis and Cultural Theory, Thresholds* (New York: St. Martin's Press, 1991), p. 12 (emphasis added).

6. Ibid., pp. 12, 13.

7. Michel Foucault, "Of Other Spaces," trans. Jay Miskowiec, *Diacritics* 16, no. 1 (1986):22. In this essay Foucault characterizes the dilemma linking looking with objectification with the notion that contemporary space is in practice still not desanctified, so that contemporary life is still governed by oppositions between public and private, leisure and work, and presumably objective and subjective.

8. Burgin, "Geometry and Abjection," p. 13.

9. Michele Montrelay, "Inquiry into Femininity," in Toril Moi, ed., *French Feminist Thought* (Oxford: Basil Blackwell, 1987), p. 233. In Montrelay, such ruin refers to the unconscious representation of castration, which, unlike conscious representation (which she claims is imaginary) "no longer refers to anything but the words which constitute it. Taken out of reality, it no longer refers to anything other than its form.... The unconscious representation is only a text" (p. 232). It may be the case that the difference here is less than Montrelay thinks; nonetheless, the point is that if such representation is ruined, its castrating effects disappear, and the representation circulates "emptily" (p. 233).

10. Burgin, "Geometry and Abjection," pp. 13, 14, 16.

11. Gilles Deleuze, *Différence et répétition* (Paris: Presses Universitaires de France, 1968). (Subsequent references are cited parenthetically in the text.)

12. See, for example, Gilles Deleuze, *Francis Bacon, Logique de la sensation*, (Paris: La Différence, 1984); also *Cinema I: The Movement-Image*, trans. Hugh Tomlinson and Barbara Habberjam (Minneapolis: University of Minnesota Press, 1986) and *Cinema II, The Time-Image*, trans. Hugh Tomlinson and Robert Galeta (Minneapolis: University of Minnesota Press, 1989).

13. See Svetlana Alpers, *The Art of Describing: Dutch Art in the Seventeenth Century* (Chicago: University of Chicago Press, 1983), p. 41. Alpers distinguishes between single-point perspective and what she calls eye-point perspective—which she thinks thrived in sixteenth-century Dutch painting—through a series of differences: a concern for objects in space versus surfaces, form versus texture, a few large objects versus many large ones, objects modeled by light and shadow versus light reflected off objects, framed versus unframed images, a clearly situated viewer versus none, the picture as an object in the world like a framed window versus the picture taking the place of the eye (pp. 44–45).

14. David Summers, *Michaelangelo and the Language of Art* (Princeton: Princeton University Press, 1981), pp. 73, 478–479.

15. H. W. Janson, *History of Art* (New York: Harry N. Abrams, 1971), p. 471.

Dorothea Olkowski

16. Julia Kristeva, *Desire in Language, A Semiotic Approach to Literature and Art*, ed. Leon S. Roudier, trans. Thomas Gora, Alice Jardin, and Leon S. Roudier (New York: Columbia University Press, 1980), p. 214.

17. Aristotle, "Metaphysics," in Richard McKeon, ed., *The Basic Works of Aristotle* (New York: Random House, 1970), X, 4, 1055a5.

18. Ibid., X, 5, 1054b25 (emphasis added).

19. Ibid., III, 3, 998b20 (emphasis added).

20. Franz Brentano, *On the Several Senses of Being in Aristotle*, trans. Rolf George (Berkeley: University of California Press, 1975), pp. 58, 59–60.

21. Aristotle, VIII, 6, 1045a36.

22. Brentano, *On the Several Senses*, p. 60.

23. Aristotle, IV, 2, 1003b (emphasis added).

24. Ibid., IV, 1, 1003b15.

25. Michel Foucault, "Theatrum Philosophicum," in *Language, Counter-memory, Practice*, trans. Donald F. Bouchard (Ithaca: Cornell University Press, 1977), p. 183. Given that Foucault's analysis occurs in the context of an essay that remarks that "perhaps one day, this century will be known as Deleuzian" (p. 165), he tends to characterize "freeing difference" (p. 185) in euphoric terms that I take to be too closely associated with those who see in Deleuze a turn to some romanticized anarchism. It is my intent to show that a form of reason operates in Deleuze's philosophy of difference, but that it is simply not the hierarchized, conceptualized reason of equivocal being.

26. Gilles Deleuze and Félix Guattari, *A Thousand Plateaus*, vol. 2 of *Capitalism and Schizophrenia*, trans. Brian Massumi (Minneapolis: University of Minnesota Press, 1987), p. 43. (Subsequent references are cited parenthetically in the text.) Deleuze and Guattari insist that there are always two kinds of articulation and two kinds of multiplicity. The proposition, therefore, is no more than an expression of the other articulation and the other multiplicity that have mostly been submitted to the domination of the model of judgment.

27. Foucault, "Theatrum Philosophicum," p. 182.

28. Summers, *Michelangelo*, p. 73.

29. Alpers, *Art of Describing*, p. 58.

30. See Brian Massumi, *A User's Guide to Capitalism and Schizophrenia: Deviations from Deleuze and Guattari* (Cambridge: MIT Press, 1992), pp. 120–121, 194–195n53. Massumi characterizes nomadism politically in terms of anarchy. I specifically avoid this insofar as it is posited here as opposed to statism and as one pole in a continuum. It seems to me that such a characterization obscures the hard-won ground of difference as what is and thus of differences each having their own essence, their own meaning. I am loath to take this risk, and I am also

Difference and the Ruin of Representation in Gilles Deleuze

unwilling to place Deleuze and Guattari back into the context of choosing between extremes. Any particular group of "anarchists" may or may not practice nomadism; it depends largely on how they position themselves with regard to difference.

31. See Jean-Clet Martin, *Variations: La philosophie de Gilles Deleuze* (Paris: Éditions Payot, 1993). Martin develops the notion of difference and multiplicities in the context of Deleuze's aesthetic and ethical formulations as a poetic organization of thought. I hope that my own approach approximates Martin's simultaneously logical and poetic analysis.

32. Alphonso Lingis, "The Society of Dismembered Body Parts," in Constantin V. Boundas and Dorothea Olkowski, eds., *Gilles Deleuze and the Theatre of Philosophy* (New York: Routledge 1994), pp. 228–229.

33. Ibid., p. 229.

34. Deleuze and Guattari name four such assemblages: the despotic signifying regime of signs (the state apparatus discussed above); the "so-called primitive *presignifying semiotic*, which is much closer to the 'natural' codings operating without signs" (exemplified by societies of hunter-nomads) (p. 147); a "countersignifying semiotic" ("fearsome, warlike, animal-raising nomads" who remain exterior to the state apparatus) (p. 148); and finally, the "postsignifying regime" effecting a "finite legislator-subject" who replaces the absolute signifying despot (p. 162).

Contributors

Margaret Atherton is professor, Department of Philosophy, University of Wisconsin, Milwaukee. Dr. Atherton is the author of *Berkeley's Revolution in Vision* and editor of *Women Philosophers of the Early Modern Period*.

Peg Birmingham is associate professor, Department of Philosophy, De Paul University, Chicago. Dr. Birmingham is coeditor, with Philippe van Haute, of *Dissensus Communis: Between Ethics and Politics*. She is writing a book on Hannah Arendt, *The Predicament of Common Responsibility*.

Rebecca Comay is associate professor, Department of Philosophy and Literary Studies, University of Toronto, Toronto, Canada. Dr. Comay is the author of *On the Line: Reflections on the Bad Infinite*, a study of Hegel and Heidegger. She is working on a book on Heidegger and Benjamin, tentatively entitled *Pausing for Breath*.

William James Earle is professor of philosophy, Baruch College and the Graduate Center of the City University of New York, and a member of the Executive Committee of the Center for Cultural Studies at the Graduate Center. Dr. Earle is the author of a guidebook to contemporary analytic philosophy and the entry on William James in the *Encyclopaedia of Philosophy*.

Yaron Ezrahi is professor, Department of Political Science, Hebrew University, and Fellow of the Israel Democracy Institute. Dr. Ezrahi is the author of *The Descent of Icarus: Science and the Transformation of Contemporary Democracy*.

David Michael Levin is professor, Department of Philosophy, Northwestern University. Dr. Levin is the author of *Reason and Evidence in Husserl's Phenomenology*, *The Body's Recollection of Being*, *The Opening of Vision*, and *The Listening Self*. He has edited *Pathologies of the Modern Self: Postmodern Studies on Narcissism, Schizophrenia, and Depression*, and *Modernity and the Hegemony of Vision*.

Sandra Rudnick Luft is professor, Department of Humanities, San Francisco State University. Dr. Luft's work includes essays on Vico, Nietzsche, Blumenberg, Heidegger, and Derrida. She is currently completing a book on Vico, relating his thought to modern and postmodern epistemologies.

Dorothea Olkowski is associate professor, Department of Philosophy, and Director of Women's Studies, University of Colorado, Colorado Springs. Dr. Olkowski is coeditor, with Constantin Boundas, of *Deleuze and the Theatre of Philosophy*. She is writing a book on the problem of representation.

James I. Porter is associate professor, Department of Classical Studies and Comparative Literature, University of Michigan, Ann Arbor. He has published mostly on ancient Greek and contemporary literary theory. He is the author of *Nietzsche's Atoms* and is coeditor of The Body in Theory: Histories of Cultural Materialism, a book series published by the University of Michigan Press. He is currently working on a book with the title *The Material Sublime: Critical Discourse in Classical Antiquity*.

Mary C. Rawlinson is associate professor, Department of Philosophy, State University of New York at Stony Brook. Dr. Rawlinson's numerous publications include studies of Husserl, Derrida, Kristeva, Irigaray, Foucault, and Proust and essays on psychoanalysis, feminism, and the philosophy of medicine.

John Russon is assistant professor, Department of Philosophy, Pennsylvania State University. Dr. Russon's publications include studies of ancient Greek philosophy, German idealism, and twentieth-century European philosophy.

P. Christopher Smith is professor, Department of Philosophy, University of Massachusetts, Lowell. Dr. Smith is the author of *Hermeneutics and Human Finitude: Toward a Theory of Ethical Understanding*. He has also translated three of Hans-Georg Gadamer's works: *Hegel's Dialectic, The Idea of the Good in Platonic-Aristotelian Philosophy*, and *Dialogue and Dialectic*.

John H. Smith is associate professor, Department of German, University of California, Irvine. Dr. Smith is the author of *The Spirit and Its Letter: Traces of Rhetoric in Hegel's Philosophy of Bildung*. He is completing a study of dialectical conceptions of the will in modern French and German thought.

Catherine Wilson is professor and chair, Department of Philosophy, University of Alberta. Dr. Wilson is the author of *Leibniz's Metaphysics* and *The Invisible World*, a study of early microscopy.

Index